Hurst's

THE HEART
10th Edition

SELF-ASSESSMENT AND BOARD REVIEW

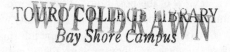

NOTICE

Medicine is an ever-changing science. As new research and clinical experience broaden our knowledge, changes in treatment and drug therapy are required. The authors and the publisher of this work have checked with sources believed to be reliable in their efforts to provide information that is complete and generally in accord with the standards accepted at the time of publication. However, in view of the possibility of human error or changes in medical sciences, neither the authors nor the publisher nor any other party who has been involved in the preparation or publication of this work warrants that the information contained herein is in every respect accurate or complete, and they disclaim all responsibility for any errors or omissions or for the results obtained from use of the information contained in this work. Readers are encouraged to confirm the information contained herein with other sources. For example and in particular, readers are advised to check the product information sheet included in the package of each drug they plan to administer to be certain that the information contained in this work is accurate and that changes have not been made in the recommended dose or in the contraindications for administration. This recommendation is of particular importance in connection with new or infrequently used drugs.

Hurst's
THE HEART
10TH EDITION

SELF-ASSESSMENT AND BOARD REVIEW

Edited by

DAVID R. FERRY, M.D.

Associate Professor of Medicine
Loma Linda University School of Medicine

Chief, Cardiology Section
Jerry Pettis Veterans Administration Medical Center
Loma Linda, California

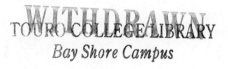
McGRAW-HILL
Medical Publishing Division

New York   Chicago   San Francisco   Lisbon   London
Madrid   Mexico City   Milan   New Delhi   San Juan   Seoul   Singapore   Sydney   Toronto

BS

McGraw-Hill
A Division of The **McGraw·Hill** *Companies*

Hurst's The Heart, 10th Edition, Self-Assessment and Board Review

1 2 3 4 5 6 7 8 9 0   VLP/VLP   0 9 8 7 6 5 4 3 2 1

ISBN 0-07-137469-8

This book was set in Times Roman by Circle Graphics.
The editor was Darlene Cooke.
The production supervisor was Lisa Mendez.
Project management was provided by Columbia Publishing Services.
The cover designer was Aimee Nordin.
Vicks was printer and binder.

This book is printed on acid-free paper.

Library of Congress Cataloging-in-Publication Data

Ferry, David R.
    Hurst's the heart, 10th edition : self-assessment and board review / David R. Ferry.
        p. ; cm.
    Includes bibliographical references and index.
    ISBN 0-07-137469-8
    1.   Cardiovascular   system—Diseases—Examinations,   questions,   etc.   2.   Heart—
Diseases—Examinations, questions, etc. I. Hurst, J. Willis (John Willis), 1920- II. Title.
    [DNLM: 1. Cardiovascular Diseases—Examination Questions. WG 18.2 F399h 2002]
    RC667 .H88 2001 Suppl.
    616.1'0076—dc21
                                                                                    2001044037

10/29/03

Dedicated to the cardiology fellows,
who indulge my need to explain things

CONTENTS

PREFACE

I would like to thank my major professors at the University of Texas Health Science Center at San Antonio for teaching me to do cardiology right. They accepted only the very best work from us fellows, from history taking and physical examination all the way through cardiac catheterization and research. Although many have moved to other positions, Drs. Robert A. O'Rourke, Michael H. Crawford, Kent L. Richards (no, Kent, I no longer snap the entire length of the pulmonary artery catheter with my fingernail to remove every microbubble—sorry), Richard A. Walsh, and Morton J. Kern (nice cath book, Mort) have made huge impacts on my life as a cardiologist.

I would also like to thank my two principal initial writers: Jennifer Blount Thorn and Tiffany Stanhiser, both medical students at Loma Linda University. Jenny is the daughter of my best friend from high school and college, and I had heard of her language skills from very early in her life. A true Jenny story: at age 4, while sitting in the bathtub, she watched bubble bath being poured into the tub and said, "Mommy, look at the soap *dissipate* in the water!" Her father told me he had to go look that word up. At any rate, I expected that Jenny would be able to identify new information in the 10th edition of *Hurst's The Heart,* but I was astounded when she began writing "preliminary" versions of the questions and answers. She had quickly grasped the fundamental issues of material she had yet to study in school, and was able to construct easily readable and logical questions and comprehensive and lucid answers. She is the primary reason why this text was sent to the publisher 6 months after the 10th edition of *Hurst's* appeared. Tiffany, who wrote the first drafts of Parts XII and XIII, was also very helpful.

I had to make a plan for the contents of this book quickly, and it seemed reasonable that we should emphasize information that was new in the 10th edition of *Hurst's.* Therefore, we have thoroughly "scouted" the 9th and 10th editions and have included in this book almost everything that represents significant advances in our understanding of cardiovascular diseases, their diagnosis, and their treatment. It is obviously important that these issues receive a preponderance of attention for clinical reasons, but this information is also very likely to be emphasized on cardiovascular disease boards.

Finally, I would like to thank my Administrative Assistant, Cheryl Redfern, for her usual heroic efforts to help me in this task. I also want to apologize to her and to my colleagues Drs. Alan K. Jacobson and Geir P. Frivold as I became ever more frantic to meet publishing deadlines. They shouldered many clinical and administrative responsibilities that I should have been doing. Thanks as well to Darlene Cooke at McGraw-Hill for her more or less patient mothering of this project. I appreciate her trust in me to be able to produce a quality text in a very short time. I wish to acknowledge Jerre Frederick Lutz, M.D., for his contribution to previous editions.

David R. Ferry, M.D.

INTRODUCTION

Hurst's The Heart, 10th Edition, Self-Assessment and Review has been designed to provide physicians with a comprehensive review of current cardiovascular knowledge with a particular emphasis on the most recent information. Although the primary audience is likely to be cardiologists who are preparing to take the American Board of Internal Medicine's Examination in Cardiovascular Disease, the book is appropriate for physicians in any stage of training who want to test their knowledge of recent advances in cardiovascular medicine.

The questions and answers have been written to relate to specific clinical decision-making problems. The choices in the question sections are those which the clinician would encounter under actual circumstances. The answers are designed not only to justify the correct response, but also to explain why the alternatives are not appropriate in this situation.

Although some of the questions reflect information that has been known for years, most of the topics are concerned with recent issues. Therefore, those seeking a thorough review of a topic such as aortic stenosis should rely on the main text of *Hurst's The Heart* and use this book to quickly identify any new information pertaining to that topic.

Finally, each question now contains the pages in *Hurst's The Heart* that concern that topic. This allows the reader to refer to the main text and then formulate a response before referring to the answer section. The traditional bibliography has been replaced by a current list of all the major practice guidelines for cardiology which have been evaluated by the National Guideline Clearinghouse (NGC), a service of the Agency for Healthcare Research and Quality (AHRQ), a subdivision of the U.S. Department of Health and Human Services. All of these guidelines and any that have been added or modified since the publication of this book can be found at *www.guideline.gov.*

PART I
BASIC FOUNDATIONS
OF CARDIOLOGY

I. BASIC FOUNDATIONS OF CARDIOLOGY

QUESTIONS

DIRECTIONS: Each question listed below contains five suggested responses. Select the **one best** response to each question.

I-1. Which of the following statements regarding the incidence or mortality of cardiovascular disease is true?

(A) coronary heart disease accounts for slightly more than 50 percent of all deaths in persons over the age of 35
(B) the recent decline in cardiovascular mortality extends almost exclusively to higher socioeconomic groups
(C) the lifetime risk of developing coronary heart disease over age 40 is 50 percent in men and 32 percent in women
(D) in 1999, the total U.S. expenditure on health care costs and lost productivity for cardiovascular disease was slightly over $150 billion dollars
(E) cardiovascular diseases, although on the decline, still account for approximately 70 percent of all deaths in the United States

(pages 3–4)

I-2. Which of the following statements regarding the differences between men and women in the incidence, prevalence, and mortality of cardiovascular diseases is true?

(A) the average age of occurrence of cardiovascular disease, excluding stroke, is 20 years later in females
(B) the prevalence of myocardial infarction for men over age 75 is 16 percent, but only 5 percent in women over age 75
(C) the first clinical symptom of coronary heart disease in women is likely to be angina, whereas in men it is more likely to be myocardial infarction
(D) coronary heart disease is the leading cause of death in men over age 45, but only the third leading cause in women
(E) after surviving acute myocardial infarction, men are less likely than women to have sudden cardiac death

(pages 3–5)

I-3. Which of the following statements concerning recently recognized coronary heart disease (CHD) risk factors is true?

(A) about 10 percent of the general population have elevated serum levels of homocysteine
(B) inadequate intake of vitamins B_6 and B_{12} and folate account for about 25 percent of elevated homocysteine levels in the general population
(C) about 50 percent of the general population have elevated levels of Lp(a) lipoprotein cholesterol
(D) small, dense low-density lipoprotein (pattern B) occurs in 11 percent of the population and in 50 percent of patients with CHD
(E) serum fibrinogen levels of greater than 200 mg/dL are definitively associated with increased CHD event rates

(page 6)

I-4. Evidence from the Framingham Study suggests that the presence of certain risk factors in women can eliminate their advantage in cardiovascular risk over men. Which one of the following factors in women is clearly associated with increased risk?

(A) left ventricular hypertrophy on electrocardiogram
(B) depression
(C) elevated homocysteine levels
(D) obesity
(E) elevated lipoprotein (a) levels

(page 6)

I-5. Which of the following statements regarding prognosis after an acute myocardial infarction (MI) is true?

(A) women are twice as likely as men to have recurrent infarction within 6 years of an MI

(B) women are twice as likely as men to develop recurrent angina after an MI

(C) men are twice as likely as women to develop disabling heart failure after an MI

(D) men are twice as likely as women to have sudden death after an MI

(E) prognosis is much better in either sex after a recognized MI as opposed to an unrecognized MI

(page 7)

I-6. Which of the following statements regarding blood pressure is true?

(A) of all the cardiovascular diseases, only coronary heart disease is more prevalent than hypertension

(B) in the United States, about 15 percent of all people ages 18 to 74 have a blood pressure greater than or equal to 140/90 mm Hg

(C) the prevalence of hypertension is the same in both blacks and whites

(D) in general, between the ages of 30 and 60, systolic blood pressure increases approximately 20 mm Hg and diastolic blood pressure increases 10 mm Hg

(E) the treatment of isolated systolic hypertension in the elderly has not been shown to decrease the risk of stroke and coronary artery disease

(page 9)

I-7. Which of the following statements regarding heart failure is true?

(A) dilated cardiomyopathy accounts for the majority of cases of heart failure

(B) after the age of 65, the annual occurrence of heart failure approaches 15 percent of the population

(C) there has been an improvement in the prognosis of patients with heart failure over the last 4 decades

(D) five-year survival rates for heart failure are approximately 25 percent in men and 40 percent in women

(E) there are an estimated 200,000 new cases of heart failure each year

(page 12)

I-8. Structures visible within the right atrium include all the following EXCEPT the

(A) thebesian valve

(B) eustachian valve

(C) sulcus terminalis

(D) moderator band

(E) coronary sinus orifice

(page 50)

I-9. Which of the following statements regarding the right ventricle is true?

(A) the right and left ventricles are ellipsoidal spheres

(B) the right ventricle is 4 to 5 mm thick compared to the left ventricle, which is 8 to 15 mm thick

(C) the trabecular muscles in the right ventricle are more coarse than those in the left ventricle

(D) the moderator band is a muscle that carries the posterior fascicle of the left bundle branch from the ventricular septum to the right ventricular endocardium

(E) the right ventricle provides very little of the inferior heart border on a frontal view of the cardiac silhouette

(pages 44–45)

I-10. Which of the following statements regarding the cardiac valves is true?

(A) the atrioventricular (AV) valves are supported by the mass of the ventricular myocardium

(B) the posterior mitral valve leaflet is rectangular and has three scallops, the middle one being the largest

(C) the AV valves and the semilunar valves are avascular structures

(D) the anterior leaflet of the mitral valve is much smaller in area than the posterior leaflet

(E) the annulus of the mitral valve is larger than that of the tricuspid valve

(pages 28–31)

I-11. Which of the following statements regarding surgery of the cardiac valves is true?

(A) the surgical repair of the mitral valve usually requires an anterior mitral annular ring

(B) because the commissural chords of the mitral valve are seldom elongated, they serve as an accurate reference point for determining the proper closing plane during mitral repair

(C) in patients with congenital bicuspid aortic valve, the aortic annulus is usually contracted

(D) structures in the posterior atrioventricular ring that could be damaged during mitral valve repair include the circumflex coronary artery and the great cardiac vein

(E) during aortic valve replacement, the right bundle branch may be injured

(page 35)

I-12. Which of the following branches virtually always arises from the right coronary artery?

(A) AV node artery
(B) sinoatrial (SA) node artery
(C) right ventricular branches
(D) posterior descending artery
(E) conus branch

(page 52)

I-13. With total occlusion of the proximal right or circumflex artery, flow to the distal posterior descending artery may be provided through the AV node by

(A) the bridging collaterals
(B) the circle of Vieussens
(C) the circle of Willis
(D) the oblique vein of Marshall
(E) Kugel's artery

(pages 51–55)

I-14. Which of the following coronary venous structures drain DIRECTLY into the right atrium?

(A) great cardiac vein
(B) middle cardiac vein
(C) small cardiac vein
(D) oblique vein of Marshall
(E) thebesian vein

(pages 51–55)

I-15. The epicardial blood supply to the anterolateral papillary muscle is provided by which of the following structures?

(A) left anterior descending coronary artery
(B) circumflex artery
(C) right coronary artery
(D) left anterior descending coronary artery and circumflex artery
(E) left anterior descending and right ventricular branches of the right coronary artery

(page 55)

I-16. Which of the following statements regarding atrial pressures and wave forms is true?

(A) mean left atrial pressure is usually slightly lower than right atrial pressure
(B) the positive *a* wave occurs during the early phase of ventricular diastole
(C) the *v* wave is caused by passive filling of the atria during ventricular systole
(D) the *a* wave is normally smaller than the *v* wave in the right atrium
(E) the *y* descent is more rapid than the simultaneous decline of ventricular pressure at the onset of ventricular filling

(page 66)

I-17. Which of the following statements regarding the excitation system is true?

(A) contraction is initiated by a slow inward Ca current through L-type Ca channels
(B) maintenance of the Na-K transmembrane gradient is not an energy-consuming process
(C) the earliest and largest component of membrane depolarization is an efflux of K ions
(D) L-type channels are also known as benzothiazipine (BZT) receptors
(E) the action potential results in a net movement of K ions into and a net movement of Na ions out of the cytoplasm

(page 67)

I-18. Which of the following statements regarding the excitation-contraction coupling system is true?

(A) a two-component structure involved in Ca transfer, known as a *dyad,* is located midway between the T-tubules
(B) the sarcoplasmic reticulum utilizes a process termed Ca-induced Ca release (CICR) to release a large store of Ca ions into the cytoplasm
(C) the CICR functions to increase the cytoplasmic concentration of calcium about fivefold
(D) a specialized pump, the SR Ca ATPase (SERCA2) serves to maintain the high cytoplasmic concentration of Ca during the contraction phase
(E) phospholamban (PLB) is a protein attached to the SERCA2 pump which, under normal circumstances, enhances the pump activity

(page 67)

I-19. Which of the following statements regarding the contractile system is true?

    (A) the alpha form of myosin heavy chains is more adapted to slower, more forceful contraction than the beta form

    (B) the giant protein molecule titin assists the myosin chains during the contraction phase

    (C) the troponins TnC, TnI, and TnT work together in complex conformational ways to bind Ca and initiate contraction

    (D) properties which are important in the process of thin filament activation include nearest-neighbor interactions and increased catecholamine levels

    (E) large changes in Ca concentrations are necessary to recruit contractile reserve

(pages 70–71)

I-20. Which of the following statements regarding the contractile system is true?

    (A) ATP hydrolysis primarily occurs during the myocyte contraction phase

    (B) the essential light chain appears to function as a lever between the thick and thin filaments

    (C) if no external restraining force (afterload) is applied, a maximum amount of force is produced by contraction

    (D) during isometric contraction, cross-bridge activity produces a minimum of force

    (E) the Frank-Starling relation (i.e., the increase in contractile performance with increasing ventricular preload) is best attributed to thick and thin filament overlap

(page 72)

I-21. Which of the following statements regarding myocyte energy metabolism is true?

    (A) under basal conditions, myocytes primarily utilize glycolysis to produce ATP

    (B) certain ionic pumps, such as SERCA2, are especially dependent on fatty acid metabolism

    (C) nitric oxide, generated by vascular endothelium, increases mitochondrial oxygen consumption

    (D) the processes that account for most of the myocardial energy consumption are cross-bridge recycling, Ca uptake by SERCA2, and basal metabolism

    (E) the rate of myocardial energy consumption is independent of loading conditions

(page 73)

I-22. Which of the following statements regarding the force-frequency relation (FFR) control mechanism of contractility is true?

    (A) the FFR functions primarily to maintain appropriate relaxation rates at the basal heart rate of about 60 beats per minute

    (B) the mechanism of FFR involves increased and more rapid Ca cycling per beat as the heart rate rises

    (C) a protein called Ca-activated calmodulin decreases Ca pumping activity by SERCA2

    (D) the FFR appears to function well in spite of myocardial stress or disease

    (E) the FFR is markedly attenuated by β-adrenergic stimulation

(page 73)

I-23. Which of the following statements regarding the extrinsic control mechanisms of contractility is true?

    (A) normal myocytes contain primarily β_2-adrenergic receptors

    (B) agonist binding to the β-adrenergic receptors decreases cytoplasmic cyclic AMP

    (C) cyclic AMP activates protein kinase A, which in turn increases Ca entry by increasing SERCA2 pumping

    (D) cholenergic stimulation has a more profound effect on contractility than β-adrenergic stimulation

    (E) cholenergic stimulation has little effect on heart rate

(page 74)

I-24. Which of the following statements regarding the non-adrenergic extrinsic control mechanisms of contractility is true?

    (A) NOS-3, the predominant form of nitric oxide (NO) synthase in the myocyte, is activated by increasing intracellular Ca levels

    (B) NO has a positive inotropic effect

    (C) the effect of NO is mediated by increased levels of cyclic AMP

    (D) atrial naturetic peptide and brain naturetic peptide are naturally occurring vasoconstrictors and diuretics

    (E) endothelin-1 and angiotensin II have a net negative inotropic effect

(page 74)

I-25. Which of the following statements regarding ventricular architecture is true?

    (A) the orientation of the muscle fibers is nearly longitudinal to the long axis of the left ventricle throughout its thickness

    (B) there is little variation in regional left ventricular wall thickness

    (C) the left ventricle contracts from the apex to the base to facilitate ventricular emptying

    (D) the interventricular septum is functionally part of the left ventricle

    (E) right ventricular function is primarily independent of interventricular septal contraction

(page 74)

I-26. Which of the following statements regarding the filling pressure and stroke volume of the left ventricle is true?

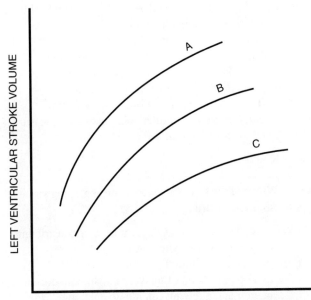

LEFT VENTRICULAR STROKE VOLUME

LEFT VENTRICULAR END DIASTOLIC PRESSURE

(A) in the Frank-Starling effect depicted in the figure above, curve C represents decreased contractility
(B) with increasing filling pressures, the normal curve B would eventually develop a descending limb
(C) substituting end diastolic volume for filling pressure would substantially change the shape of the curves above
(D) identical curves would result from alterations in diastolic compliance
(E) with a normal heart, maximal cardiac output is limited by pumping capacity, not the ability of the systemic circulation to provide adequate venous return

(page 75)

I-27. Which of the following statements regarding ventricular systole is true?

(A) it is possible to define a load-independent contractility
(B) in isotonic contraction, the developed force and afterload are constant
(C) in isometric contraction, tension is generated and shortening occurs
(D) in the Laplace relation, left ventricle wall stress (pressure × external radius) is divided by twice the wall thickness
(E) ejection fraction is independent of loading conditions

(page 76)

I-28. Which of the following statements regarding the elastance concept of ventricular contractile function is true?

(A) the concept of elastance has to do with considering ventricular function as similar to a spring with constant stiffness
(B) the slope (E_{max}) of the end systolic pressure-volume relationship changes according to positive or negative inotropic interventions
(C) E_{max} has been shown to represent a load-independent marker of contractility
(D) in the concept of mechanoenergetics, total mechanical energy consists of heart rate and potential energy
(E) the pressure-volume area inside the pressure-volume curve consists of the sum of external work and afterload

(page 78)

I-29. Which of the following statements regarding the assessment of systolic ventricular performance is true?

(A) the maximal rate of pressure rise (max dP/dt) is especially sensitive to changes in afterload
(B) max dP/dt is useful in quantifying long-term changes in contractility
(C) mean circumferential fiber shortening velocity is a good measure of intrinsic contractile performance, assuming normal afterload
(D) the maximal ventricular power index takes into account the work done by the ventricle and the rate at which it is generated
(E) preload recruitable stroke work is the relationship between the stroke work and the end diastolic pressure

(page 79)

I-30. Which of the following statements regarding diastolic function is true?

(A) ventricular relaxation is complete at the time of the opening of the atrioventricular valve
(B) the sole determinant of the rate of the isovolumic pressure fall is the myocyte relaxation rate
(C) during the rapid filling period of the ventricle, pressure in the atrium and ventricle both fall initially, but the atrial pressure falls more rapidly than the ventricular pressure
(D) restoring forces generate kinetic energy during contraction
(E) once relaxation is complete, the end diastolic pressure-volume relationship is the prime determinant of ventricular pressure

(pages 79–82)

I-31. Which of the following statements regarding the short-term modulation of ventricular function is true?

(A) there is some lengthening of the relaxation phase in conjunction with the positive force-frequency relation

(B) paracrine modulation has more prominent effects on contraction than on relaxation

(C) neurohumoral modulation is a result of variations of both sympathetic and parasympathetic stimulation

(D) interaction between the right and left ventricles is not involved in the short-term modulation of ventricular function

(E) increases in coronary artery flow have an inverse effect on systolic performance

(page 82)

I-32. Which of the following statements regarding capillary exchange is true?

(A) extracellular fluid is reabsorbed into the capillary lumen by oncotic pressure

(B) a negative Q_f value indicates net filtration

(C) the movement of fluid from the extracellular compartment through the capillary wall is known as ultrafiltration

(D) the metabolic and myogenic factors in the microcirculation that are involved in transcapillary exchange play a role in determining downstream resistance

(E) vascular endothelial growth factor is a peptide that starts a signal-transduction event which eventually results in decreased permeability

(page 83)

I-33. Which of the following statements regarding peripheral resistance is true?

(A) according to Poiseuille's equation, resistance to flow is inversely proportional to the tube length

(B) doubling the inner radius of a tube results in a fourfold increase in flow

(C) lumen diameter is the most powerful determinant of vascular resistance

(D) the vessels that primarily regulate and determine peripheral resistance are the large arteries

(E) in a serial arrangement of tubes, resistance tends to be located primarily with the smaller arteries

(pages 83–84)

I-34. Which of the following statements regarding blood flow autoregulation is true?

(A) autoregulation is the ability of an organ to maintain a constant blood flow despite changes in systemic pressure

(B) increased blood flow serves as a stimulus for vasoconstriction through shear stress-induced release of vasoactive substances from the endothelium

(C) autoregulation is a well-developed means for blood flow regulation in all organs

(D) during exercise, metabolic factors such as potassium and hydrogen ions, or adenosine released either directly or indirectly, cause the constriction of vascular smooth muscle

(E) effective autoregulation is determined by the ability of arteries to dilate with increased pressure and to constrict with decreased pressure

(pages 85–86)

I-35. Which of the following statements regarding vascular smooth muscle is true?

(A) vascular smooth muscle is capable of constricting only in response to chemical signals

(B) increased transmural pressure causes a hyperpolarization of the vascular smooth muscle membrane, allowing calcium to enter and bring about cell contraction

(C) calcium-induced activation of sodium channels may be an important feedback mechanism for membrane hyperpolarization in myogenic behavior

(D) endothelial denudation results in an altered response to cholinergic stimulation

(E) vasoactive molecules derived from the endothelium are released solely in response to physical stimuli

(pages 86–87)

I-36. Which of the following statements regarding the autonomic regulation of peripheral blood flow is true?

(A) the maintenance of arterial and venous tone is by sympathetic innervation only during stressful conditions

(B) the nucleus tractus solitarius has an excitatory influence on the rostral ventral lateral medulla

(C) sympathetic denervation produces widespread effects on cerebral and coronary circulation

(D) the adrenal medulla releases epinephrine in response to activation of sympathetic postganglionic afferents

(E) the parasympathetic nervous system produces a minor effect on total resistance

(pages 87–88)

I-37. Which of the following statements regarding coronary circulation is true?

(A) the left circumflex branch of the left coronary artery usually gives rise to the posterior descending artery

(B) venous blood from coronary circulation returns to

the cardiac chambers through arteriosinusoidal channels

(C) most coronary blood flow occurs during systole

(D) the most important role in autoregulation is played by myogenic and metabolically mediated responses

(E) during times of increased metabolic demand, the release of adenosine is an important mediator of autoregulation

(page 88)

I-38. Which of the following findings concerning molecular biology is true?

(A) each individual strand of DNA in the double helix consists of a unique code containing different information from its partner strand

(B) when DNA is subjected to high temperatures, it is possible to separate the individual strands of the double helix

(C) one nucleotide codes for one amino acid

(D) restriction enzymes are used to join DNA fragments together

(E) the enzyme reverse transcriptase is necessary for the transcription of DNA to mRNA

(pages 95–96)

I-39. Which of the following statements regarding nucleic acids is true?

(A) it is estimated that 95 percent of DNA codes for protein

(B) a nucleotide consists of a nitrogenous base, a five-carbon sugar, and a phosphate group

(C) the pyrimidine bases are adenine and guanine

(D) the enzyme RNA polymerase always initiates replication of DNA from the 3′ end of the strand and continues toward the 5′ end

(E) covalent bonds are responsible for the pairing of complementary bases

(page 96)

I-40. Which of the following statements regarding the transcription of DNA is true?

(A) transcription is the production of protein from an mRNA template

(B) transcription takes place in the cytoplasm

(C) the 5′ cap of a molecule of mRNA makes it more stable, thus increasing longevity in the cytoplasm

(D) when mRNA undergoes splicing, the exons are removed and the introns are joined together

(E) small nuclear ribonucleoproteins are important in the splicing of mRNA

(pages 96–97)

I-41. Which of the following statements regarding the translation of mRNA is true?

(A) the term *degeneracy* refers to the fact that some amino acids contain more than one codon

(B) the codon AUG is the stop codon which also codes for the amino acid methionine

(C) GTP provides the energy source for the covalent joining of a transfer RNA and an amino acid

(D) the final modifications to a protein are completed during translation

(E) generally mRNA is very stable and can survive in the cytoplasm for long periods of time

(pages 98–100)

I-42. Which of the following statements regarding the structure of genes is true?

(A) the coding region, which is the region that codes for protein, is located on the first portion of the mRNA molecule

(B) *upstream* is a term referring to everything located 3′ to the first nucleotide to be transcribed

(C) the transcription initiation site is located 5′ to the sequence to be transcribed

(D) polymerase II has a strong affinity for DNA and will bind it readily

(E) the average exon is much larger than the average intron

(page 100)

I-43. Which of the following statements regarding gene regulation is true?

(A) genes that are heavily methylated are targets for immediate transcription

(B) transcription of the housekeeping genes in a cell is a highly regulated process

(C) promoter sequences may be located either upstream or downstream from the coding region on a DNA molecule

(D) only adjacent sequences of primary mRNA may be spliced together to produce a mature mRNA molecule

(E) the poly(A) tail is located on the 3′ region of the mRNA

(pages 101–102)

I-44. Which of the following statements regarding recombinant DNA technology is true?

(A) a restriction map from a segment of DNA requires the use of DNA ligase in its construction

(B) complementary DNA is produced using the retrovirus enzyme, reverse transcriptase

   (C) in electrophoresis, fragments of DNA migrate towards the negative electrode

   (D) the Southern blotting technique is used to transfer proteins from a gel electrophoresis to a solid support medium

   (E) one restriction endonuclease can recognize and cleave several different nucleotide sequences

(pages 102–104)

I-45. Which of the following statements regarding gene libraries is true?

   (A) creating a genomic library requires the use of a restriction endonuclease

   (B) the use of a plasmid is not appropriate in the creation of a gene library

   (C) a genomic library is created from mRNA using reverse transcriptase

   (D) the complementary DNA library derived from the heart will be identical to one derived from the liver

   (E) the yeast artificial chromosome is a particularly good vector and is often used to clone DNA for a library

(pages 105–106)

I-46. Which of the following statements regarding the polymerase chain reaction (PCR) is true?

   (A) only a short 15- to 30-base-pair sequence at the start of the DNA fragment to be amplified must be known to perform a PCR

   (B) DNA polymerase must be added between each cycle of amplification

   (C) the use of a restriction endonuclease, such as Hind-III, is necessary to perform PCR

   (D) the first step of a PCR involves raising the temperature to 95°C to allow the DNA to denature and separate into two strands

   (E) several thousand copies of the RNA or DNA to be studied are needed to perform a PCR

(pages 106–107)

I-47. Which of the following statements regarding cytoskeletal proteins is true?

   (A) microtubules are composed of polymers of the protein actin

   (B) microfilaments are especially involved in the movement and organization of cellular organelles

   (C) intermediate filament subunit proteins are globular, forming a beads-on-a-string type arrangement

   (D) intermediate filaments are specific for different cells and tissue types

   (E) the main function performed by microtubules is the transmission of force

(pages 108–110)

I-48. Which of the following statements regarding cellular growth is true?

   (A) growth that is associated with an increase in the number of a certain type of cell is termed hypertrophy

   (B) most growth in an adult heart is constitutive

   (C) a growth factor that is released in an autocrine mechanism is secreted from the cell and affects the growth of adjacent cells

   (D) an effector molecule that acts on translation is a long-acting growth regulator

   (E) signaling proteins relaying an external stimulus will dampen the stimulus through phosphorylation of downstream signal molecules

(pages 110–111)

I-49. Which of the following statements regarding cardiac growth is true?

   (A) the myocardium's growth in response to injury is an important determinant of morbidity and mortality

   (B) when hypertrophy takes place in the heart, new sarcomeres are added in series

   (C) the growth seen in the heart following injury is similar to the developmental growth in utero and during puberty

   (D) supernatants taken from a homogenized hypertrophied ventricle and perfused into a normal heart induce no change in transcription in the normal heart

   (E) fetal proteins are expressed only in embryonic cells while in utero

(pages 111–112)

I-50. Which of the following statements regarding hypertrophy and cardiac growth is true?

   (A) all stages of cardiac growth require contractile activity as a stimulus

   (B) cardiac growth is always a balance of hypertrophy and hyperplasia

   (C) isotonic exercises, such as running or biking, produce eccentric hypertrophy in the heart

   (D) the same molecular, biochemical, and physiologic changes are seen in both pathologic and physiologic hypertrophy

   (E) the volume overloading seen in mitral or aortic regurgitation results in concentric ventricular hypertrophy

(pages 115–116)

I-51. Which of the following statements regarding stretch-induced growth factors of the growth signal transduction pathway is true?

(A) protein kinase C (PKC) is an important modulator of cytosolic calcium through its interaction with the sarcoplasmic reticulum

(B) G-protein, produced in response to stretching of a cardiomyocyte, activates membrane-bound phospholipase C

(C) mitogen-activated protein kinase (MAPK) is activated only through receptor protein tyrosine kinases

(D) the important transcription factors, c-jun and c-myc, are substrates of PKC phosphorylation

(E) transfection of an antisense nucleotide into MAPK has been shown to cause cardiomyocyte hypertrophy

(pages 116–117)

I-52. Which of the following statements regarding non-stretch-induced growth factors is true?

(A) thyroid hormone acts directly on transcription factors to cause hypertrophy

(B) components of the signal transducers and activators of transcription (STAT) pathway are elevated in patients with congestive heart failure

(C) stimulation of cell-membrane serine-threonine kinases cause either a hyperplastic or hypertrophic response in neonatal cardiomyocytes

(D) acidic fibroblast growth factors bring about an increase in protein synthesis, causing cell hypertrophy

(E) cytokines of the interleukin-6 family activate the cardiomyocyte transmembrane receptor, gp130, which results in phosphorylation of STAT

(pages 117–118)

I-53. Which of the following statements regarding proteins in the heart is true?

(A) the efficiency of protein synthesis is measured by determining how much RNA has been produced per gram of tissue

(B) collagen can be synthesized by vascular smooth muscle cells

(C) the activity of matrix metalloproteinases is decreased in dilated cardiomyopathy

(D) the critical determinant for cardiac hypertrophy has been shown to be the capacity for protein synthesis

(E) dephosphorylation of phospholamban results in disinhibition and leads to increased calcium uptake by the sarcoplasmic reticulum

(pages 119–120)

I-54. Which of the following statements regarding the hypertrophied heart is true?

(A) the most common electrical abnormality seen in a hypertrophied heart is a decrease in the duration of the action potential

(B) in compensated cardiac hypertrophy, the effective number of active cross bridges per unit of myocardium is preserved, but there is an increase in the rate of cross-bridge cycling

(C) in severe hypertrophy, the increases in calcium and calcium-activated currents are important in prolonging the action potential

(D) the ratio of capillaries to myocytes seen in patients and animals with hypertrophied hearts from a pressure overload is no different from that seen in a normal heart

(E) it is believed that myocardial stunning comes from either hydroxy-free radical generation, a decrease in calcium or both of these mechanisms

(pages 120–122)

I-55. Which of the following statements regarding the progression from compensated hypertrophy to heart failure is true?

(A) studies have shown that there is a depression of steady-state mRNA levels in both compensated and decompensated hypertrophy

(B) abnormal signal transduction plays a role in the development of heart failure, but not in cardiac hypertrophy

(C) a disturbance in cardiomyocyte calcium homeostasis is a feature of compensated hypertrophy

(D) underexpression of protein kinase C isoform B produces cardiac hypertrophy and failure

(E) there are a number of signaling molecules that are involved in both hypertrophy and apoptosis

(pages 122–123)

I-56. Which of the following statements regarding the structure of vessel walls is true?

(A) the internal elastic membrane is located between the media and the adventitia

(B) the orientation of the smooth muscle cell is generally helical in large, elastic arteries

(C) pericytes are cells which serve a contractile function and are found in muscular arteries

(D) smooth muscle cells acquire a contractile phenotype in response to vascular insults

(E) smooth muscle cells are normally found in the intimal layer

(page 127)

I-57. Which of the following statements regarding the physiology of the endothelial cell is true?

(A) the expression of "scavenger" low-density lipoprotein receptors, which take up oxidized LDL, is regulated to parallel the growth of the endothelial cell

(B) heparin sulfates bind the enzyme lipoprotein lipase to the endothelial cell surface

(C) endothelial cells present an entirely antithrombogenic surface

(D) water-soluble macromolecules generally pass through tight junctions in the endothelial cells

(E) caveolae formation is likely a major mechanism for edema formation in response to histamine

(pages 128–129)

I-58. Which of the following statements regarding the physiology of the vascular smooth muscle cell is true?

(A) under normal conditions, the vascular smooth muscle cell responds to hormonal stimulation with growth or hypertrophy

(B) the final signal generated in a smooth muscle cell following a stimulus by a calcium-mobilizing vasoactive agonist is hydrolysis of the phosphoinositides

(C) angiotensin II produces a sustained contraction in vascular smooth muscle cells

(D) classic growth factors cause hypertrophy of vascular smooth muscle cells

(E) evidence shows that tyrosine phosphatases, by inhibiting the phosphorylation of tyrosine, can offset the mitogenic effects of growth factors

(pages 130–131)

I-59. Which of the following statements regarding endothelium-derived relaxing factor (EDRF) is true?

(A) after nitric oxide (NO) crosses the smooth muscle cell membrane, it binds to adenylate cyclase and enhances cyclic ATP formation

(B) an increase in intracellular calcium causes the release of EDRF/NO

(C) electrons flowing to tetrahydrobiopterin rather than to oxygen cause the uncoupling of NO synthase which occurs in a variety of diseased states

(D) NO is produced by smooth muscle cells

(E) the expression of endothelial NO synthase is altered by pretranslational modification

(pages 132–134)

I-60. Which of the following statements regarding endothelial control of vascular tone is true?

(A) endothelin-1 is involved in nitroglycerin tolerance

(B) prostacyclin, which relaxes vascular smooth muscle by increasing the intracellular cyclic AMP level, is secreted by smooth muscle cells

(C) adenine nucleosides bind to P1 receptors that are coupled to phosphoinositide hydrolysis

(D) the endothelin-B receptor is predominantly found on vascular smooth muscle

(E) endothelium-derived hyperpolarizing factor is thought to contribute to the rebound phenomenon seen upon the sudden discontinuance of nitroglycerin that has previously been given for several days

(pages 134–135)

I-61. Which of the following statements regarding the control of vascular growth by the endothelium is true?

(A) when agents such as cortisone or γ-interferon bind to heparin, they stimulate angiogenesis

(B) the experimental removal of the endothelium allows the initiation of the mitogenic response

(C) heparin, if administered during the first three days of vascular injury, causes a complete inhibition of angiogenesis

(D) one possible mechanism by which endothelial cells maintain smooth muscle cell quiescence is by inducing tyrosine kinase activity in the smooth muscle cells

(E) fibroblast growth factor is secreted from endothelial cells to stimulate smooth muscle cell growth

(pages 135–137)

I-62. Which of the following statements regarding the interactions between leukocytes and endothelial cells is true?

(A) cytokines, thrombin, and histamine differentially regulate expression of chemoattractant proteins and adhesion molecules, thus allowing the accumulation of different types of leukocyte classes at sites of inflammation

(B) cytokines released at the site of vascular injury cause endothelial cell contraction, thus increasing permeability

(C) chemoattractant proteins and leukocyte adhesion molecules are involved in angiogenesis

(D) E-selectin and GMP-140 bind active leukocytes

(E) histamine can stimulate the endothelial cell release of chemoattractant proteins and expression of adhesion molecules

(page 137)

I-63. Which of the following statements regarding the effects of oxidative stress on vascular disease is true?

(A) increased production of reactive oxygen species (ROS) throughout the body causes a harmful effect on the vascular wall known as oxidative stress

(B) endothelial cells produce ROS through the same mechanism as neutrophils

(C) free radical production in the vasculature is largely a result of the production of superoxide anions by lipoxygenases

(D) the uncoupling of the enzyme endothelial nitric oxide synthase seems to play an important role in several diseases, including hypertension and diabetes

(E) angiotensin II, mediated by superoxide anions, causes a substantial amount of vascular smooth muscle hypertrophy

(page 138)

I-64. Which of the following statements regarding endothelial cell dysfunction and atherosclerosis is true?

(A) the endothelial dysfunction seen in atherosclerosis is primarily related to the stimulation of endothelial contraction, leading to a vasospastic tendency

(B) studies have shown the low-density lipoprotein (LDL) and cytokines downregulate endothelial nitric oxide synthase by converting the enzyme to its inactive form

(C) cholesterol feeding in animals has been shown to increase reactive oxygen production leading to a dysfunctional endothelium

(D) dysfunctional endothelium stops its production of growth inhibitory factors, directly leading to intimal proliferation

(E) a central role in atherogenesis is played by oxidative stress and by oxidatively modified LDL

(page 139)

I-65. Which of the following statements regarding restenosis following angioplasty is true?

(A) vitamins E and C may reduce the risk of restenosis because of their ability to decrease the vascular smooth muscle cell growth factors

(B) the primary problem associated with the removal of the endothelial surface in angioplasty is that the paracrine hormonal environment is altered

(C) the hormonal influences from the infiltration and activation of macrophages in response to the

denuded vessel wall are partially responsible for the response of the vessel to injury by angioplasty

(D) the cytoskeleton of a differentiated smooth muscle cell is similar to that of a cultured cell

(E) the outpouring of fibroblast growth factor in the initial response to deep injury to smooth muscle cells seems to depend on platelet factors

(page 141)

I-66. Which of the following statements regarding the Human Genome Project is true?

(A) there are between 20,000 and 30,000 genes in a human

(B) the project is scheduled to be completed in 2010

(C) the National Institutes of Health and the Department of Health have conducted all the research for the Human Genome Project

(D) not only genes are sequenced, but the intervening sequences are determined as well

(E) all the mRNA from one cell must be extracted to be able to sequence the DNA from that cell

(pages 148–149)

I-67. Which of the following statements regarding functional genomics is true?

(A) knowledge of the protein composition of most genes parallels the identification of genes

(B) the first genome that was completely sequenced was that of *Treponema pallidum*

(C) the most important reason for sequencing the genomes of single-celled organisms is that genetic information can more easily be obtained from them than from humans

(D) advances are needed in the technology used to determine the functions of human genes

(E) *Caenorhabditis elegans* is a single-celled organism that has been important in determining the human genome

(page 149)

I-68. Which of the following statements regarding gene bank networks and DNA microchips is true?

(A) the difficulty accessing research from other scientific labs has slowed the process of genetic sequencing

(B) data is entered into GenBank as individual labs complete research on a particular gene

(C) the DNA microchip is promising because it offers the ability to detect gene mismatches in hybridization

(D) mutations in genes are now detected quickly and easily

(E) the inability for genes to be analyzed as families has made it more tedious to determine the function of certain genes

(pages 149–150)

I-69. Which of the following statements regarding the restorative biology possible with genetic advances is true?

(A) investigators have found several abundant sources of stem cells in the human body
(B) transfection of a stem cell with MyoD has been shown to commit that cell to becoming a cardiomyocyte
(C) it is currently illegal to obtain embryonic stem cells from aborted fetal tissue
(D) research has proven that differentiated adult cells have great potential to change into other cell types
(E) stem cells can be obtained from bone marrow, liver tissue, and skeletal muscle

(page 150)

I-70. Which of the following statements regarding polygenic disorders is true?

(A) positional cloning involves determining the location of a diseased gene by comparing how the inheritance of a certain chromosome segment coincides with the familial inheritance of disease
(B) Mendelian inheritance has a great possibility of use for common diseases such as diabetes, coronary artery disease, and stroke
(C) a score of 10 on a δ *sib* would show no familial contribution to the risk of having a certain disease
(D) one of the benefits of using single nucleotide polymorphisms (SNPs) to determine the location of diseased genes is that they can be used to compare individuals of different genetic backgrounds
(E) the locations of all SNPs have recently been determined

(pages 151–153)

I-71. Which of the following statements regarding the bioethical considerations of genetic testing is true?

(A) the Human Genome Project has not taken into account the ethical, legal, and societal implications of genetic testing
(B) the current working group recommendations regarding genetic information state that under no conditions are employers allowed access to an employee's or a potential employee's genetic information
(C) at present, there is no specification that genetic counseling needs to accompany genetic testing
(D) there is currently a shortage of medical geneticists

and genetic counselors available to meet the present demand for their services
(E) it is customary to screen high school athletes for their risk of familial hypertrophic cardiomyopathy

(pages 153–154)

I-72. Which of the following statements regarding viral vectors is true?

(A) a limitation of adenoviral vectors is that in order to integrate and express their viral genome, they require actively dividing human cells
(B) retroviral vectors have been effective vectors for cardiovascular applications
(C) transient gene expression and the inflammatory and immune responses of the host have limited the effectiveness of adenoviral vectors
(D) retroviral vectors have been shown to infect a broad range of cell lines
(E) adeno-associated viral vectors can accept the largest transgene insert of the known viral vectors

(pages 157–158)

I-73. Which of the following statements regarding nonviral vectors is true?

(A) the direct injection of plasmid DNA into skeletal or cardiac muscle has resulted in stable transfection to a large number of cells
(B) cationic liposomes bind to a specific site on the cell membrane and are then uptaken by receptor-mediated endocytosis
(C) antisense oligonucleotides (ASOs), once inside the nucleus, are transcribed into the mRNA of the desired protein
(D) the nuclear protein high-mobility group 1 (HMG-1) enhances its integration into the host nucleus by binding the transfected DNA
(E) ASOs are not yet good agents for gene therapy, as only small quantities of them can be obtained

(pages 158–159)

I-74. Which of the following statements regarding the experimental applications of antisense oligonucleotides (ASOs) is true?

(A) administration of ASOs against c-myb to the intimal layer of a rat carotid artery inhibited the intimal proliferation that commonly occurs following balloon injury
(B) vein grafts offer an opportunity for combining in vivo gene-transfer techniques with ex vivo application of a transfection medium

(C) genetic engineering can decrease the ability of the graft to mount a hyperplastic response following acute injury

(D) following vein graft combined with gene therapy, medial hyperplasia is seen rather than neointima formation

(E) genetic therapies will likely not have an effect on the proatherogenic environment of a normal graft wall

(page 160)

I-75. Which of the following statements regarding vascular remodeling following gene transfer is true?

(A) fibroblast growth factor 1 overexpression in porcine arteries has been shown to result in substantial production of an extracellular matrix as well as intimal and medial hyperplasia

(B) Herpes simplex virus thymidine kinase indirectly disrupts replication of DNA in the G1 phase of the cell cycle

(C) transforming growth factor β1 overexpression in vessels may promote vascular healing following injury, without extensive cellular intimal hyperplasia

(D) the bystander effect leads to increased expression of the genes that are being inhibited in adjacent transfected cells

(E) expression of human platelet-derived growth factor BB in porcine arteries stimulates angiogenesis in the neointima, showing its possible involvement in the neovascularization of atherosclerotic plaques

(pages 161–162)

I-76. Which of the following statements regarding clinical trials with gene therapy is true?

(A) blockade of the cell cycle with the dominant negative transcription decoy E2F leads to arrest of the S phase of the cell cycle

(B) inhibition of the cell cycle by transfecting human bypass vein grafts with E2F decoy oligodeoxynucleotide is a safe and feasible method of treatment

(C) in a study for treating myocardial ischemia, recombinant aFGF has been injected into the left anterior descending artery of patients undergoing coronary bypass surgery

(D) the use of transforming growth factor β1 to reduce the extent of myocardial infarction following coronary artery inclusion has so far shown it to be ineffective

(E) it has been determined that a vector must be used to deliver DNA to myocardial tissue, as direct injection has proven impossible

(pages 163–164)

I-77. Which of the following statements regarding embryo patterning is true?

(A) the initial patterning of the embryo, dividing the heart into dorsal-ventral and left-right axes, begins the morphogenesis of the heart

(B) control of development by the embryonic genome begins after the first replication cycle

(C) retinoic acid exerts the greatest effect on the arterial pole of the heart tube and the smallest effect on the venous pole

(D) asymmetry is first seen in the embryo during the trophoblast stage

(E) the primitive streak gives positional information to ectodermal cells

(page 168)

I-78. Which of the following statements regarding the molecular factors involved in cardiogenesis is true?

(A) it is thought that the expression of eHAND determines the formation of the left ventricle

(B) homeobox (Hox) genes are generally downregulated during early development

(C) *Nkx-2* factors are proteins that have been shown to activate translation in the mouse

(D) the murine Hox gene, *Nkx-2.5/Csx,* is expressed only during early cardiogenic differentiation

(E) the Hox code is the combined effect on development by all Hox genes expressed in a particular area

(pages 169–171)

I-79. Which of the following statements regarding molecular factors and their effect on cardiac development is true?

(A) cardiac-restricted ankyrin repeat protein (CARP) gene, which lies upstream of the Hox gene *Nkx-2.5,* encodes a nuclear coregulator of gene expression

(B) it has been suggested that GATA-4 directs and controls CARP expression

(C) GATA-4 is expressed only in the endocardium

(D) MEF2 genes are highly expressed in only the early heart progenitor cells and are probably key regulators of the differentiation program of the heart

(E) the cardiac alpha-actin gene is activated by the combination *Nkx-2.5* and SRF proteins

(pages 171–172)

I-80. Which of the following statements regarding cardiac development is true?

  (A) Sonic hedgehog expression on the right side of Hensen's node is enhanced, while expression on the left side is repressed
  (B) there is a genetic basis for chemical signals that direct the left-right asymmetry seen in the heart
  (C) neural crest cells receive developmental information from surrounding structures following their migration
  (D) myofibrils are aligned in parallel as they are formed in embryonic myocytes
  (E) all segments of a mature heart are present in the primitive linear heart tube although they are not in the mature orientation

(pages 172–173)

I-81. Which of the following statements regarding heart tube development is true?

  (A) laminin and type IV collagen are responsible for setting up migratory pathways through the cardiac jelly
  (B) cells of the cardiac jelly eventually make up the fibrous skeleton of the cardiac valves
  (C) as the tubular heart grows, it bends to the left and anteriorly
  (D) the outflow tract of the heart while in the heart tube formation is connected only to the right ventricle
  (E) the formation of a d-loop results in ventricular inversion along with transposition of the great arteries

(pages 173–175)

I-82. Which of the following statements regarding myocardial trabeculation is true?

  (A) rapid cell division of endothelial cells along the endocardial tube and rapid reabsorption of cardiac jelly results in myocardial ridges and trabeculae
  (B) myocardial trabeculation generally extends toward the future apex of the heart
  (C) there are no distinct morphologic differences between the trabeculation of the right and left ventricles in the embryonic heart
  (D) in noncompaction of the ventricular myocardium, there is always right ventricular involvement regardless of whether the left ventricle is involved or not
  (E) there is generally low familial recurrence with noncompaction of the ventricular myocardium

(pages 176–177)

I-83. Which of the following statements regarding atrial septation and the development of the pulmonary veins is true?

  (A) septum secundum is made up of an active growth of myocardium and endocardial cushions
  (B) fenestrations in the myocardial portion of the secondary septum result in the secondary foramen
  (C) fusion of the endocardial cushions and the leading edge of mesenchyme results in the closure of ostium primum
  (D) after atrial septation is complete, the pulmonary pit becomes recognizable
  (E) atrial septal defect (ASD) at the fossa ovalis, or secundum-type ASD, is due to a malformation of secondary atrial septum

(pages 178–179)

I-84. Which of the following statements regarding the myocardialization of the heart is true?

  (A) absence of myocardialization results in malformations involving failure of conal cushion fusion
  (B) the communication remaining between the right and left ventricles is bordered by the muscular ventricular septum, the fused endocardial cushions, and the conal septum
  (C) the mesenchymal cap from the atrial septum primum fuses with the concave side of the fused endocardial cushions
  (D) in ventricular septal defect, there is a cleft in the anterior mitral valve cusp
  (E) in a partial atrioventricular valve canal defect, there is both interatrial and interventricular communication

(page 180)

I-85. Which of the following statements regarding the development of the heart valves and the aortic arch is true?

  (A) the endocardial cushions develop in the areas where there is rapid relaxation and contraction
  (B) in the early stages of cushion development, it is possible to distinguish the superior, inferior, and lateral cushions
  (C) tricuspid valve atresia probably occurs as a result of an abnormality in delamination of the myocardium
  (D) the primitive pulmonary arteries branch from the fifth aortic arch
  (E) the anomalous subclavian artery is frequently seen in the setting of an interrupted aortic arch

(pages 182–184)

I-86. Which of the following statements regarding coronary artery development is true?

(A) coronary smooth muscle cells and coronary endothelial cells derive from the proepicardium, a cell cluster found on the dorsal wall of the sinus venosus

(B) cells derived from the myocardial cell layers contribute to the coronary network

(C) epicardially-derived cells control the development of the elastic lamina and the branching pattern of the coronary artery

(D) the coronary vasculature matures using both angiogenesis and vasculogenesis

(E) coronary vascular endothelial growth occurs following the development of the epicardium

(page 184)

I. BASIC FOUNDATIONS OF CARDIOLOGY

ANSWERS

I-1. **The answer is C.** *(Ch. 1)* Cardiovascular diseases are the major cause of death in the United States. In 1991, they accounted for 43 percent of the total deaths in the United States. These cardiovascular diseases include hypertension, coronary artery disease, cerebral vascular disease, and occlusive peripheral vascular disease. Cardiovascular disease is the leading cause of death in men after the age of 40 and in women after the age of 65. In addition, coronary heart disease accounts for slightly more than one-fourth of all deaths in persons over the age of 35. Since 1940, there has been a downward trend in mortality from cardiovascular diseases, and this decline has been universal: death rates have declined in both sexes, all races, all age groups, and in every geographic area in the United States. The greatest declines have been seen in young adults and in higher socioeconomic subgroups. Cardiovascular diseases cause approximately 70 percent of all deaths in patients beyond the age of 75. The estimated U.S. expenditures in 1999 for both health care and lost productivity was approximately $280 billion.

I-2. **The answer is C.** *(Ch. 1)* Coronary heart disease is the leading or one of the leading causes of death in men and women in every racial and ethnic group. However, extensive differences are found between men and women regarding the incidence, prevalence, and mortality of coronary heart disease. For instance, the death rate for coronary heart disease is approximately five times higher in men than in women from the ages of 25 to 34. However, that ratio declines to 1.5 by ages 75 to 84. Men usually have the first occurrence of coronary heart disease 10 years earlier than women. In addition to the differences in incidence and prevalence, the clinical presentation and prognosis of coronary heart disease also vary between men and women. Women are more likely to have angina as their first coronary presentation, whereas men are more likely to have a myocardial infarction. Following a myocardial infarction, sudden cardiac death is almost twice as prevalent in men as in women.

I-3. **The answer is D.** *(Ch. 1)* In the general population, 29 percent of people have a vitamin B intake that is deficient enough to elevate homocysteine levels to more than 14 μmol/L. The inadequate intake of vitamins B_{12} and B_6 and folate account for more than 67 percent of elevated homocysteine levels seen in the general populations. It is estimated that 25 percent of the population have lipoprotein cholesterol LP(a) values that are greater than 20 mg/dL. Small, dense low-density lipoprotein (pattern B) is seen in 11.1 percent of the population but is seen in 50 percent of patients with coronary heart disease. Fibrinogen is another risk factor, with serum levels greater than 300 mg/dL occurring in 30 percent of the population.

I-4. **The answer is A.** *(Ch. 1)* The presence of certain risk factors in women can eliminate an advantage in cardiovascular risk compared with men according to the Framingham Study. The male-female gap in incidence closes with advancing age. After menopause, risk escalates two- to threefold with a higher infarction and sudden death rate. A high total/HDL cholesterol of 7.5 or greater eliminates the female advantage. Diabetes has twice the impact on risk in women, eliminating the advantage. Left ventricular hypertrophy on ECG has a greater impact on risk in women. A high triglyceride/HDL ratio correlates with dyslipidemic hypertension.

I-5. **The answer is A.** *(Ch. 1)* Within the 6 years that follow an MI, men have an 18 percent risk of a recurrent infarction, while women have a 35 percent risk. During this time period,

27 percent of men and 14 percent of women develop angina. Approximately 22 percent of men are disabled with cardiac failure following an MI, while this figure is 46 percent in women. Sudden death will be experienced by 6 percent of women and 7 percent of men after an MI. Following an unrecognized MI, the prognosis is nearly as bad and is sometimes much worse.

I-6. The answer is D. *(Ch. 1)*   Hypertension is the most prevalent of all cardiovascular diseases and one of the most powerful contributors to mortality and morbidity from cardiovascular causes. It is estimated that approximately 30 percent of the U.S. population between the ages of 18 and 74 have a blood pressure greater than or equal to 140/90 mm Hg. The number of people in the United States with mild hypertension, defined as a diastolic pressure of 90 to 104 mm Hg, was approximately 25 million in 1989. The number of patients in the United States with isolated systolic hypertension, defined as a systolic blood pressure greater than 160 mm Hg and a diastolic blood pressure less than 95 mm Hg, was approximately 4 million. The prevalence of hypertension increases with age and is highest in the black population. Although in some populations around the world, blood pressure does not increase with age, in most affluent populations there is a rise. In general, between the 3rd and the 6th decades, the systolic pressure rises 20 mm Hg and the diastolic pressure rises approximately 10 mm Hg. Treatment of systolic hypertension in the elderly was efficacious against the incidence of stroke and coronary heart disease in the Systemic Hypertension in the Elderly Program.

I-7. The answer is D. *(Ch. 1)*   Despite improvement in the overall survival of patients with cardiovascular diseases, there has been no significant change in the prognosis of patients with congestive heart failure over the last 4 decades. This dismal fact remains despite dramatic improvements in the clinical armamentarium used for this condition. Hypertension remains the dominant cause of congestive heart failure and alone or in combination with coronary heart disease accounts for the vast majority of patients with congestive heart failure. The National Heart, Lung, and Blood Institute estimates that 2 to 3 million Americans have heart failure. The incidence increases with age and the annual occurrence rate may approach 1 percent of the population for those greater than age 65. There are an estimated 400,000 new cases of heart failure each year. The overall 5-year survival rates are approximately 25 percent for men and 40 percent for women. It is postulated that the lack of improvement in survival of patients with congestive heart failure may be due to improved survival among patients with angina and subsequent myocardial infarction that eventually progresses to heart failure. This increases the prevalence of heart failure in the population and inflates the absolute numbers of patients dying from heart failure.

I-8. The answer is D. *(Ch. 2)*   Venous blood from the head and upper extremities returns to the right atrium via the superior vena cava while blood returns from the lower extremities to the right atrium via the inferior vena cava. There is no valve at the ostium of the superior vena cava, but a rudimentary valve called the eustachian valve guards the inferior vena cava. The coronary venous return enters the right atrium via the coronary sinus, which is guarded by the thebesian valve. On the posterior external surface of the right atrium, a ridge, the sulcus terminalis, extends from the superior to inferior vena cava. The moderator band joins the lower ventricular septum to the anterior papillary muscle in the right ventricle.

I-9. The answer is B. *(Ch. 2)*   The right ventricle has a crescent-shaped cavity and is 4 to 5 mm thick since it is designed to pump against low-resistance pulmonary arteries. The left ventricle is smooth and 8 to 15 mm thick as it is designed to pump against high resistance, but it still contains the ridge-like trabeculae carneae like the right ventricle. The right bundle does course through the moderator muscle band to the right ventricular endocardium. The right ventricle is an anterior structure, which comprises most of the inferior surface of the heart on a frontal roentgenogram, while the right atrium makes up most of the right heart border on the frontal cardiac silhouette.

I-10. The answer is B. *(Ch. 2)*   The four cardiac valves are anchored to their valve rings, or annuli. The fibrous skeleton of the heart is formed by these four joined rings at the base of the heart. The posterior mitral leaflet is rectangular and has three leaflets, with the middle one being the largest. The atrioventricular valves and the semilunar valves are all avascular structures. The mitral leaflets are similar in area, with the anterior leaflet being twice the height of the posterior leaflet, but having half of its annular length. The mitral valve annulus is smaller than the tricuspid annulus.

I-11. The answer is B. *(Ch. 2)* Mitral repair techniques are currently based on the principle of asymmetric annular dilatation. Mitral valve annuloplasty reduces the mitral valve inlet by reducing the posterior leaflet circumference. This is the rationale behind the use of a partial posterior annuloplasty ring. Due to the fact that the commissural chords of the mitral valve are seldom elongated, they serve as accurate reference points for determining the proper closing plane for the leaflets during surgical repair. Structures which could be damaged during mitral valve surgery include the left circumflex coronary artery, which travels in the left atrioventricular groove near the anterolateral commissure, and the coronary sinus, coursing within the left atrioventricular groove adjacent to the annulus of the posterior mitral leaflet. In patients with bicuspid valves, the annular diameter is usually enlarged. During aortic valve replacement, the left bundle branch may be damaged.

I-12. The answer is C. *(Ch. 2)* In about 50 percent of humans, the conus artery arises separately in the right sinus of Valsalva rather than as a right coronary branch. The sinoatrial node artery arises from the proximal right coronary in 50 to 60 percent of cases. The posterior descending and atrioventricular node arteries arise from the circumflex artery in 10 to 15 percent of cases. The right coronary branch gives rise to arteriographically identified right ventricular branches.

I-13. The answer is E. *(Ch. 2)* Kugel's artery arises from the proximal right coronary artery or left circumflex artery; it courses through the posterior atrial septum to join the AV artery and retrograde fills the posterior descending artery. This vessel is usually seen with a total proximal occlusion of the right coronary artery or the circumflex artery. Kugel's artery arises from either the proximal right or left circumflex artery and gives collateral flow through the AV nodal artery to the distal right or left circumflex artery, whichever gives rise to the AV nodal artery (85 percent from the distal right and 15 percent from the distal circumflex artery). Kugel's collateral occurs when the artery which gives rise to the AV nodal artery is occluded. Bridging collaterals connote a total occlusion with ipsilateral local collateralization around the focal occlusion. Occlusion of the proximal right coronary artery may be accompanied by excellent collateralization of the right ventricular branch from a large wraparound left anterior descending vessel (circle of Vieussens).

I-14. The answer is E. *(Ch. 2)* The coronary sinus is the major venous drainage of the left ventricle. The coronary sinus receives its blood supply from the great, middle, and small cardiac veins; the posterior veins of the left ventricle; and the oblique vein of Marshall. Thebesian veins are tiny venous channels that drain the myocardium directly into either the right atrium or right ventricle.

I-15. The answer is D. *(Ch. 2)* The left anterior descending coronary artery provides most of the blood supply to the anterolateral papillary muscle while the right coronary artery supplies the posteromedial papillary muscle. The left circumflex artery provides blood to both papillary muscles.

I-16. The answer is C. *(Ch. 3)* Mean left atrial pressure is normally higher than that of the right atrium. The positive *a* wave resulting from atrial contraction is followed by a decline in pressure as the atria relax. This is the time when ventricular contraction begins. The *v* wave is caused by the passive filling of the atria while the AV valves are closed. The *a* wave is larger than the *v* wave in the right atrium, while the *v* wave is larger than the *a* wave in the left atrium. The pressure decline following the *v* wave is the *y* descent that begins with AV valve opening and is more gradual than the simultaneous decline in ventricular pressure occurring at the onset of filling.

I-17.   The answer is A.   *(Ch. 3)*   Contraction is initiated by a relatively slow, inward Ca current through voltage-sensitive, L-type Ca channels. The resting potential is maintained by a trans-sarcolemmal Na-K-ATPase, using the energy gained from ATP hydrolysis to pump Na ions out of the cytoplasm. The earliest and largest component of membrane depolarization is caused by a rapid influx of Na. L-type channels are also termed dihydropyridine receptors. A net movement of Ca ions into and a net movement of Na ions out of the cytoplasm characterizes the action potential.

I-18.   The answer is B.   *(Ch. 3)*   At the end of each collar in the sarcoplasmic reticulum is a cistern that closely abuts a T-tubule, which creates a dyad or triad structure. The sarcoplasmic reticulum uses a process termed Ca-induced Ca release (CICR), which takes place within or near the dyad, to release a large store of Ca ions into the cytoplasm. The CICR results in a cytoplasmic Ca concentration increase from a diastolic value of 0.1 μM to 10 μM, thus giving a 100-fold increase. The SERCA2 pump removes free Ca ions rapidly from the cytoplasm, thus making the intracellular Ca increase transient. Although the SERCA2 pump is partially self-regulating, phospholamban, a key modulator of cardiac responses to adrenergic signaling, also regulates the SERCA2 pump.

I-19.   The answer is C.   *(Ch. 3)*   The alpha form of myosin heavy chain has both higher ATPase activity as well as a more rapid cross-bridge formation and velocity than the beta form. Titin is closely associated with myosin on one end and is anchored in the Z-line on the other end. It plays an important role in determining the passive viscoelasticity of the myocyte. TnC, TnI, and TnT, the subunit proteins of troponin, work together to bind calcium and initiate contraction. Important factors in thin filament activation are the nearest-neighbor interactions and the strong binding of actin to myosin. Cardiac muscle is highly cooperative, which functionally means that contractile reserve can be recruited with modest changes in Ca concentration.

I-20.   The answer is B.   *(Ch. 3)*   ATP hydrolysis occurs during the transition from force production to the detached/weakly bound states. The essential light chain does appear to function as a lever arm between the thick and thin filaments. If no afterload is applied, the maximum amount of displacement and work is performed, without any force generation. During an isometric contraction, the cross-bridge energy is almost exclusively used for force generation. The Frank-Starling relation (i.e., the increase in contractile performance with increasing ventricular preload) is best explained by length-dependent activation at the sarcomere level. This displaces the previous theory of the Frank-Starling relation being explained by thick and thin filament overlap.

I-21.   The answer is D.   *(Ch. 3)*   Myocytes preferentially take up and oxidize fatty acids to generate their ATP under basal conditions. SERCA2 and certain other ion pumps may be especially dependent on glycolytic ATP. Myocardial oxygen consumption (VO_2) is decreased by nitric oxide generated by the vascular endothelium. Cross-bridge recycling, Ca uptake by SERCA2, and basal metabolism account for most of the myocardial energy. The rate of energy consumption is heavily dependent on loading conditions and resulting work and power generation.

I-22.   The answer is B.   *(Ch. 3)*   The duration of the myocardial twitch contraction is such that at a basal rate of 60 beats per minute, relaxation would be incomplete at the rates achieved during exercise and would cause impaired diastolic filling. The mechanism of the FFR causes increased and more rapid Ca cycling per beat as frequency increases, which prevents this problem from occurring. Ca-activated calmodulin increases SERCA2 activity in response to increased Ca concentration. The FFR depends on the intactness of multiple elements of Ca handling, shown by the fact that it is depressed when the myocardium is diseased or subject to chronic stress. The FFR is markedly amplified in response to increased β-adrenergic stimulation.

I-23. The answer is C. *(Ch. 3)* Normal myocytes predominantly contain β_1 receptors. Agonist binding to the β-adrenergic receptors increases the concentration of cytoplasmic cyclic AMP. Cyclic AMP activates protein kinase A, which, in turn, increases Ca entry by increasing SERCA2 pumping. Cholinergic stimulation has a much weaker effect on contractility than adrenergic stimulation. Cholinergic responses are important modulators of heart rate.

I-24. The answer is A. *(Ch. 3)* NOS-3 is the predominant form of NO in the myocyte. It is activated by increasing levels of intracellular calcium. NO has a negative inotropic effect, which is mediated by cyclic GMP. Atrial naturetic peptide and brain naturetic peptide are produced in the atria and ventricles and are vasodilators and diuretics. The integrated responses to agents such as endothelin-I and angiotensin II have a net positive inotropic effect.

I-25. The answer is D. *(Ch. 3)* The orientation of myocyte bundles changes from the subepicardium to the subendocardium. The bundles progress from nearly longitudinal (to the long axis of the ellipsoid) in the subepicardium to roughly circumferential in the middle two-thirds of the wall to longitudinal again in the subendocardium. There are variations in the ventricular wall thickness to equalize regional wall stress. Left ventricular contraction proceeds from the base to the apex with a wringing motion characterized by a counterclockwise rotation. Interventricular septal fibers are continuous with those of the left ventricle free wall. A significant fraction of the right ventricle's mechanical output is related to energy transferred from the left ventricle through the interventricular septum.

I-26. The answer is D. *(Ch. 3)* Curve A represents increased contractility. There is no descending limb in the function curve in a normal heart. A function curve relating end diastolic volume to mechanical output is a more accurate representation of the Frank-Starling effect, but filling pressure is usually used as it is more easily obtained in a clinical setting. Regardless of which measure is used, changes in contractile performance result in upward or downward shifts of the curve, not changes in the shape of the curve. Alterations in diastolic compliance would produce an identical curve because the effects are indistinguishable from alterations in contractile performance. A normal heart can pump adequate amounts of blood to meet the body's needs under stressful conditions. Maximal cardiac output is limited by the ability of the systemic venous system to return blood to the heart.

I-27. The answer is B. *(Ch. 3)* Contractility is used as a comparative concept to define differences of intrinsic contractile performance that cannot be accounted for by differences in loading conditions. It is, however, impossible to measure contractility in an intact heart. The developed force and afterload are constant in isotonic contraction. In isometric contraction, tension is generated but no shortening occurs. Ejection fraction is sensitive to alterations in preload and afterload, which is why it is used to measure ventricular contractile function.

I-28. The answer is B. *(Ch. 3)* The elastance concept is based on the observation that the ventricle behaves like a spring with a time-varying elastance that increases from a minimum at end diastolic to a maximum at end systolic. The slope (E_{max}) of the end systolic pressure-volume relationship changes with acute positive and negative inotropic interventions. It was initially thought that E_{max} could be an index of contractility that was load independent, but those initial conclusions have since been modified. In the concept of mechanoenergetics, total mechanical energy consists of external work and potential energy. The total mechanical energy is the area under the pressure-volume curve, termed the pressure-volume area.

I-29. The answer is C. *(Ch. 3)* The maximal rate of pressure rise (max dP/dt) varies with preload and is very sensitive to changes in intrinsic contractile performance. Max dP/dt is useful to quantify acute changes in contractility. The mean circumferential fiber shortening velocity is a good measure of intrinsic contractile performance if the afterload is normal or can be accounted for. Maximal ventricular power index is important because it takes into account both the work done by the ventricle and the time over which it is generated. Preload recruitable stroke work is the relationship between end diastolic volume and stroke work.

I-30.   The answer is E.   *(Ch. 3)*   Ventricular relaxation does not finish completely until after atrioventricular valve opening. The rate of the isovolumic pressure fall is determined by the myocyte relaxation rate, the load on the myocardium, and a normal temporal and spatial activation sequence. During the rapid filling period of the ventricle, pressure in the atrium and ventricle both fall initially, but the ventricular pressure falls more rapidly than the atrial pressure. Restoring forces generate potential energy during contraction in the form of a deformation of a myocyte. Once relaxation is complete, the end diastolic pressure-volume relationship is the prime determinant of ventricular pressure.

I-31.   The answer is C.   *(Ch. 3)*   There is some shortening of the relaxation phase in conjunction with the positive force-frequency relation. Paracrine factors tend to have more prominent effects of relaxation than on contraction. The most important short-term neurohumoral modulation is a result of sympathetic and parasympathetic stimulation variations. The interaction between the ventricles plays a role in short-term modulation of the ventricle's function. Increases in coronary artery flow augment systolic performance and may also cause a decrease in passive compliance.

I-32.   The answer is A.   *(Ch. 3)*   Oncotic pressure, the force associated with increasing concentration of a solute along the length of a capillary, pulls extracellular fluid back into the capillary through a process called resorption. A positive Q_f value indicates net filtration. Ultrafiltration is a process where fluid moves through the capillary wall into the extracellular compartment. The metabolic and myogenic factors in the microcirculation that are involved in transcapillary exchange play a role in determining upstream resistance and thus the pressure within a capillary bed.

I-33.   The answer is C.   *(Ch. 3)*   Poiseuille's equation is

$$R = \frac{8\eta L}{\pi r^4}$$

Resistance is proportional to the tube length. A doubling of the inner radius of a tube would result in a 16-fold increase in flow. The diameter of the lumen is the most powerful determinant of vascular resistance. The small arteries and arterioles primarily determine peripheral resistance. In a serial arrangement of tubes, total resistance is the sum of individual resistance elements, thus the larger vessels contribute to the resistance.

I-34.   The answer is A.   *(Ch. 3)*   Autoregulation is the ability of an organ to maintain a constant blood flow despite changes in systemic pressure. Increased blood flow is a stimulus for vasodilation through shear stress-induced release of vasoactive substances from the endothelium. Although all organs maintain the ability to autoregulate, this ability is particularly well developed in the cerebral, coronary, and renal circulations. Metabolic factors such as adenosine and potassium and hydrogen ions released during exercise induce hyperpolarization and relaxation of vascular smooth muscle. Effective autoregulation is determined by an artery's ability to constrict to increased and dilate to decreased pressure in order to keep a relatively constant flow.

I-35.   The answer is D.   *(Ch. 3)*   Vascular smooth muscle (VSM) can constrict in response to pressure or stretch. Transmural pressure leads to the depolarization of the VSM membranes. L-type Ca channels are activated that allow extracellular Ca to enter the VSM cell. Ca-induced activation of K channels may be an important feedback mechanism for membrane hyperpolarization in myogenic behavior. The loss of the endothelium abolishes relaxation to acetylcholine. The endothelium releases vasoactive molecules in response to physical and chemical stimulation.

I-36.   The answer is E.   *(Ch. 3)*   The sympathetic nervous system contributes to arterial and venous pressure under both normal and stressful conditions. The nucleus tractus solitarius has an inhibitory effect on the rostral ventral lateral medulla. Cerebral and coronary circulations, most likely because of their intrinsic autoregulatory abilities, are relatively unaffected by sympathetic denervation. Large amounts of epinephrine are released by the adrenal medulla during intense sympathetic activity. The parasympathetic nervous system contributes a very minor effect to total resistance.

I-37.   The answer is E.   *(Ch. 3)*   The right coronary artery usually supplies the blood flow to the inferior left ventricle. The left circumflex branch of the left coronary artery only provides the blood flow in about 10 percent of cases. Venous blood from coronary circulation returns to the cardiac chambers mostly through the coronary sinus, but can also return through arteriosinusoidal channels. Most of the coronary blood flow occurs during diastole. The washout of metabolites plays the most important role in autoregulation. Myogenic and metabolically mediated responses play a much smaller role. During times of increased metabolic demand, the release of adenosine is an important mediator of autoregulation.

I-38.   The answer is B.   *(Ch. 4)*   Each individual strand of DNA in the double helix contains the same information as its partner strand. When DNA is subjected to high temperatures, the two strands of the double helix can be separated. One amino acid is coded for by a three-nucleotide codon. Restriction enzymes recognize specific sequences in the DNA and cut at those locations. DNA ligase is the enzyme used to join DNA fragments together. The enzyme RNA polymerase II is needed for the transcription of DNA to mRNA. Reverse transcriptase is the retroviral enzyme used to make DNA from RNA.

I-39.   The answer is B.   *(Ch. 4)*   It is estimated that only 5 percent of DNA is used to code for protein. A nucleotide is made up of a nitrogenous base, a five-carbon sugar, and a phosphate group. The pyrimidine bases are cytosine and thymine. Adenine and guanine are the purine bases. RNA polymerase always initiates replication of DNA from the 5′ end and travels in the 3′ direction. Hydrogen bonds are responsible for the pairing of complementary bases.

I-40.   The answer is E.   *(Ch. 4)*   Transcription is the production of RNA from a DNA template. Transcription takes place in the nucleus. The 5′ cap is important for the initiation of translation. The poly(A) tail makes the mRNA more stable in the cytoplasm. When the mRNA undergoes splicing, the introns are removed and the exons are joined together. Small nuclear ribonucleoproteins are important in mRNA splicing.

I-41.   The answer is A.   *(Ch. 4)*   The term *degeneracy* refers to the fact that more than one codon codes for some amino acids. The codon AUG is the start codon and also codes for methionine. ATP provides the energy source for the covalent joining of a transfer RNA to an amino acid. The final modifications to a protein are done after translation. mRNA is not very stable and can survive in the cytoplasm for only a few minutes to a few hours.

I-42.   The answer is C.   *(Ch. 4)*   The coding region is located on the central part of the mRNA molecule. Sequences regulating translation are located on the 5′ region of the molecule and regulatory sequences and coding signals for stability in the cytoplasm are located on the 3′ region. Upstream refers to everything that is 5′ to the sequence to be translated. The initiation site for transcription is located 5′ to the coding sequence. Polymerase II has a very low affinity for DNA and will bind it only with the help of transcription factors, thus presenting regulatory opportunity. The average exon is only about 300 base pairs long, while introns are much larger.

I-43.   The answer is E.   *(Ch. 4)*   Genes that are heavily methylated are generally not transcribed. The methylation makes them insensitive to DNase. Transcription of the housekeeping genes takes place in a constitutive manner. Enhancer sequences can be located either upstream or downstream from the coding region. The promoter region is located just upstream from the coding region. An exon can either be spliced with the adjacent exon, or several exons can be excluded when it joins an exon downstream. This contributes to the great variety of proteins that can be made from a single gene. The poly(A) tail is located at the 3′ region of the mRNA and contributes to its stability in the cytoplasm.

I-44.   The answer is B.   *(Ch. 4)*   A restriction map is made using restriction endonucleases to cut DNA into a segment containing the fragment of interest. Complementary DNA is created from mRNA using the retroviral enzyme reverse transcriptase. Phosphate groups give DNA a net negative charge, thus DNA migrates toward the positive electrode during electrophoresis. Southern blotting is used to transfer DNA from a gel to a nylon membrane. Northern blotting is used to transfer mRNA, and Western blotting is used for transferring proteins. A restriction endonuclease recognizes and cuts a specific nucleotide sequence.

I-45.   The answer is A.   *(Ch. 4)*   A genomic library is created by cutting DNA using restriction endonucleases. A plasmid is a vector that can be used in cloning and is thus appropriate for use in the creation of a gene library. A complementary DNA (cDNA) library is created using reverse transcriptase to create DNA from mRNA. This library will contain the DNA that a certain cell is actively transcribing. The DNA in a cDNA library will differ from one cell to another, as each cell only needs to use a certain portion of its DNA to carry out its function. A genomic library contains all the DNA in a cell, not just the DNA being actively transcribed. The yeast artificial chromosome can accommodate a large DNA insert, but is very difficult to work with on a routine basis.

I-46.   The answer is D.   *(Ch. 4)*   To perform PCR you must know short sequences at the beginning and at the end of the DNA fragment. The first step of PCR involves raising the temperature to 95°C to separate the two DNA strands. Most polymerases would denature at this high temperature. However, Taq1 DNA polymerase, taken from *Thermus aquaticus,* which is thermostable, is used. This enzyme will not denature at high temperatures, and thus polymerase does not need to be re-added between cycles. Restriction enzymes are not necessary in PCR. The usefulness of PCR comes from the fact that it can be performed starting only one copy of the DNA or RNA needed and in a few hours, millions of copies will be generated.

I-47.   The answer is D.   *(Ch. 4)*   Microtubules are made up of globular subunits. They function in the movement and organization of cellular organelles. Microfilaments are composed of actin filaments and serve to transmit force throughout the cytoplasm. Intermediate filaments are extended molecules that form ropelike polymers. They are highly specific for each cell and tissue type.

I-48.   The answer is B.   *(Ch. 4)*   Growth that is by an increase in cell number is termed *hyperplasia.* Growth that is by an increase in cell size is termed *hypertrophy.* Most of the growth seen in the adult heart is constitutive, or hypertrophic, because the cells have lost their ability to proliferate. Growth factors released in a paracrine mechanism affect the growth of adjacent cells. Factors that are secreted in an autocrine mechanism bind to receptors on the same cell that secreted it. Effector molecules that act on transcription factors have a sustained change in growth. Those that act on translation have a more transient effect. Signaling proteins use both kinases and phosphatases to transmit a signal. The kinases will phosphorylate and amplify the signal. The phosphatases, by dephosphorylation, will dampen the signal.

I-49. The answer is A. *(Ch. 4)* The response of the myocardium to injury, whether it is myocardial infarction or valvular disease, plays a major role in determining morbidity and mortality. When there is hypertrophy in the heart, new sarcomeres are added in parallel, giving rise to thickened walls in the cardiac chambers. The growth seen in the heart in utero or during puberty is orchestrated from a variety of hormonal stimuli, such as growth hormones. In the response to injury, the growth stimulus is localized to the affected organ. A hypertrophied ventricle contains growth factors, and thus when supernatants taken from it are perfused into a normal heart, the normal heart begins to initiate transcription in response to the growth factors. Cardiac myocytes are able to re-express several fetal proteins in their normal growth response.

I-50. The answer is C. *(Ch. 5)* The earliest stage of cardiac growth in utero, occurs in the absence of contractile activity. Mechanical forces become increasingly important following this period. Cardiac growth is a mix of hyperplasia and hypertrophy during the embryonic period and for a few weeks following birth. Adult myocytes, however, are terminally differentiated and cannot re-enter the cell cycle. This makes their growth possible only through hypertrophy. Eccentric hypertrophy is a normal ratio of wall thickness to dimension. This type of hypertrophy occurs during isotonic exercises. There is a large difference between the molecular, biochemical, and physiologic changes seen in pathologic and physiologic hypertrophy. Concentric ventricular hypertrophy results from pressure overloading, for example, as seen in systemic hypertension or aortic coarctation. Volume overloading conditions, like mitral or aortic regurgitation, result in eccentric hypertrophy.

I-51. The answer is B. *(Ch. 5)* G-protein, produced in response to stretch of a cardiomyocyte, activates membrane-bound phospholipase C. In this important signaling pathway, phospholipase C hydrolyzes phosphatidylinositol bisphosphate into diacylglycerol and inositol triphosphate. Diacylglycerol activates PKC. PKC phosphorylates a number of downstream proteins and transcription factors, while inositol triphosphate plays an important role in modulation of cytosolic calcium through its interaction with the sarcoplasmic reticulum. MAPKs, which are activated later in the pathway, are serine-threonine protein kinases. c-jun and c-myc are the transcription factors that are phosphorylated at the end of the signaling pathway. Transfection of an antisense nucleotide into MAPK was shown to prevent cardiomyocyte hypertrophy.

I-52. The answer is E. *(Ch. 5)* Thyroid hormone-induced hypertrophy is an indirect effect of the T^3-mediated increased oxygen consumption that results in increased cardiac work and hypertrophy. The cytokines interleukin-1 and tumor necrosis factor alpha are elevated in patients with congestive heart failure. Stimulation of cell-surface tyrosine-kinase receptors can elicit a hyperplastic or hypertrophic response in neonatal cardiomyocytes. Acidic fibroblast growth factors (FGFs) produce a hyperplastic response while the basic FGFs stimulate increased protein synthesis, resulting in hypertrophy. Cytokines of the interleukin-6 and cardiotrophin family activate the cardiomyocyte transmembrane receptor, gp130, resulting in the phosphorylation of signal transducers and activators of transcription.

I-53. The answer is B. *(Ch. 5)* The efficiency of protein synthesis is measured as moles of amino acid incorporated per milligram of cellular RNA per hour. The capacity is measured by determining the number of milligrams of RNA per gram of tissue. Vascular smooth muscle cells have the ability to produce collagen. In dilated cardiomyopathy, the activity of matrix metalloproteinases is increased. The critical determinant for cardiac hypertrophy is an increased capacity for protein synthesis. The phosphorylation of phospholamban results in disinhibition and leads to an enhancement of calcium uptake by the sarcoplasmic reticulum.

I-54. The answer is D. *(Ch. 5)* The most common electrical abnormality seen in a hypertrophied heart is a prolongation of the action potential. In compensated cardiac hypertrophy, the effective number of active cross bridges per unit of myocardium remains the same, but the rate of cross-bridge cycling is reduced. In severe hypertrophy, the prolongation of the action potential is most importantly determined by a decrease in the potassium currents Ikl and Ito. In mild hypertrophy, increases in calcium and calcium-activated currents are important in prolongation of the action potential. The ratio of capillaries to myocytes seen in patients and animals with hypertrophied hearts from a pressure overload is no different than that seen in a normal heart. Since myocyte area is increased, there is an increase in nutrient diffusion distance in the hypertrophied heart. It is believed that myocardial stunning results from either hydroxy-free radical generation, calcium overload, or both mechanisms.

I-55.   The answer is E.   *(Ch. 5)*   Studies have shown that there is a depression in steady-state mRNA levels and sarcoplasmic reticulum ATPase and phospholamban proteins only in decompensated hypertrophy. These findings are not seen in compensated hypertrophy. There is evidence that abnormal signal transduction plays a role in the development of both cardiac hypertrophy and heart failure. A derangement of calcium homeostasis in the cardiomyocyte is a feature of decompensated hypertrophy and failure. Overexpression of the calcium-sensitive protein kinase C isoform B produces cardiac hypertrophy and heart failure. There are a number of signaling molecules that produce both hypertrophy and apoptosis. This complicates the issue of whether apoptosis may contribute to the heart failure phenotype.

I-56.   The answer is B.   *(Ch. 6)*   The internal elastic membrane is located between the intima and the medial. The smooth muscle is generally oriented in a helical arrangement in large, elastic arteries and in concentric arrangement in muscular arteries. Pericytes are smooth muscle-like cells that serve a synergistic and nutritive function. These cells are apposed to occasional endothelial cells. In normal arteries, smooth muscle cells are generally in the contractile phenotype and acquire the synthetic phenotype in response to injury. Smooth muscle cells are cells are found in the media.

I-57.   The answer is B.   *(Ch. 6)*   The expression of "scavenger cells," which uptake oxidized low-density lipoprotein, is unaffected by the growth state of the endothelial cell. Heparin sulfates bind the enzyme lipoprotein lipase, an enzyme that hydrolyzes triglycerides into fatty acids, to the surface of the endothelial cell. Endothelial cells normally present an antithrombotic surface, but are capable of synthesizing and secreting prothrombotic factors under the influence of cytokines and inflammatory agents. These actions result in an antithrombotic/thrombotic balance. Water-soluble macromolecules are generally transported by vesicular transport. Edema formation is thought to result from a contractile response of the endothelium in response to agonists. This contractile response results in a shape change that opens gap junctions between the cells.

I-58.   The answer is E.   *(Ch. 6)*   Under normal conditions, the vascular smooth muscle responds to hormonal stimulation with contraction or relaxation. The first signals generated within a smooth muscle cell following stimulation involve hydrolysis of the phosphoinositides. Angiotensin II induces a transient constriction of many vessels. Norepinephrine and vasopressin usually induce a sustained contraction. Classic growth factors cause hyperplasia, while hypertrophy results in response to long-term stimulation with vasoconstrictor-type agents. There is evidence that tyrosine phosphatases can counteract the mitogenic effects of growth factors by inhibiting the phosphorylation of specific substrates by tyrosine.

I-59.   The answer is B.   *(Ch. 6)*   After NO crosses the smooth muscle cell membrane, it binds to the heme moiety of guanylate cyclase, thus enhancing the formation of cyclic GMP. The release of endothelium-derived relaxing factor/NO is in response to an increase in intracellular Ca^{2+}. In the absence of tetrahydrobiopterin or L-arginine, electrons flow to oxygen, resulting in the formation of superoxide anion. This is termed the *uncoupling* of NO synthase. NO is released from the endothelium. Endothelial NO synthase expression is altered by changing the half-life of mRNA.

I-60.   The answer is A.   *(Ch. 6)*   Endothelin-1 (ET-1) is involved in nitroglycerin tolerance as well as being a growth factor for smooth muscle and a chemoattractant for monocytes.

Prostacyclin, which relaxes vascular smooth muscle by increasing intracellular cyclic AMP content, is released by the endothelium. Adenine nucleosides bind to P1 receptors that activate cyclic AMP and lead to relaxation. Adenine nucleotides stimulate P2 receptors that are coupled to phosphoinositide hydrolysis. The ET-B receptor is found on endothelial cells. Subthreshold concentrations of ET-1 enhance vasoconstriction to a number of agents and is thought to lead to the rebound phenomenon that occurs after the discontinuance of nitroglycerin that has previously been administered for several days.

I-61. The answer is B. *(Ch. 6)* When agents such as γ-interferon or cortisone bind to heparin, they inhibit angiogenesis. Experimental removal of the endothelium has allowed the initiation of the mitogenic response and the regrowth of normal endothelium inhibits further proliferation. Heparin can inhibit vascular smooth muscle cell mitogenesis and migration and reduce neointimal proliferation during the first three days after injury, although the inhibition is not complete. This incomplete inhibition shows that there are other endothelial factors involved. A possible mechanism for how endothelial cells can aid in maintaining smooth muscle quiescence is induction of tyrosine phosphatase activity in smooth muscle cells. FGF does not contain the signal peptide that usually causes transport out of the cell, thus it is probably not secreted by endothelial cells. However, FGF is present in endothelial cells and may be released upon cell lysis or death.

I-62. The answer is A. *(Ch. 6)* Cytokines, thrombin, and histamine differentially regulate expression of chemoattractant proteins and adhesion molecules, which allow leukocyte accumulation on the vascular surface. Histamine released at the site of vascular injury causes endothelial cells to contract and results in increased permeability. Chemoattractant proteins and leukocyte adhesion molecules are involved in atherogenesis. E-selectin and GMP-140 bind only resting, nonactivated neutrophils. Cytokines stimulate the endothelial cell release of chemoattractant proteins and adhesion molecules.

I-63. The answer is D. *(Ch. 6)* Increased production of ROS in the vascular wall is referred to as oxidative stress. The existence of all the neutrophil substrates has been shown in endothelial cells, although it is not clear that they function together in the same way to produce ROS as they do in neutrophils. An important source of free radicals in the vasculature is the lipoxygenases. Lipoxygenases do not produce superoxide anions, but instead react directly with unsaturated fatty acids to form a lipid radical. The uncoupling of the enzyme endothelial nitric oxide synthase seems to play an important role in several diseases, including hypercholesterolemia, hypertension, and diabetes. Angiotensin II, mediated by hydrogen peroxide, causes a substantial amount of vascular smooth muscle hypertrophy.

I-64. The answer is E. *(Ch. 6)* The endothelial dysfunction seen in atherosclerosis has been defined as an impairment of endothelial-dependent relaxation. This leads to the vasospastic tendency that is seen in vessels. Studies have shown that LDL and cytokines downregulate endothelial nitric oxide synthase (eNOS) by destabilizing the eNOS RNA. Studies with cholesterol fed animals have shown a manifestation of a dysfunctional endothelium as there is a recruitment of monocytes and macrophages into the vessel wall. Dysfunctional endothelium in atherosclerosis shifts its production of growth factors from growth-inhibitory factors to growth-promoting factors, thus leading to intimal proliferation. Oxidative stress and oxidatively-modified LDL play a central role in atherogenesis.

I-65. The answer is C. *(Ch. 6)* Vitamins C and E, which are antioxidants, may reduce the risk of restenosis. This theory is based on the observation that superoxide is increased in vessels following balloon injury. Removal of the endothelium does alter the paracrine hormonal environment, although the major problem associated with it is that it exposes a thrombogenic surface. The hormonal influences from the infiltration and activation of macrophages in response to denuded vessel wall are partially responsible for the vessel response to injury by angioplasty. The cytoskeleton of a proliferating smooth muscle cell (SMC) is similar to that of a cultured cell. The cytoskeleton of a proliferating SMC is different, however, from a differentiated SMC. The initial outpouring of fibroblast growth factor in response to deep injury does not seem to depend on platelet factors, but appears to be directly related to removal of the endothelium.

I-66.   **The answer is D.**   *(Ch. 7)*   It is estimated that there are between 50,000 and 100,000 genes in the human genome. The Human Genome Project was completed in 2000. The National Institutes of Health and the Department of Health did 60 to 70 percent of the gene sequencing, with the remainder done by the Sanger Institute in Cambridge, England and some other international partners. The research involved both sequencing the genes as well as all the intervening sequences. All the mRNA from a cell had to be extracted to develop a genomic physical map, using sequence tagged sites.

I-67.   **The answer is D.**   *(Ch. 7)*   Very little is known about the protein composition of most genes and thus also little is known about their function. With the current technology available, it would take a century to determine the function of genes. This area requires a boost from improved technology and increased awareness. The first genome that was completely sequenced was *Haemophilus influenzae,* which was done in 1995. The most important reason for sequencing the genomes of single-celled organisms is that the information we obtain offers the potential for diagnosis and treatment of human infectious diseases. *Caenorhabditis elegans* was the first multicellular organism for which the genome has been sequenced.

I-68.   **The answer is C.**   *(Ch. 7)*   GenBank is a computerized network of gene banks established to allow for efficient input and access to all current information for free. Investigators input their research into GenBank everyday. The DNA microchip is a promising advance because it would offer the ability to detect gene mismatches in hybridization. It is not currently possible to easily detect mutations in genes. An emerging contribution from bioenergetics is the concept that genes with a common functioning pathway can be grouped into families. Genes with similar functions will have a common motif. This common motif can then be applied to genes of unknown function to determine their function.

I-69.   **The answer is E.**   *(Ch. 7)*   Investigators have been fairly unsuccessful in obtaining stem cells from most organs in the body. Transfection of a stem cell with MyoD has been shown to induce a skeletal muscle phenotype in fibroblasts and some other cell types. Embryonic stem cells are currently obtained from fetal tissue from abortions and miscarriages as well as from embryos used for in vitro fertilization that could not be implanted by fertility clinics. Differentiated adult cells have little or no potential to be able to differentiate into other cell types. It is possible to obtain limited numbers of stem cells from bone marrow, liver tissue, and skeletal muscle.

I-70.   **The answer is A.**   *(Ch. 7)*   Positional cloning proceeds in several stages, one of which is determining the location of a diseased gene by comparing how the inheritance of a certain chromosome segment coincides with the familial inheritance of disease. Common diseases, such as coronary artery disease, diabetes, and stroke, are multifactorial in nature, and thus Mendelian inheritance is not a very powerful means to determine risk of disease. A score of 10 on a δ *sib* would show that all familial factors together increase the risk of disease 10-fold. One of the limitations of using SNPs to determine the location of diseased genes is that patients and controls must have a well-matched genetic background. It is anticipated that the locations of all SNPs will be known within the next 5 years.

I-71.   **The answer is D.**   *(Ch. 7)*   The National Institutes of Health has allocated 5 percent of the Human Genome Project (HGP) budget and the U.S. Department of Energy has allocated 3 percent of their HGP budget to go towards the formal initiative on the ethical, legal, and societal implications of the HGP. There are a few instances where an employer may have access to the genetic information of an employee or a potential employee. There is currently a shortage of medical geneticists and genetic counselors available to meet the growing demand for their services. High school athletes are not currently genetically screened for their risk of familial hypertrophic cardiomyopathy.

I-72. **The answer is C.** *(Ch. 8)*   Adenoviral vectors infect nondividing cells and do not integrate into the host's genome. Retroviral vectors have not been effective for cardiovascular applications because they require actively dividing cells for integration and expression of their genome. The usefulness of using an adenoviral vector has been limited due to transient gene expression and the inflammatory and immune responses of the host. Adeno-associated viral vectors are able to infect a broad range of cell lines. These vectors, however, accept only a limited size gene insert of 4 to 5 kb.

I-73. **The answer is D.** *(Ch. 8)*   The direct injection of plasmid DNA into cardiac or skeletal muscle gives a stable transfection of only a small percentage of cells. It is postulated that cationic liposomes are taken up by the cell using the following mechanisms: 1) spontaneous capture of negatively charged polynucleotides with cationic lipids in a condensation reaction, 2) fusion with the membrane or an endosome, and 3) increased cellular uptake due to interactions between positively charged complexes with the negatively charged biological membrane. ASOs are designed to be complementary to the coding sequence of a target RNA. Once they are inside the cell, they bind to the complimentary RNA and decrease its translation. ASOs are attractive agents for gene therapy as they can be synthesized in large quantities and do not require a viral component for entry into the cell. High-mobility group 1 is a nuclear protein that binds DNA and enhances the integration of transfected DNA into the nucleus.

I-74. **The answer is B.** *(Ch. 8)*   Administration of antisense oligonucleotides against c-myb to the adventitial layer of a rat carotid artery inhibited neointimal hyperplasia following balloon injury. Vein grafts present a good opportunity to combine in vivo gene-transfer techniques with ex vivo application of a transfection medium. Genetic engineering can alter the ability of a graft to mount a hyperplastic response following acute injury yet leave intact the ability to respond to chronic hemodynamic stress via a hypertrophic response. After a vein graft with gene therapy, there is a shift from neointimal hyperplasia to medial hypertrophy. The ability to inhibit cell cycle progression with gene therapy is very likely to have an effect on the proatherogenic environment of a normal graft wall.

I-75. **The answer is C.** *(Ch. 8)*   Fibroblast growth factor 1 overexpression in porcine arteries was associated with intimal thickening of transfected vessels as well as neocapillary formation in the expanded intima. Herpes simplex virus thymidine kinase (HSVtk) encodes for the enzyme thymidine kinase, which phosphorylates gangciclovir or acyclovir into a metabolite that disrupts DNA replication in the S phase of the cell cycle. It is possible that overexpression of transforming growth factor β1 could promote healing after vascular injury without extensive cellular intimal hyperplasia. The bystander effect is when a by-product of a chemical reaction diffuses into adjacent cells and allows for incorporation of it into those cells. For instance, the cell cycle can be inhibited in cells surrounding ones that have received the HSVtk. Human platelet-derived growth factor BB transfected into porcine arteries developed intimal hyperplasia with increased numbers of intimal smooth muscle cells.

I-76. **The answer is B.** *(Ch. 8)*   Blockade of the cell cycle with the dominant negative transcription decoy E2F leads to arrest of the G1 phase of the cell cycle. A safe and feasible method in inhibition of the cell cycle is by transfecting human bypass vein grafts with E2F decoy oligodeoxynucleotides. In a study to treat myocardial ischemia, recombinant aFGF was injected into the anastomosis site of the left internal mammary artery and the left anterior descending artery of patients undergoing coronary bypass surgery. Intracardiac myoblast grafts that were transfected with transformity growth factor β1 showed increased DNA synthesis in vascular endothelial cells that is consistent with a sustained angiogenic response. Direct injection of DNA into myocardial tissue has been shown to be effective for the local delivery of a transgene into the heart.

I-77. **The answer is C.** *(Ch. 9)* The initial patterning of the embryo determines the three axes of the heart: dorsal-ventral, left-right, and anterior-posterior. The embryonic genome does not take control of development until after the second cell cycle. The maternal genome controls the first two cycles. Retinoic acid exerts the greatest effect on the arterial pole of the heart and the least effect on the venous pole. Asymmetry in the embryo is seen in the blastodisc stage, when the primitive streak defines the anterior-posterior axis and the position of the yolk sac defines the dorsal-ventral axis. Hensen's node contains retinoic acid and may confer positional information on mesodermal cells. The mesoderm is formed as ectodermal cells migrate through the primitive streak that runs adjacent to Hensen's node.

I-78. **The answer is A.** *(Ch. 9)* dHAND expression in the heart tube is restricted to the conotruncus and the future right ventricle, and it is thus thought that its expression is necessary in the formation of the right ventricle. eHAND expression is thought necessary for the formation of the left ventricle. Hox genes are usually upregulated during early differentiation and appear in a time-dependent sequence. *Nkx-2* factors in the mouse have been shown to activate transcription. The murine Hox gene, *Nkx-2.5/Csx,* is expressed before cardiogenic differentiation and continues through adulthood. *Hox code* is a term that denotes that a particular combination of Hox genes are active in a particular region and are thus specifying the developmental fate of that region.

I-79. **The answer is E.** *(Ch. 9)* Cardiac-restricted ankyrin repeat protein (CARP), which lies downstream of the Hox gene *Nkx-2.5,* codes for a nuclear regulator for cardiac gene expression. *Nkx-2.5* controls CARP expression in part through GATA-4, which has been found in cardiac mesoderm and gut epithelium. MEF2 genes are highly expressed in both early heart and skeletal muscle progenitor cells. MEF2 has been implicated as a key regulator of both heart and skeletal muscle differentiation programs. The cardiac alpha-actin gene are not activated by *Nkx-2.5* only, but instead are activated by a combination of *Nkx-2.5* and SRF proteins.

I-80. **The answer is B.** *(Ch. 9)* Sonic hedgehog (Shh) expression on the right side of Hensen's node is repressed by the secreted morphogen activin. Shh expression on the left side induces nodal expression in the lateral plate mesoderm. The chemical signals that direct the left-right asymmetry in the developing heart have a genetic basis. Several types of unlinked mutations have been found that affect the left-right laterality in mice and humans. Neural crest cells carry the information for the formation of structures to the specific site where they migrate. The information is thus defined at the origin of the neural crest cell, rather than at the destination site. Myofibrils appear to be disarrayed in an embryonic myofibril and become organized as development proceeds. In mature myocardium, the sarcomeres are aligned in parallel to lines of stress. It is important to remember that the primitive linear heart tube does not contain all of the segments present in the mature heart.

I-81. **The answer is D.** *(Ch. 9)* Fibronectin most likely sets up the migratory pathways for the primordial endothelial cells through the cardiac jelly. The endocardium is transdifferentiated in the endocardial cushions. These cells eventually make up part of the fibrous skeleton of the cardiac valves. The tubular heart bends to the right and anteriorly as it grows, resulting in a d-loop configuration. The formation of an l-loop results in ventricular inversion and transposition of the great arteries. The outflow tract of the heart in the heart tube formation is connected only to the right ventricle.

I-82. **The answer is A.** *(Ch. 9)* The rapid cell division of endothelial cells along the endocardial tube and the rapid resorption of cardiac jelly results in myocardial ridges and trabeculae. Myocardial trabeculation begins at the apex and extends proximally and distally. Due to the distinct morphological differences between the developing heart chambers, the right and left ventricles can be identified in an embryonic heart. Noncompaction of the ventricular myocardium is a rare, familial disease. The familial recurrence of this disease is high. Noncompaction of the ventricular myocardium always affects the left ventricle. Right ventricular involvement may or may not be present.

I-83.   The answer is C.   *(Ch. 9)*   The primary atrial septum (septum primum) forms from active growth of a myocardial septum. Multiple fenestrations in the myocardial portion of the primary septum result in the secondary foramen. Fusion of the endocardial cushions and the leading edge of mesenchyme result in the closure of ostium primum. The pulmonary pit, where the future pulmonary vein will enter, becomes recognizable before atrial septation is complete. ASD at the fossa ovalis is due to a malformation of the primary atrial septum. This defect is often referred to as secundum-type ASD.

I-84.   The answer is B.   *(Ch. 9)*   Most of the malformations involved with the absence of myocardialization involve malalignment of the outlet septum with the muscular interventricular septum. These malformations result in ventricular septal defects. The communication between the right and left ventricles is bordered by the muscular ventricular septum, the fused endocardial cushions and the conal septum. The mesechymal cap of the atrial septum primum fuses with the convex side of the endocardial cushions. In ventricular septal defect, there is no cleft in the anterior mitral valve cusp because the endocardial cushions fuse normally. In a partial AV valve canal defect, there is only an interatrial communication, known as an ostium primum-type artrial septal defect. In complete AV valve canal defect, there is both an interatrial and interventricular communication.

I-85.   The answer is E.   *(Ch. 9)*   The endocardial cushions develop in areas with slow contraction and relaxation. In the early stages of endocardial cushion development, it is only possible to distinguish the inferior AV cushion and the superior AV cushion. Ebstein's anomaly of the tricuspid valve is most likely due to an abnormality of myocardial delamination. Tricuspid and mitral valve atresia probably result from abnormal formation and/or premature fusion of the endocardial cushion tissue bordering the AV canal. The primitive pulmonary arteries branch from the sixth arch. The fifth aortic arch is rudimentary in mammals. An anomalous subclavian artery is frequently present with an interrupted aortic arch.

I-86.   The answer is D.   *(Ch. 9)*   Coronary endothelial cells and coronary smooth muscle cells are derived from the proepicardium. This is a cluster of cells attached to the ventral wall of the sinus venosus. The coronary network is formed from epicardially-derived cells that have transdifferentiated and migrated into the myocardial layers. Neural crest cells control the development of the coronary arterial branching system and the elastic lamina. The coronary vasculature matures using the processes of both angiogenesis and vasculogenesis. The growth of the coronary vascular endothelium parallels the development of the epicardium.

PART II
GENERAL EVALUATION
OF THE PATIENT

II. GENERAL EVALUATION OF THE PATIENT

QUESTIONS

DIRECTIONS: Each question listed below has five suggested responses.
Select the **one best** response to each question.

II-1. Which of the following statements regarding chest pain is true?

(A) the warm-up phenomenon occurs when a patient's angina threshold increases during a second exercise effort
(B) chest pain that is described as "stabbing" or "shooting" and reaches its maximum intensity almost instantly is indicative of classical angina
(C) a patient describing chest pain with a clenched fist held over the sternal area indicates chest pain of a pulmonary origin
(D) angina pectoris is defined as chest pain or discomfort that results from an imbalance between myocardial oxygen supply and demand
(E) associated symptoms such as nausea, vomiting, or diaphoresis generally indicate chest pain of a psychogenic origin

(pages 196–197)

II-2. Which of the following statements regarding angina is true?

(A) the term *linked angina* applies to episodes of angina caused by gastrointestinal factors that are related to an increase in cardiac work
(B) a patient with coronary artery spasm superimposed on coronary atherosclerosis characteristically has exertional angina
(C) syndrome X is a heterogeneous grouping of patients who suffer from a wide spectrum of chest pain and have a variety of vascular and smooth muscle hypersensitive constrictor responses
(D) the history alone is generally quite specific for predicting the presence of coronary artery disease in patients with rest angina
(E) males are more likely than females to have angina in the presence of arteriographically normal coronary arteries

(page 197)

II-3. Which of the following pulmonary causes of chest pain is most easily confused with myocardial infarction?

(A) spontaneous pneumothorax
(B) pulmonary embolism
(C) pneumonia
(D) pulmonary infarction
(E) pleurisy

(page 199)

II-4. Which of the following statements concerning respiratory symptoms is true?

(A) the occurrence of dyspnea 2 to 3 h after going to bed that is relieved by sitting upright and does not return upon falling back asleep is seen in patients with left heart failure
(B) dark or clotted blood may be present in the sputum of patients with mitral stenosis
(C) a recent dramatic increase in dyspnea is more likely related to lung disease than it is to heart disease
(D) the sputum of a patient with acute pulmonary edema is usually bloody
(E) Cheyne-Stokes respirations may occur in patients with central nervous system disease, but not in patients with heart failure

(page 200)

II-5. Which of the following signs or symptoms are most likely cardiac in origin?

(A) edema mainly affecting the face and arms
(B) fatigue and weakness
(C) syncope associated with incontinence and followed by confusion and/or drowsiness
(D) fever, chills, or sweats in a patient with a new heart murmur and a recent history of dental work
(E) pain localized to the temporal area

(pages 199–202)

II-6. Which of the following signs indicative of congenital disorders is associated with mitral valve prolapse?

(A) hypoplastic deltoids, skeletal anomalies of the forearm, and bradydactyly

(B) cleft-palate, micrognathia, and low-set ears

(C) short stature, short neck, barrel chest, widely spaced teeth, and cloudy cornea

(D) epicanthal folds, low-set ears, widely spaced eyes, and mental retardation

(E) blue sclera, disproportionately long legs, and a thumb that protrudes past the ulnar side of the hand when clenching the hand around the flexed thumb

(page 203–205)

II-7. Which of the following signs is seen in a disorder associated with pulmonic stenosis?

(A) nontender, hemorrhagic lesions found on the palms and the soles

(B) café-au-lait spots and mental retardation

(C) the CREST syndrome (calcinosis, Raynaud's phenomena, esophageal involvement, sclerodactyly and telangiectasia)

(D) ulnar deviation of the fingers, subluxation of the metacarpophalangeal joints, and a "swan neck" deformity

(E) a combination of polyarthritis, abdominal pain, and diarrhea

(pages 209–212)

II-8. Which of the following statements regarding the measurement of blood pressure is true?

(A) in children, the diastolic pressure should be recorded as the point where sounds become inaudible

(B) the auscultatory gap is a period of silence between Korotkoff phases II and III

(C) there is generally a good correlation between indirect and direct measurements of blood pressure in the arm

(D) the period during which sounds become crisper and increase in intensity is Korotkoff phase II

(E) if the cuff is immediately reinflated for several pressure determinations, the systolic pressure may be falsely elevated

(pages 219–220)

II-9. Which of the following statements regarding the arterial pulse is true?

(A) the resistance encountered in peripheral arteries varies with heart rate

(B) palpation of the carotid artery is more accurate than peripheral vessels for assessing the severity of aortic regurgitation

(C) a reflected wave occurring during systole decreases ventricular afterload

(D) palpation of the carotid artery is used to assess cardiac performance

(E) in the normal proximal aortic pulse, the tidal wave represents the impulse generated from left ventricular ejection

(pages 222–224)

II-10. The figure below depicts aortic pressure. Which of the following statements is true?

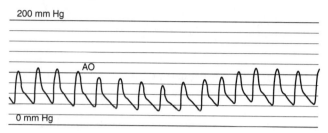

(A) this patient has aortic regurgitation

(B) this patient has aortic stenosis

(C) this patient has cardiac tamponade

(D) this patient has hypertrophic cardiomyopathy

(E) this is a normal patient

(pages 224–225)

II-11. Which of the following statements regarding the arterial pulse is true?

(A) a bisferiens pulse occurs in patients with left ventricular failure

(B) pulsus alternans can be best distinguished by palpating a distal artery rather than the carotid artery

(C) the dicrotic pulse is most prominent in the elderly and in patients with hypertension

(D) pulsus paradoxus is frequently seen with constrictive pericarditis

(E) a parvus et tardus pulse is never associated with a systolic ejection murmur

(pages 224–226)

II-12. Which of the following statements regarding the venous pulse is true?

(A) the abdominojugular test is useful in patients with superior vena cava obstruction

(B) the *v* wave results from the tricuspid valve bulging into the atrium during right ventricular systole

(C) the most common cause of Kussmaul's sign is constrictive pericarditis

(D) a giant *a* wave is most likely seen with pulmonic stenosis or pulmonary hypertension

(E) in a patient with an atrial septal defect, the *a* and *v* waves are often equal in size, and there is an increase in venous pressure

(pages 227–229)

II-13. From the right atrial pressures depicted in the following figure, which of the following statements is true?

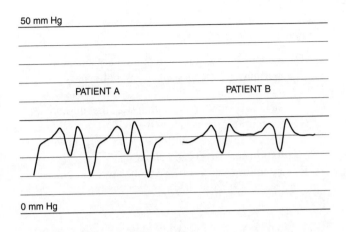

(A) Patient B is more likely than Patient A to have Kussmaul's sign

(B) Patient B is more likely than Patient A to have an early diastolic sound

(C) Patient B is more likely than Patient A to have calcification of the diaphragm on chest x-ray

(D) Patient B is more likely than Patient A to have pulsus paradoxus

(E) Patient B is unlikely to have a pericardial effusion

(pages 227–229)

II-14. Which of the following signs in the retina accompany decompensated retinal circulation in hypertension?

(A) papilledema

(B) copper or silver "wiring"

(C) neovascularization

(D) microaneurysms

(E) flame hemorrhages

(pages 232–234)

II-15. Which of the following statements regarding inspection and palpation of the precordium is true?

(A) the point of maximal impulse and the cardiac apex impulse are synonymous

(B) an abnormal pulsation in the sternoclavicular joint in patients with chest pain may be associated with aortic regurgitation

(C) high-frequency movements, such as ejection sounds and valve closure sounds, are best assessed by palpation with the finger pads

(D) a systolic thrill in the third, fourth, or fifth intercostal space is characteristic of a ventricular septal defect

(E) a sustained apex impulse indicates left ventricular dilation

(pages 236–239)

II-16. Which of the following statements regarding the first heart sound (S_1) is true?

(A) paradoxical splitting of S_1 is seen with a right bundle branch block

(B) there is decreased intensity of S_1 with mitral valve prolapse

(C) there is increased intensity of S_1 in patients with Lown-Ganong-Levine syndrome

(D) there is increased intensity of S_1 in patients with mitral valve calcification and severe mitral stenosis

(E) S_1 is increased in intensity in patients with left bundle branch block

(page 241)

II-17. In relation to the figure below, recorded using a high-fidelity catheter, which of the following statements is true?

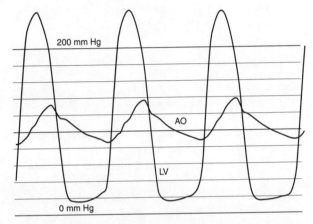

(A) the left ventricular end-diastolic pressure remains unaffected by this condition

(B) in the congenital form of this condition, an ejection sound would most likely be heard at the apex

(C) normal splitting of the second heart sound would be present

(D) this patient would have a bisferiens pulse

(E) a thrill, if present, would be felt in the fourth or fifth left intercostal space

(page 259)

II-18. In relation to the figure below, recorded using a high-fidelity catheter, which of the following statements is true?

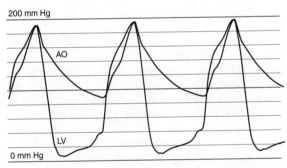

(A) this patient would have a hyperkinetic arterial pulse

(B) only one murmur would be heard in this condition, a systolic ejection murmur in the right second intercostal space

(C) the pulse pressure is narrow

(D) the left ventricular end-diastolic pressure is normal

(E) this figure depicts an acute condition

(page 270)

II-19.   Which of the following statements regarding a mid-systolic click is true?

(A)   a midsystolic click is heard in aortic stenosis
(B)   this sound is associated with a midsystolic, crescendo-decrescendo murmur heard in the second right and second left intercostal spaces
(C)   there is only one pathologic condition associated with a midsystolic click
(D)   the click occurs just as the valves begin to prolapse
(E)   the Valsalva maneuver will move the click closer to S_1

(page 247)

II-20.   Which of the following statements regarding the second heart sound (S_2) is true?

(A) A_2 and P_2 are due to the clapping together of the valve leaflets
(B)   a wide splitting of S_2 would be heard in a patient with mitral regurgitation
(C) P_2 is normally loudest at the left fifth intercostal space
(D)   left bundle branch block would result in wide physiologic splitting of S_2
(E)   in wide physiologic splitting, A_2 and P_2 move closer together during inspiration

(pages 248–252)

II-21.   Which of the following patients would be most likely to have a pathologic third heart sound (S_3)?

(A)   a patient with constrictive pericarditis
(B)   an otherwise healthy young adult
(C)   a patient with mitral stenosis
(D)   a patient with chronic mitral regurgitation
(E)   a patient with severe valvular aortic stenosis

(pages 254–255)

II-22.   Which of the following situations represents a pathologic murmur?

(A)   a high-frequency murmur with a musical quality, heard loudest at the apex of a 52-year-old man with systolic hypertension
(B)   a vibratory systolic murmur heard along the left sternal border at the third or fourth interspace in a 7-year-old boy
(C)   a supraclavicular bruit that begins shortly after S_1 and extends to S_2 in a 55-year-old man
(D)   a low- to medium-pitched murmur with a blowing quality heard along the left sternal border in a 15-year-old girl
(E)   a bruit heard loudest above the clavicles, shortly after S_1, that is diamond-shaped and of brief duration, in a 10-year-old boy

(pages 260–261)

II-23.   Which of the following statements is characteristic of the murmur associated with a ventricular septal defect?

(A)   the murmur can mimic a pulmonary ejection murmur in patients with severe pulmonary hypertension
(B)   there is respiratory variation with the murmur
(C)   the murmur radiates into the axilla
(D)   there is reversed splitting of S_2 in patients with significant left-to-right shunting
(E)   the murmur is best heard at the apex

(page 266)

II-24.   Which of the following statements is true of an Austin-Flint murmur?

(A)   this murmur is present in patients with mitral stenosis
(B)   there is a mid-diastolic component to this murmur
(C)   this murmur is introduced with an opening snap
(D)   vasodilating agents, such as amyl nitrate, will increase the murmur
(E) S_1 is increased in intensity

(page 270)

II-25.   Which of the following conditions would have a continuous murmur best heard in the left infraclavicular area and the second left intercostal space?

(A)   mammary souffle
(B)   cervical venous hum
(C)   patent ductus arteriosus
(D)   sinus of Valsalva aneurysms
(E)   coronary artery fistula

(pages 271–272)

II-26.   Which of the following statements concerning ventricular depolarization and repolarization is correct?

(A)   the sequence of ventricular repolarization is from epicardium to endocardium with positive charges in front of the negative charges
(B)   the sequence of ventricular repolarization is from endocardium to epicardium with positive charges in front of the negative charges
(C)   the sequence of ventricular depolarization is from epicardium to endocardium with negative charges in front of the positive charges
(D)   the sequence of ventricular depolarization is from endocardium to epicardium with positive charges in front of the negative charges
(E)   the sequence of ventricular depolarization both begins and terminates in the endocardium with positive charges leading negative charges

(page 282)

II-27. What condition is present in the following electrocardiogram (ECG)?

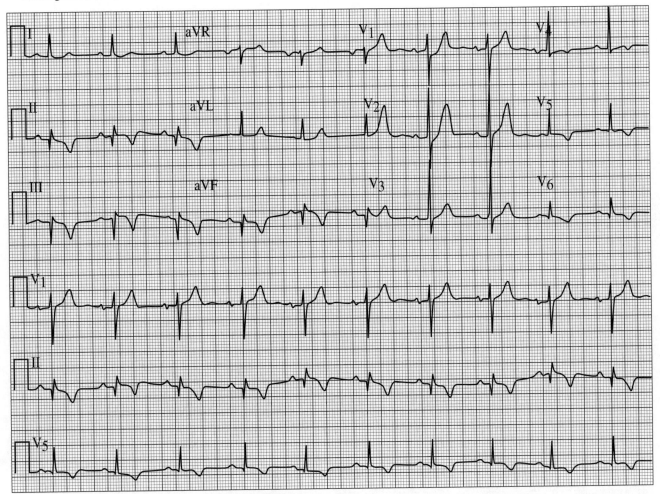

- (A) acute inferior myocardial infraction (MI) with
      posterolateral extension
- (B) acute pericarditis
- (C) acute inferior MI with reciprocal anterior changes
- (D) early repolarization
- (E) hyperkalemia

(page 289)

II-28.   In the following ECG, which of the following is most
likely the cause of the abnormality seen in the tracing?

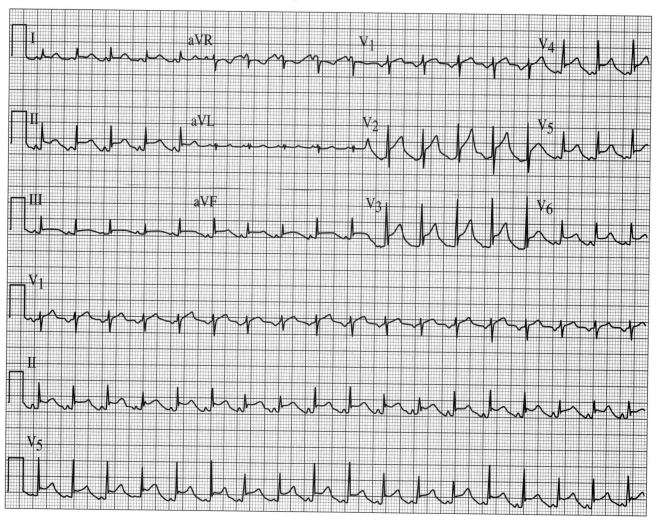

(A) acute myocardial infarction
(B) left bundle branch block
(C) left ventricular hypertrophy
(D) early repolarization
(E) acute pericarditis

(page 290)

II-29. What condition is present in the following ECG?

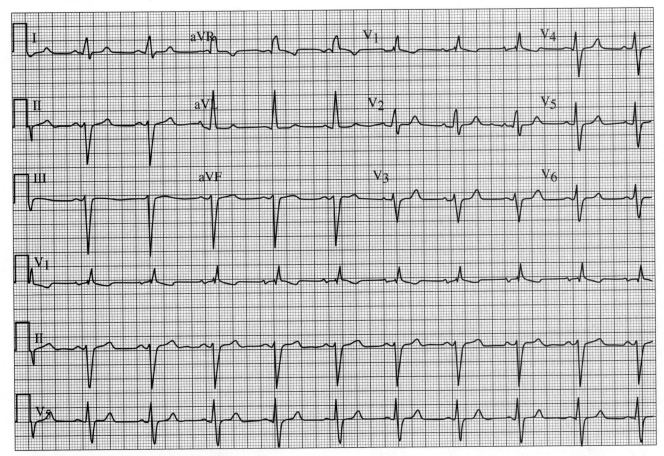

(A) right bundle branch block (RBBB) alone
(B) left bundle branch block (LBBB)
(C) RBBB and left anterior fascicular block
(D) RBBB and left posterior fascicular block
(E) left anterior fascicular block alone

(page 294)

II-30. What condition is present in the following ECG?

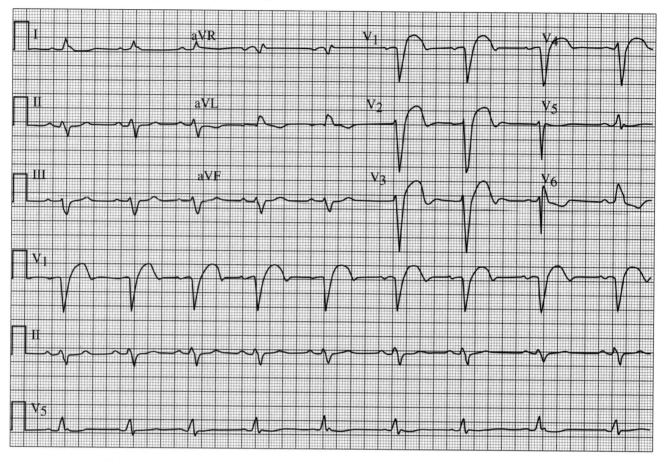

- (A) right bundle branch block alone
- (B) left bundle branch block alone
- (C) right bundle branch block with an acute inferior infarction
- (D) left bundle branch block with an acute anterior infarction
- (E) hyperkalemia

(page 296)

II-31. Which of the following statements regarding the associated ECG is true?

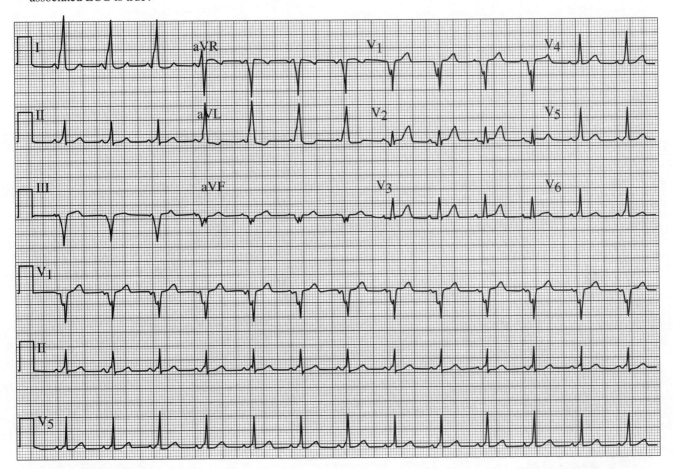

(A)   old inferior MI
(B)   left anterior fascicular block
(C)   left ventricular hypertrophy
(D)   hypercalcemia
(E)   a loud S₁

(page 298)

II-32. What condition is present in the following ECG?

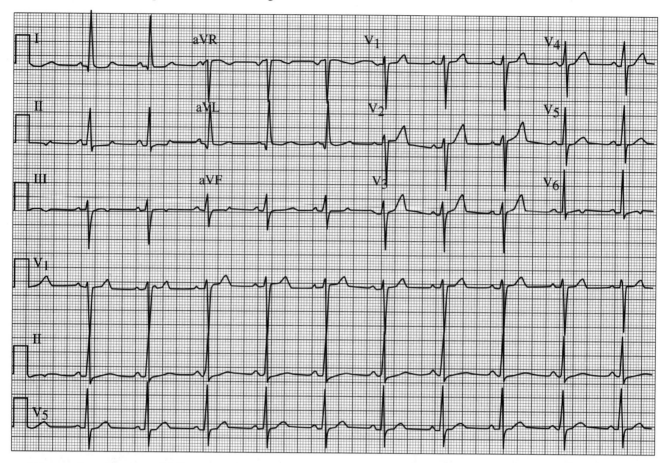

(A) previous anteroseptal MI
(B) right ventricular hypertrophy from chronic lung disease
(C) left ventricular hypertrophy
(D) left posterior fascicular block
(E) incomplete right bundle branch block

(page 302)

II-33. What condition is present in the following ECG?

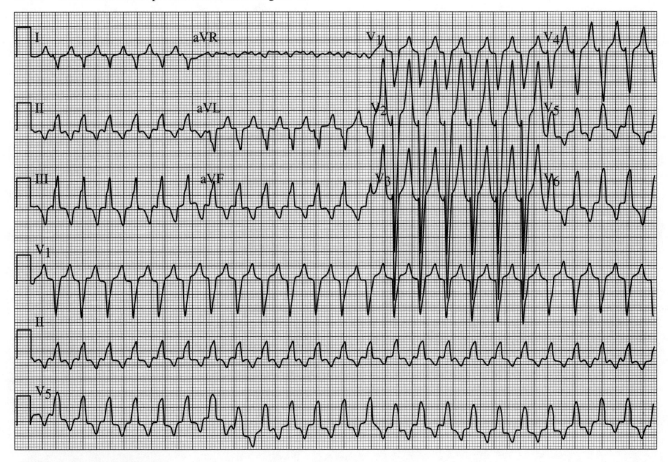

(A) severe hyperkalemia
(B) left bundle branch block
(C) ventricular tachycardia
(D) severe hypothermia
(E) Wolff-Parkinson-White syndrome

(page 302)

II-34. The following radiograph represents which pathologic finding?

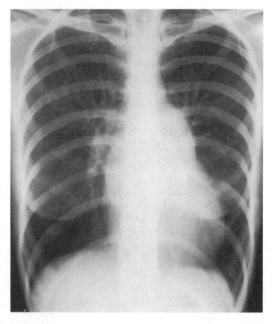

(A) localization
(B) lateralization
(C) cephalization
(D) collateralization
(E) centralization

(page 316)

II-35. The following radiograph demonstrates what pathologic finding?

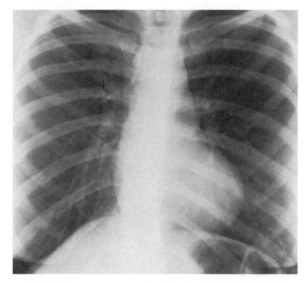

(A) tetralogy of Fallot
(B) acute myocardial infarction
(C) coarctation of the aorta
(D) pulmonary emboli
(E) left ventricular aneurysm

(page 316)

II-36. The following radiograph represents which pathologic finding?

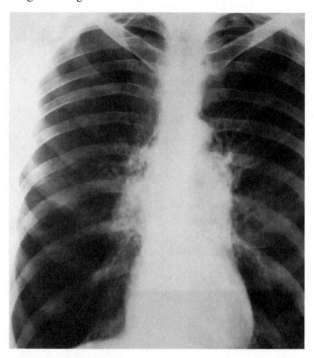

(A) cardiac tamponade
(B) chronic left heart failure
(C) mitral stenosis
(D) constrictive pericarditis
(E) emphysema with right heart failure

(page 316–339)

II-37. Which of the following statements regarding the positioning of the heart is true?

(A) levocardia with situs solitus has an extremely high incidence of cyanotic congenital cardiac lesions
(B) the majority of patients with dextroversion have congenitally corrected transposition of the great arteries
(C) patients having dextrocardia with situs inversus have an extremely high incidence of congenital heart disease
(D) patients with cardiac malpositions and situs ambiguus who have polysplenia usually die in infancy
(E) in patients with dextroversion, there is a low, 2 percent incidence of congenital heart disease

(pages 319–321)

II-38. Which of the following statements regarding abnormalities seen in roentgenograms is true?

(A) in straight-back syndrome, the prominence of the pulmonary trunk is still a good indicator of right ventricular enlargement

(B) a "3 sign" on the aorta and an "E sign" on the esophagus depict an aortic aneurysm

(C) coarctation of the aorta is the most common cause of rib notching

(D) generalized dilatation of the ascending aorta is a hallmark of valvular aortic stenosis

(E) a diminution in the size of the pulmonary trunk and an increase in the size of the aorta in a roentgenogram indicates a leftward rotation of the heart

(pages 321–323)

II-39. Which of the following statements regarding pulmonary blood flow is true?

(A) patients with severe obstructive emphysema demonstrate cephalization of the pulmonary vascularity

(B) when the artery-bronchus ratio is 1:3, there is increased blood flow to the lungs

(C) patients with mitral stenosis show lateralization of blood flow

(D) there should normally be equal amounts of blood flow in the base and the apex of the lung

(E) intravascular pressure exceeding the oncotic pressure of the blood is responsible for the cephalization of pulmonary vascularity

(pages 327–330)

II-40. Which of the following pathologic conditions is characterized by a normal heart and alveolar pulmonary edema in a butterfly pattern?

(A) chronic right-sided heart failure

(B) acute right-sided heart failure

(C) chronic left-sided heart failure

(D) acute left-sided heart failure

(E) combined right-sided and left-sided heart failure

(pages 332–334)

II-41. Which of the following statements represents a benefit of ultrasound?

(A) sound energy is poorly transmitted through air and bone

(B) when the beam is directed parallel or nearly parallel to the interface, little or no sound energy will be reflected

(C) harmonic imaging transmits sound at one frequency and receives it at a higher frequency

(D) some structures reflect such strong signals that they are transmitted again back into the field

(E) the ultrasound beam diverges with distance from the transducer and always has a finite width

(page 345)

II-42. Which of the following statements regarding the standard two-dimensional examination is true?

(A) the long-axis plane of the heart is best viewed in the apical and subcostal positions

(B) the long-axis plane of the heart is best viewed in the suprasternal and subcostal positions

(C) The short-axis plane is best viewed in the subcostal and suprasternal positions

(D) the short-axis plane is best viewed in the parasternal and subcostal positions

(E) the four-chamber views are best obtained in the suprasternal and apical positions

(page 351)

II-43. Which of the following statements regarding Doppler echocardiography is true?

(A) the transducer must be placed perpendicular to blood flow in order to obtain accurate velocity determinations

(B) the Doppler principle is based on the fact that the frequency of sound changes proportional to the velocity and direction of the moving object that it strikes

(C) a normal laminar flow will manifest as a broad signal which is multitoned, dissonant, and harsh, due to the varying velocities between blood cells near the wall and blood cells in the lumen

(D) flow shown above the baseline represents flow away from the transducer

(E) Doppler echocardiography is able to give abundant information regarding cardiac structure

(pages 356–363)

II-44. Which of the following statements regarding mitral valve Doppler inflow patterns is true?

(A) under conditions of restrictive filling of the left ventricle, the E wave velocity is equal to that of the *a* wave

(B) mitral valve inflow velocities are altered only by the intrinsic diastolic properties of the left ventricle

(C) pseudonormalization of the mitral inflow pattern refers to a relative increase in E wave velocity in patients with impaired relaxation due to elevated left atrial pressures

(D) in patients with impaired relaxation, there is an augmentation of the mitral E wave velocity due to the reduction in diastolic compliance of the left ventricle and subsequent decreased early mitral inflow

(E) it is not currently possible to distinguish between a normal and a pseudonormal mitral inflow pattern

(page 367)

II-45. Which of the following statements regarding trans-esophageal echocardiography (TEE) is true?

(A) TEE is useful for the diagnosis of infective endocarditis

(B) the three views recommended in a TEE study include posterior to the base of the heart, above the heart, and posterior to the left atrium

(C) TEE is of particular value because of the view it provides of the left ventricle

(D) when the transducer is in the esophagus, posterior structures appear at the bottom of the image

(E) TEE is useful for the Doppler interrogation of the pulmonary arteries

(pages 375–376)

II-46. Which of the following conditions can be diagnosed after intravenous injection of agitated saline solution?

(A) aortic regurgitation
(B) patent foramen ovale
(C) mitral regurgitation
(D) coronary artery disease
(E) aortic stenosis

(page 376)

II-47. Which of the following statements regarding aortic regurgitation (AR) recorded by echocardiography is true?

(A) 2D and M-mode echocardiography provide direct evidence of the presence and severity of AR

(B) AR jet velocity, as recorded by continuous-wave (CW) Doppler, is maximal in mid-diastole

(C) severe, acute AR can cause a systolic mitral regurgitation

(D) the analysis of the size and shape of the flow disturbance by CW Doppler correlates directly with the severity of the AR

(E) the M-mode finding of premature diastolic closing of the mitral valve indicates acute, severe AR

(page 386–389)

II-48. Which of the following statements regarding echocardiographic findings in mitral stenosis is true?

(A) 2D ultrasound findings in patients with mitral stenosis are not helpful in making a diagnosis

(B) changes in mitral valve motion due to stenosis are not seen by echocardiography

(C) an increase in the E-F slope correlates with the severity of the stenosis

(D) Doppler estimates of mitral valve area are indirect and less accurate than those derived by planimetry of the mitral valve orifice

(E) a score of greater than nine on the echocardiographic scoring system indicates that

percutaneous catheter balloon mitral commissurotomy should not be performed

(pages 390–394)

II-49. Which of the following statements regarding pulmonary hypertension and right ventricular function is true?

(A) accurate calculations of right ventricular volume can be made using 2D echocardiography

(B) in right ventricular pressure overload, the interventricular septum flattens during diastole and returns to its normal curvature during systole

(C) in severe pulmonary hypertension with elevated right atrial pressure, the inferior vena cava should decrease in diameter during inspiration

(D) the presence of a high velocity tricuspid regurgitation jet in Doppler echocardiography can indicate pulmonary hypertension

(E) pulsed-wave Doppler shows a lengthening of the acceleration time of flow through the pulmonic valve in pulmonary hypertension

(pages 402–403)

II-50. Which of the following statements regarding echocardiography and infective endocarditis is true?

(A) echocardiography provides indirect evidence of vegetations

(B) in patients with suspected endocarditis, the most reasonable approach begins with transthoracic echocardiography (TTE) as the first screening

(C) M-mode recordings produce the best evidence of infective endocarditis

(D) TTE provides a more sensitive measurement than TEE for detection of vegetations

(E) echocardiographic evaluation is valuable in its ability to discern between active vegetations and healed vegetations

(pages 406–410)

II-51. Which of the following statements regarding MI and echocardiography is true?

(A) echocardiography is valuable in excluding transmural infarctions

(B) a postinfarction left ventricular aneurysm is recognized by echocardiography by its highly localized nature and the presence of a narrow neck connecting it to the ventricle

(C) calculation of a wall motion score by echocardiography has identified patients who are at a low risk for complications

(D) echocardiography usually detects postinfarction free wall rupture of the ventricle

(E) acquired ventricular septal defects are characterized by discrete orifices and are readily visualized by echocardiography following an MI

(pages 411–414)

II-52. Which of the following statements regarding stress echocardiography is true?

  (A) dobutamine stress echocardiography has a very weak negative predictive value
  (B) the sensitivity and specificity of stress echocardiography is lower than that of comparable nuclear imaging modalities
  (C) when compared to traditional exercise ECG testing, exercise echocardiography has a significantly higher false positive rate
  (D) a biphasic wall motion response during dobutamine is indicative of hibernating myocardium
  (E) stress echocardiography uses three basic types of stress: exercise, mental, and pharmacologic

(pages 415–417)

II-53. Which of the following statements regarding the cardiomyopathies is true?

  (A) an abnormal "speckled" pattern or "ground-glass" appearance of the myocardium on 2D echocardiography is seen in hypertrophic cardiomyopathy
  (B) systolic anterior motion of the mitral valve is a characteristic of restrictive cardiomyopathy
  (C) four-chamber dilatation is a common finding of dilated cardiomyopathy
  (D) hypertrophic cardiomyopathies are characterized by infiltration of the myocardium by fibrotic tissue
  (E) midsystolic closure of the aortic valve is seen dilated cardiomyopathy

(pages 417–420)

II-54. Which of the following statements regarding cardio-vascular shunts is true?

  (A) an ostium secundum atrial septal defect (ASD) is characterized by the lack of interatrial septal tissue between the defect and the base of the interventricular septum
  (B) 2D echocardiography is the most useful imaging method for detecting a ventricular septal defect (VSD)
  (C) ostium primum defects are usually accompanied by other abnormalities
  (D) color-flow Doppler is not useful in the diagnosis of a patent ductus arteriosus
  (E) contrast found in the left atrium in the absence of MR, distinguishes an isolated VSD from an ASD

(page 421)

II-55. Which of the following conditions is associated with a long, linear, freely mobile structure viewed by echocardiography in the right atrium at the mouth of the inferior vena cava?

  (A) the Chiari network
  (B) an aneurysm of the interatrial septum
  (C) lipomatous hypertrophy of the interatrial septum
  (D) persistence of the eustachian valve
  (E) enlargement of the right ventricular moderator band

(pages 429–431)

II-56. Which of the following statements regarding intra-cardiac thrombi is true?

  (A) thrombi that originate in the right atrium tend to be serpentine and mobile
  (B) left atrial thrombi form in the setting of low cardiac output
  (C) spontaneous echo contrast (or "smoke") occurs exclusively in the left atrium
  (D) left atrial thrombi are generally of heterogeneous echo density
  (E) left ventricular thrombi are always laminar and fixed

(pages 431–433)

II-57. Which of the following statements regarding the pericardium is true?

  (A) the normal pericardium is easily visualized by echocardiography
  (B) electrical alternans is created by the heart swinging back and forth within the pericardial space in the setting of a moderate or large effusion
  (C) an echolucent space seen anterior to the right ventricle with echocardiography most likely represents pericardial fluid
  (D) the apical position is best for deciphering between pericardial and pleural effusions on echocardiography
  (E) cardiac ultrasound readily detects constrictive pericarditis

(pages 435–436)

II-58. A 27-year-old medical student approaches her doctor to discuss a training program. She wishes to understand how the cardiovascular system responds to a strenuous exercise program. Which of the following statements is true?

  (A) there will be no change to her resting heart rate
  (B) the percentage of maximum oxygen uptake (VO_2 max) is the best overall measure of efficiency
  (C) vagal tone at rest is decreased
  (D) if only the legs are used in vigorous training exercises, the whole body will benefit from the circulatory adaptive changes that improve muscle performance
  (E) trained muscles need less oxygen per unit of work performed than untrained muscles

(pages 465–467)

II-59. Which of the following statements represents a normal blood pressure response to maximal exercise?

(A) the systolic blood pressure rises ≥ 10–20 mm Hg
(B) the diastolic blood pressure increases
(C) the systolic blood pressure does not rise with increasing treadmill workload
(D) patients with the lowest maximal systolic blood pressure have the lowest risk of coronary artery disease
(E) the post-exercise systolic blood pressure may decrease below the pre-exercise level

(pages 466–467)

II-60. Which of the following patients could safely undergo exercise testing?

(A) a patient with unstable angina
(B) a patient with active endocarditis
(C) a patient with mild aortic stenosis
(D) a patient with an acute myocardial infarction
(E) a patient with severe aortic stenosis

(page 474)

II-61. Which of the following vessels would be cannulated in a trans-septal catheterization to enter the left atrium?

(A) median cubital vein
(B) brachial artery
(C) common femoral artery
(D) right femoral vein
(E) internal jugular vein

(pages 481–482)

II-62. Which of the following statements regarding pressure measurements obtained at catheterization is true?

(A) in pulmonic stenosis, the right ventricular pressure curve is peaked or triangular
(B) left ventricular end-diastolic pressure (LVEDP) is recorded at the upstroke of the *a* wave
(C) a decreased LVEDP reflects a dilated failing left ventricle
(D) during diastole, pulmonary artery wedge pressure provides an accurate estimate of left atrial pressure
(E) fluid-filled catheter recording systems are used to obtain high-fidelity phasic pressure curves from the ventricles and the great arteries

(pages 484–485)

II-63. Which of the following left ventricular responses would be seen in a patient with poor left ventricular reserve during a hand grip maneuver?

(A) no change in left ventricular stroke work and an increase in LVEDP
(B) a decrease in left ventricular stroke work and an increase in LVEDP

(C) a decrease in left ventricular stroke work and no change in LVEDP
(D) no change in either left ventricular stroke work or LVEDP
(E) an increase in left ventricular stroke work and an increase in LVEDP

(page 486)

II-64. The curve below represents the injection of an indicator dilution substance into the right atrium and sampling a peripheral arterial site. What is demonstrated in this figure?

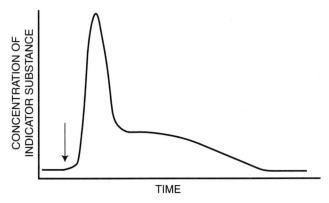

(A) a normal recirculation curve
(B) an early recirculation curve
(C) no recirculation curve
(D) a very late recirculation curve
(E) unintelligible results since the recirculation prevents the indicator substance from being detected by the catheter

(page 488)

II-65. A view of which of the following structures can be seen by 30° axial right anterior oblique and 40° cranial angulation in angiography?

(A) the four heart chambers
(B) the anterior two-thirds of the ventricular septum
(C) the right ventricular infundibulum
(D) the pulmonary artery and its bifurcation
(E) the posterior third of the ventricular septum

(page 494)

II-66. Which of the following statements represent the most frequently expected complication following cardiac catheterization?

(A) death
(B) myocardial infarction
(C) cerebral emboli
(D) an arterial complication at the insertion site
(E) ventricular fibrillation

(pages 496–497)

II-67. Which of the following statements regarding coronary blood flow is true?

(A) pressure gradients at rest provide an accurate characterization of the ischemic potential of a stenosis

(B) the fraction flow reserve (FFR) reflects a reduction in myocardial perfusion from a stenosis pressure gradient

(C) the FFR is dependent upon hemodynamic and microcirculatory factors

(D) intracoronary injection of adenosine produces a more sustained hyperemia than intravenous injection

(E) a major limitation to relative coronary flow reserve (rCFR) is patients with three-vessel coronary disease with no suitable reference vessel

(pages 513–515)

II-68. Which of the following methods would best assess the extent of myocardial salvage following thrombolytic therapy administered during an acute myocardial infarction?

(A) ^{99m}technetium methoxy isobutyl isonitrile [^{99m}Tc-MIBI (sestamibi)]

(B) ^{99m}Tc-teboroxime

(C) planar imaging with ^{201}thallium

(D) dobutamine stress echocardiography

(E) left ventriculography

(page 527)

II-69. Which of the following statements regarding ^{99m}Tc-teboroxime tracer is true?

(A) it is chemically similar to the cationic complexes, which include ^{99m}Tc-MIBI

(B) it exhibits low myocardial extraction

(C) it washes out slowly from the myocardium

(D) regional washout rates are related to regional myocardial blood flow

(E) ^{99m}Tc-teboroxime tracer is used in single-detector systems

(pages 527–528)

II-70. Which of the following statements regarding pharmacologic stress testing and myocardial perfusion single photon emission computed tomography (SPECT) is true?

(A) the diagnostic accuracy of pharmacologic stress testing is somewhat less than that of exercise testing

(B) dobutamine is used only for patients who have asthma

(C) caffeine blocks the cellular re-uptake of adenosine

(D) dipyridamole blocks adenosine binding, thus eliminating the effect on coronary vasodilation

(E) dobutamine is the first choice agent for use in myocardial perfusion scintigraphy

(pages 532–533)

II-71. Which of the following statements regarding non-perfusion myocardial SPECT is true?

(A) loss of effective sympathetic innervation in heart failure patients can be documented by meta-^{125}I-iodobenzylguanidine (MIBG)

(B) ^{123}I-labeled compounds are used exclusively for fatty acid imaging in the United States

(C) ^{123}I-iodophenyl pentadecanoic acid (IPPA) washes out of ischemic myocardium faster than out of normal myocardium

(D) MIBG is taken up more readily in regionally denervated myocardium

(E) in ischemia, denervation occurs prior to myocardial necrosis

(pages 533–534)

II-72. Which of the following statements regarding the diagnostic accuracy of myocardial perfusion SPECT in predicting coronary artery disease (CAD) is true?

(A) patients with a probability of CAD of < 15 percent should be referred only for a standard exercise tolerance test (ETT)

(B) patients having a probability of CAD of 15 to 50 percent should first be tested with a stress SPECT

(C) patients having a probability of CAD of >85 percent do not need to have a stress SPECT

(D) sensitivity is the proportion of patients without disease who are correctly detected by the test as normal

(E) the referral bias seen in SPECT testing leads to an overestimation of specificity

(page 536)

II-73. Which of the following statements regarding nuclear testing in special populations is true?

(A) diabetics with mildly to moderately abnormal scans show a higher rate of event-free survival than those without diabetes

(B) myocardial perfusion SPECT is not a good predictor of cardiac events in patients with left bundle branch block

(C) ^{201}Tl imaging in nondiabetic women under age 45 often yields false positive results

(D) exercise thallium imaging is not accurate in predicting high-risk populations in patients over the age of 65

(E) nuclear testing in noncardiac surgery patients is recommended only in those with a low risk of a cardiac event at the time of the procedure

(pages 545–547)

II-74. Which of the following statements regarding the assessment during early hospitalization for acute coronary syndromes is true?

(A) myocardial perfusion scintigraphy cannot accurately predict whether patients presenting late after chest pain should have thrombolytic therapy or percutaneous coronary intervention (PCI)

(B) rest myocardial perfusion SPECT combined with resting left ventricular function provides information on myocardial stunning

(C) patients with LBBB should not have myocardial perfusion scintigraphy to determine whether they should have thrombolytic therapy or PCI

(D) myocardial perfusion scintigraphy is too expensive to be used as a before and after therapy measure of the efficacy of the therapy

(E) there is no evidence that there is a relation between the size of a very early myocardial perfusion defect and subsequent mortality from an acute MI

(pages 552–553)

II-75. Which of the following statements regarding ultrafast computed tomography is true?

(A) it is a promising diagnostic technique for the detection of coronary artery disease in symptomatic patients

(B) it is a better diagnostic tool for evaluating native heart valves than echocardiography

(C) it is not useful for rapid diagnosis of dissecting aneurysms of the thoracic aorta

(D) it cannot be used for evaluating the pericardium

(E) it has been shown to predict accurately the patency of bypass grafts

(pages 577–578)

II-76. Which of the following statements regarding ultrafast computed tomography (CT) and coronary calcification is true?

(A) the specificity of ultrafast CT for predicting patients without obstructive CAD is high

(B) coronary calcification is present in most patients with significant CAD

(C) young patients with acute myocardial infarction frequently have calcification present in the coronary artery

(D) the degree of calcification is not related to age

(E) patients with asymptomatic CAD have a more rapid progression of coronary artery calcification than symptomatic patients

(pages 570–572)

II-77. For diagnosis of which of the following conditions is CT scanning the modality of choice?

(A) tetralogy of Fallot

(B) pericardial cyst

(C) intracardiac tumors

(D) myxoma

(E) pericardial effusion

(pages 580–584)

II-78. Which of the following statements regarding principles of nuclear magnetic resonance is true?

(A) as nuclei return to the B_0 axis following the radiofrequency pulse, they regain the original energy that they possessed

(B) T1 and T2 relaxation properties are uniform throughout all tissues of the body

(C) special magnetic resonance systems, dedicated only to the cardiovascular system, are needed for general cardiovascular imaging

(D) the magnetic field must remain uniform over the field of interest to obtain an image

(E) there is no signal in the presence of rapidly flowing blood

(pages 590–592)

II-79. The presence of which of the following items in a patient would be safe for undergoing magnetic resonance imaging (MRI)?

(A) a prosthetic heart valve

(B) a pacemaker

(C) an intracranial aneurysm clip

(D) an automated implantable cardiovascular defibrillator

(E) a cochlear prosthesis

(pages 594–595)

II-80. Which of the following statements regarding MRI is true?

(A) the fibrous tissue of the pericardium gives a higher signal intensity

(B) MRI shows evidence of regurgitation, but cannot assess the volume of regurgitant flow

(C) echocardiography provides a better estimate of the morphology of valve leaflets than MRI

(D) echocardiography and MRI detect pericardial effusions, but echocardiography is a better detector of small fluid collections

(E) hypertrophy confined to the apex is difficult to visualize with MRI

(pages 600–601)

II-81. Which of the following statements regarding white and black blood imaging techniques is true?

   (A) an ECG-gated fast spin echocardiography in black blood imaging requires 128 heartbeats

   (B) the signal-to-noise ratio is lower in conventional gradient echo than in segmented k-space techniques

   (C) the patient holds his/her breath throughout conventional gradient echocardiography in white blood imaging

   (D) conventional echo gated spin in black blood imaging is sensitive to respiratory motion

   (E) total scan time in segmented k-space scans is proportional to the number of views per segment

(pages 610–611)

II-82. Which of the following statements regarding coronary artery imaging is true?

   (A) flow velocity of the coronary arteries is easily determined with MRI

   (B) magnetic resonance angiography (MRA) can be superior to coronary angiography in identifying anomalous coronary arteries

   (C) following a coronary stent placement, it is recommended to wait several days before doing an MRI

   (D) saphenous vein grafts are difficult to visualize with MRA

   (E) MRI is not effective in deciphering between normal vessel wall components and atherosclerotic plaque

(pages 619–622)

II-83. Which of the following statements regarding positron-emitting tracers of myocardial tissue function is true?

   (A) women demonstrate higher myocardial blood flow (MBF) during rest and hyperemia

   (B) a water perfusable tissue index (PTI) of .75 indicates a normal myocardium

   (C) a near normal PTI has a strong predictive value of a normal myocardium

   (D) one of the benefits of using [^{13}N]ammonia to study MBF is its short half-life that allows repeated studies in 10-min time intervals

   (E) a decline in the size and slope of the rapid-clearance phase of [^{11}C]palmitate indicates a switch from the use of glucose to free fatty acids

(pages 630–632)

II-84. Which of the following functions has positron emission tomography been mainly used for in cardiology?

   (A) identification of cardiomyopathies

   (B) identification of pericardial effusions

   (C) identification of intracardiac tumors

   (D) identification and characterization of valvular disease

   (E) identification of viable myocardium in patients with CAD

(page 632)

II-85. Which of the following features differentiates reversible from irreversible impairment of contractile function of the myocardium?

   (A) abnormal systolic wall motion

   (B) reduced MBF

   (C) persistent metabolic activity

   (D) electrocardiographic abnormalities

   (E) non-recruitable contractile reserve

(page 637)

II. GENERAL EVALUATION OF THE PATIENT

ANSWERS

II-1. The answer is D. *(Ch. 10)* The warm-up phenomenon describes a situation in which exertion that previously produced angina does not provoke pain when attempted again. Chest pain that is described as "stabbing" or "shooting" and reaches maximum intensity quickly is generally of musculoskeletal origin. A patient describing chest pain by holding a fist over the sternal area (Levine's sign) is frequently indicative of ischemic pain. The definition of *angina pectoris* is chest pain or discomfort that usually results from a temporary imbalance between myocardial oxygen supply and demand. Symptoms such as nausea, vomiting, or diaphoresis that are associated with chest pain often accompany acute myocardial infarction, particularly involving the inferior or posterior wall of the left ventricle.

II-2. The answer is C. *(Ch. 10)* The term *linked angina* applies to patients with known CAD who have episodes of angina caused by gastrointestinal factors that are *not* related to an increase in cardiac work. A patient having coronary artery spasm superimposed on coronary atherosclerosis usually presents with rest angina. Syndrome X is a heterogeneous group of patients suffering from a wide spectrum of chest pain and having vascular and smooth muscle hypersensitive constrictor responses. For rest angina, the predictive value of the history is not as beneficial as it is for exertional angina. For reasons that are not clear, females are more likely to have angina in arteriographically normal coronary arteries.

II-3. The answer is B. *(Ch. 10)* Pulmonary embolism (PE) may occasionally simulate the pain of MI. The associated signs of dyspnea, tachypnea, and intense cyanosis are more likely in PE than with an MI. The differential diagnosis should be made by the clinical setting, ECG, echocardiography, and cardiac enzymes. Spontaneous pneumothorax generally occurs in men in their 3rd or 4th decade who are otherwise healthy. The clinical onset of spontaneous pneumothorax is characterized by abrupt, agonizing, unilateral pain with severe shortness of breath. Pain from pneumonia, pulmonary infarction, and pleurisy results from pleural irritation. The discomfort generally varies with breathing and is often accompanied by reduced inspiratory effort.

II-4. The answer is A. *(Ch. 10)* The occurrence of dyspnea 2 to 3 h after falling asleep, which is relieved by sitting upright and does not return after falling back asleep is called paroxysmal nocturnal dyspnea (PND) and occurs in patients with left heart failure. It is thought to result from the increase in central blood volume in the supine position. Frequently, however, PND indicates transient heart failure caused by an episode of ischemia. Dark or clotted blood is seen in the sputum of patients with pulmonary embolism. The sputum of patients with mitral stenosis contains bright red pulmonary venous blood from the rupture of submucosal pulmonary venules. The sputum of a patient with acute pulmonary edema is usually pink and frothy. A dramatic and recent increase in dyspnea is more likely associated with heart failure than lung disease. Cheyne-Stokes respirations are seen in patients with advanced heart failure and in patients with central nervous system disease.

II-5. The answer is D. *(Ch. 10)* Edema that affects mostly the face and arms is most likely to be due to a venous or lymphatic obstruction in the chest or neck, such as from carcinoma of the lung. The most common cause for fatigue and weakness is anxiety and depression. Although syncope of cardiac origin can cause incontinence, the presence of drowsiness or confusion following the event suggests a seizure disorder. Fever, chills, or sweats in a patient with a heart murmur who has had recent dental work suggests a diagnosis of infective endocarditis. Pain localized to the temporal region is most likely temporal arteritis and is often associated with polymyalgia rheumatica and abnormal vision.

II-6.   The answer is E.   *(Ch. 10)*   The patient in (A) has Tabatznik's syndrome, which is associated with atrial fibrillation. The patient in (B) has third and fourth pharyngeal pouch syndrome and may have truncus arteriosus. The patient in (C) has Morquio's syndrome, which is associated with aortic regurgitation. The patient in (D) has Down syndrome and frequently has a ventricular septal defect or an endocardial cushion defect. The patient in (E) has Marfan's syndrome, which is associated with mitral valve prolapse.

II-7.   The answer is B.   *(Ch. 10)*   Nontender hemorrhagic lesions found on the palms and soles are Janeway lesions and are associated with infective endocarditis. Café-au-lait spots and mental retardation are linked to pulmonic stenosis in Watson's syndrome. The CREST syndrome is a variant of scleroderma and is associated rarely with thickening of the edges of the mitral, aortic, and tricuspid valve as well as thickening and shortening of the mitral chordae. Ulnar deviation of the fingers, the "swan neck" deformity, and subluxation of the metacarpophalangeal joints are seen in rheumatoid arthritis. The most commonly seen valvular manifestations of rheumatoid arthritis are granulomatous aortic or mitral valve disease resulting in valvular regurgitation. The combination of polyarthritis, abdominal pain, and diarrhea are seen in Whipple's disease. Complications of this disease may include aortic and mitral regurgitation and endocarditis.

II-8.   The answer is C.   *(Ch. 10)*   In children, the diastolic blood pressure should be recorded at the point where a muffling of the sounds occurs (Korotkoff phase IV). The auscultatory gap is a period of silence between Korotkoff phases I and II. Generally good correlation exists between indirect and direct blood pressure measurements in the arm. The sounds become crisper and increase in intensity during Korotkoff phase III. If blood pressure is measured in the same arm repeatedly, a false decrease in systolic pressure may be recorded.

II-9.   The answer is D.   *(Ch. 10)*   The resistance encountered in peripheral arteries is not affected by heart rate. Peripheral arteries are better predictors of the severity of some cardiac diseases (e.g., aortic regurgitation) than the carotid arteries. Thus the importance of pistol shot or water hammer peripheral pulses is evident. A reflected wave during systole increases systolic pressure, thus increasing ventricular afterload. This is probably the reason that blood pressure is usually higher when measured in the legs as opposed to the arms. Palpation of the carotid artery is preferred for assessing cardiac performance, since it corresponds more closely to actual central aortic pressure. In the normal proximal aortic pulse, the tidal wave may represent the echo of the percussion wave from the upper part of the body.

II-10.   The answer is C.   *(Ch. 10)*   The figure demonstrates pulsus paradoxus, which is typical in patients with cardiac tamponade. A patient with pure aortic regurgitation would demonstrate a wide pulse pressure and perhaps a bisferiens pulse. The pulse in aortic stenosis is characterized by a slow rise and a decreased volume, or a *parvus et tardus* pulse. Hypertrophic cardiomyopathy frequently demonstrates a bisferiens pulse.

II-11.   The answer is B.   *(Ch. 10)*   A bisferiens pulse (a positive wave in systole) occurs in patients with severe aortic regurgitation with or without mild aortic stenosis. It can also be encountered in other conditions associated with rapid left ventricular ejection such as exercise, hypertrophic cardiomyopathy, fever, or a patent ductus arteriosus. Pulsus alternans can be best assessed by palpating a distal artery rather than a carotid artery, as there is normally a slightly wider pulse pressure. The dicrotic pulse (one peak in systole and the second in diastole) is most common in young or middle-aged patients with impaired left ventricular performance. The dicrotic wave diminishes with age, hypertension, diabetes, and atherosclerosis. Pulsus paradoxus is common in cardiac tamponade, but is rarely encountered in constrictive pericarditis. A parvus et tardus pulse occurs with severe aortic stenosis, which almost always has a long systolic ejection murmur.

II-12. **The answer is D.** *(Ch. 10)* The abdominojugular test is useful in determining patients who have right ventricular failure. Patients with right ventricular failure are unable to compensate for increased venous return and demonstrate elevated neck veins until the abdominal pressure is released. The *v* wave results from increased blood volume return in the venae cavea and the right atrium against a closed tricuspid valve during ventricular systole. The *c* wave results from the tricuspid valve bulging into the atrium during RV isovolumic systole. The most common cause of Kussmaul's sign is right-sided heart failure, but it is also a typical finding in constrictive pericarditis. A giant *a* wave is most likely seen in pulmonic stenosis or pulmonary hypertension. In a patient with an ASD, the *a* and *v* waves are often equal in size, but an increase in venous pressure would be unusual. In patients with constrictive pericarditis, equal *a* and *v* waves can be seen, but there will also be an increase in venous pressure and rapid *x* and *y* descents.

II-13. **The answer is D.** *(Ch. 10)* Patient A has constrictive pericarditis. This patient would have Kussmaul's sign as well as perhaps an early diastolic sound (pericardial knock.) Patient A may also show calcification on his chest x-ray. This finding was more common when tuberculosis was responsible for the majority of cases of constriction. Patient B has cardiac tamponade. Pulsus paradoxus is common with cardiac tamponade but unusual in patients with constrictive pericarditis. Echocardiography would show a pericardial effusion in virtually all cases of tamponade.

II-14. **The answer is E.** *(Ch. 10)* Decompensated retinal circulation in hypertensive patients shows observable edema, cotton-wool spots, flame hemorrhages, or swelling of the optic disk. Papilledema is the form of optic disk edema seen with increased intracranial pressure. Copper or silver "wiring" is seen with arteriosclerotic changes. Microaneurysms represent abortive attempts at revascularization seen in diabetes, retinal venous obstructive disease, sickle cell disease, Behçet's disease, sarcoidosis, and other forms of uveitis. In neovascularization, new vessels originate from capillaries from the venous side of circulation and are associated with fibrosis.

II-15. **The answer is D.** *(Ch. 10)* The point of maximal impulse and the apical impulse are not necessarily synonymous, as the maximal precordial motion may be produced by a hypertrophied right ventricle, a dilated aorta, or other conditions. In a patient with chest pain and an abnormal pulsation in the sternoclavicular area, aortic dissection should be considered. The finger pads are best used for assessing low-frequency movements. High-frequency movements, such as ejection sounds or valve closures, should be assessed with the hand held firmly against the chest wall. A systolic thrill in the third, fourth, or fifth intercostal space is characteristic of a VSD. A sustained apical impulse indicates left ventricular hypertrophy or depressed left ventricular systolic function. A diameter of the apical impulse of 3 cm or more has been shown to correlate extremely well with left ventricular enlargement.

II-16. **The answer is C.** *(Ch. 10)* The intensity of the S_1 is determined by six factors: (1) the integrity of valve closure, (2) mobility of the valve, (3) velocity of valve closure, (4) status of ventricular contraction, (5) transmission characteristics of the thoracic cavity and thorax, and (6) physical characteristics of the vibrating structures. Patients with mitral valve prolapse have increased mobility of the valve and, therefore, an increase in intensity of S_1. The converse is seen in patients with severe long-standing mitral stenosis and valvular calcification. In this circumstance, S_1 is diminished or absent. Lown-Ganong-Levine syndrome is characterized by short PR intervals; the ventricle has a short time to fill, and the leaflets are separated maximally at the beginning of ventricular systole, resulting in a loud S_1. With left bundle branch block (LBBB), there is electrical delay of left ventricular systole, and therefore S_1 is decreased in intensity and delayed. Delay in onset of right ventricular contraction with right bundle branch block (RBBB) can lead to wide splitting of S_1.

II-17. **The answer is B.** *(Ch. 10)* This figure is from a patient with aortic stenosis. Due to decreased compliance from left ventricular hypertrophy, the end-diastolic ventricular pressure is high (around 20 mm Hg). In congenital aortic stenosis, an ejection sound is commonly heard at the apex. The heavily calcified valves encountered in older patients with acquired aortic stenosis rarely cause ejection sounds. The delayed closure of the aortic valve frequently produces paradoxical splitting of the second sound. In advanced aortic stenosis, A_2 may be absent altogether. This patient would have a parvus et tardus pulse. A bisferiens pulse is primarily encountered in patients with increased aortic flow, such as aortic regurgitation, certain forms of hypertrophic cardiomyopathy, fever, and exercise. There may be a palpable thrill in the right second intercostal space, the suprasternal notch, or over the carotid arteries.

II-18. **The answer is A.** *(Ch. 10)* This figure is from a patient with chronic aortic regurgitation (AR). As long as left ventricular function is preserved, the arterial pulse would be a hyperkinetic due to the increase in stroke volume and the rate of left ventricular ejection. There are up to three murmurs present in chronic AR: a diastolic decrescendo murmur, an early-peaking systolic flow murmur, and frequently a mid-diastolic rumble (the Austin-Flint murmur). There is a wide pulse pressure due to the large stroke volume ejected in systole and the regurgitant flow during diastole. The left ventricular end-diastolic pressure is substantially elevated. This pressure recording represents chronic rather than acute AR, as the latter would show tachycardia, hypotension, a narrow pulse pressure, and equalization of diastolic pressures.

II-19. **The answer is E.** *(Ch. 10)* A midsystolic click is heard in mitral valve prolapse but can also be heard in patients with left-sided pneumothorax, adhesive pericarditis, atrial myxomas, left ventricular aneurysm, aneurysm of the membranous ventricular septum associated with a ventricular septal defect, and incompetent heterograft valves. The murmur associated with mitral valve prolapse is a late systolic murmur that crescendos to S_2. The click occurs at the point of maximal valve prolapse. Any maneuver that decreased left ventricular volume, like the Valsalva maneuver, will move the click closer to S_1.

II-20. **The answer is B.** *(Ch. 10)* A_2 and P_2 are not due to the clapping of the valve leaflets, but rather to the sudden deceleration of retrograde flow of the blood column as the elastic limits of the tensed valve leaflets are reached. Wide splitting of S_2 is heard in a patient with mitral regurgitation due to early aortic closure. P_2 is normally loudest in the left second intercostal space, but may be heard more widely in pulmonary hypertension. Left bundle branch block would cause delayed emptying of the left ventricular, and therefore a narrow splitting of S_2. A_2 and P_2 move further apart during inspiration in physiologic splitting because the increased right heart volume delays emptying of the right ventricular. In reversed splitting, A_2 and P_2 move closer together during inspiration.

II-21. **The answer is D.** *(Ch. 10)* A diastolic sound associated with constrictive pericarditis is more likely to represent a pericardial knock. The pericardial knock occurs earlier than a typical S_3, and is almost always a higher frequency sound. An S_3 can be normal in a healthy young adult, but if the S_3 continues with increasing age, it is probably pathologic. A patient with mitral stenosis would have an opening snap, a high frequency sound in early diastole. Chronic left ventricular volume overload, particularly with left heart failure, is the setting in which an S_3 typically occurs. Chronic mitral regurgitation is one of these situations. A patient with severe valvular aortic stenosis would most likely have an S_4.

II-22. **The answer is C.** A high-frequency murmur with a musical quality heard at the apex in an adult over 50 can indicate a tortuous, dilated sclerotic aortic root. This murmur is best classified as a systolic ejection murmur without associated abnormalities of the cardiovascular system. The vibratory systolic murmur heard along the left sternal border, Still's murmur, is common in children ages 3 to 8. A supraclavicular murmur in adults that extends until S_2 likely indicates organic carotid obstruction. This murmur is frequently accompanied by a history of transient ischemic attacks. A similar murmur, although shorter in duration, is a common finding in normal individuals, particularly children and adolescents. The low to medium pitched blowing murmur heard along the left sternal border is common in children, adolescents, and young adults. This is termed an *innocent pulmonic systolic murmur* because it is heard in the pulmonic area, although it is thought to be aortic in origin.

II-23.   **The answer is A.**   *(Ch. 10)*   When the defect is large and right ventricular and left ventricular pressures are equal [Eisenmenger's ventricular septal defect (VSD)], there will be no murmur across the defect. There will, however, be a short pulmonary ejection murmur of severe pulmonary hypertension. The murmur of VSD does not vary with respirations and can thus be differentiated from tricuspid regurgitation (Corvallo's sign). The murmur of VSD also does not radiate into the axilla and can thus be differentiated from mitral regurgitation. The murmur is best heard along the fourth, fifth, and sixth intercostal spaces. There is wide physiologic splitting in patients with a VSD and delayed pulmonic closure due to significant left-to-right shunting.

II-24.   **The answer is B.**   *(Ch. 10)*   The mid-diastolic and late diastolic Austin-Flint murmur has many characteristics of mitral stenosis, yet it is seen in patients with aortic regurgitation and no evidence of mitral stenosis. The Austin-Flint murmur is introduced by an S_3, rather than an opening snap. The S_1 is either of normal or decreased intensity. Vasodilating agents, such as amyl nitrate, that reduce the degree of aortic regurgitation, make the Austin-Flint murmur decrease in intensity.

II-25.   **The answer is C.**   *(Ch. 10)*   The condition that would have a continuous murmur in the left infraclavicular area and the second left intercostal space is a patent ductus arteriosus. Mammary souffle is best heard between the second and sixth intercostal spaces. A cervical venous hum is heard in the supraclavicular fossa just lateral to the sternocleidomastoid muscle. Sinus of Valsalva aneurysms are heard maximally along the lower sternal border or xiphoid over the area corresponding to the fistulous tract. Coronary artery fistulas are heard either to the left or right of the lower sternal area.

II-26.   **The answer is D.**   *(Ch. 11)*   The correct sequence of ventricular depolarization is from endocardium to epicardium. Depolarization consists of a moving wave of positive charges in front of negative charges. The sequence of ventricular repolarization occurs from epicardium to endocardium with negative charges in front of positive charges.

II-27.   **The answer is A.**   *(Ch. 11)*   This ECG shows extremely elevated ST segments in the inferior leads, moderate elevated ST segments in leads V_{5-6}, ST-segment depression in V_{1-2}, and a tall R wave in V_2. This represents an acute inferolateral MI with posterior extension. The latter is differentiated from "reciprocal" ST-segment depression by the very abnormally shaped ST segments in V_{1-2}, and particularly the tall R wave in V_2. Acute pericarditis would have diffuse ST-segment elevation. Early repolarization would never have ST-segment elevation of this magnitude, and would not explain the anterior ST-segment depression. Hyperkalemia produces peaked T waves, particularly in the anterior leads, ST-segment elevation (because the tall T wave "pulls up" the ST segment), and QRS widening.

II-28.   **The answer is E.**   *(Ch. 11)*   This ECG demonstrates diffuse ST-segment elevation. Acute MI is characterized by ST-segment elevation which is "convex upward" or in the shape of a tombstone. These changes are localized to the site of infarction, Q waves usually develop or the height of the R wave is decreased, and these changes occur in the clinical setting of an acute coronary syndrome. Left bundle branch block has a widened QRS complex (> 120 msec), and monophasic R waves and prolonged intrinsicoid deflection time in leads I and V_6. Left ventricular hypertrophy is characterized by increased voltage of the R or S wave in various leads, and ST-segment elevation usually confined to leads V_{1-3}. Early repolarization usually occurs in healthy young asymptomatic people and is characterized by "convex downward" ST-segment elevation, and sometimes a small but distinctive hump on the down slope of the R wave in the left chest leads. Frequently, however, early repolarization is a diagnosis of exclusion. Acute pericarditis is characterized by diffuse ST-segment elevation, typically in all of the leads (ST-segment depression in a V_R), tachycardia, and frequently PR-segment depression in the inferior limb leads. Acute pericarditis usually presents with a typical clinical syndrome of fever and pleuritic chest pain.

II-29. **The answer is C.** *(Ch. 11)* This ECG shows typical RBBB with a wide QRS complex (> 120 ms), an RSR′, and a delayed intrinsicoid deflection time in leads V_{1-2}. There is also left anterior fascicular block with a far left axis deviation (> −45°), an intraventricular conduction defect (> 105 ms QRS duration), and tiny Q waves in I and a V_1. LBBB is characterized by a wide QRS complex (> 120 ms), and monophasic R waves and prolonged intrinsicoid deflection time in leads I and V_6. Left posterior fascicular block is characterized by right axis deviation (> 100°), deep S wave in I and a small Q wave in III, a minor interventricular conduction defect (> 90 ms QRS duration), and lack of other causes of right axis deviation.

II-30. **The answer is D.** *(Ch. 11)* This ECG shows an acute anterior MI occurring in a patient with underlying LBBB. It is difficult if not impossible to diagnose an old MI in the presence of LBBB, but the acute ST segment elevation and even the development of new Q waves can frequently be detected in an acute ischemic event. Hyperkalemia would have a prolonged PR interval, a wide QRS complex, tall peaked T waves, and a prolonged QT interval. In progressive hyperkalemia the P wave flattens and then disappears.

II-31. **The answer is E.** *(Ch. 11)* The ECG shows the Wolff-Parkinson-White (WPW) syndrome with a very short PR interval and a typical slurred delta wave at the beginning of the QRS complex in several leads. Infarcts cannot be interpreted reliably in WPW because the delta wave may appear as a Q wave in various leads. The delta wave can radically alter the electrical axis, invalidating the diagnosis of left anterior fascicular block. Left ventricular hypertrophy (LVH) cannot be determined by traditional voltage criteria because of the distortion of the QRS complex. Hypercalcemia produces a short QT interval. Most conditions with a short PR interval produce a loud S_1 because the mitral and tricuspid leaflets are wide open when ventricular systole begins, causing the leaflets to shut rapidly and forcefully.

II-32. **The answer is C.** *(Ch. 11)* There are voltage criteria for LVH in the limb leads I and aVL. There is delayed precordial transition and slight ST-segment elevation in V_1 and V_2, most likely due to LVH.

II-33. **The answer is A.** *(Ch. 11)* This ECG shows a very wide QRS complex with an undetermined rhythm associated with severe hyperkalemia. The next stage of this condition would be an even more sine wave-like appearance and then asystole. LBBB should have some underlying discernable rhythm and morphology criteria for LBBB. The very wide, bizarre QRS complexes are unlikely to represent ventricular tachycardia or accelerated idioventricular rhythm. Hypothermia produces a peculiar slur on the downstroke of the QRS complex (the so-called "Osborn" waves). This ECG is not consistent with WPW.

II-34. **The answer is C.** *(Ch. 12)* This roentgenogram shows cephalization of the pulmonary vasculature, showing dilatation of the upper vessels with constriction of the lower vessels.

II-35. **The answer is A.** *(Ch. 12)* This radiographic shows a "boot-shaped" heart and decreased pulmonary blood flow consistent with tetralogy of Fallot. If heart failure accompanies an acute MI, the chest x-ray is characterized by pulmonary edema (often in a "butterfly" pulmonary pattern), engorgement of the hilum and upper pulmonary vessels, peribronchial cuffing, and perhaps Kerley B lines at the bases. Coarctation of the aorta produces a deformed descending aorta, rib notching, displacement of the esophagus on barium swallow, and left ventricular enlargement. A large pulmonary embolism produces dilation of the proximal pulmonary artery on the affected side and a paucity of pulmonary vasculature laterally. A left ventricular aneurysm is identified by a bulge along the left cardiac border.

II-36.   The answer is E.   *(Ch. 12)*   Chronic obstructive lung disease produces over inflated lungs, flattening of the diaphragms, pulmonary bullae, and a small, vertically oriented heart. Right heart failure from pulmonary hypertension is suggested by large proximal pulmonary arteries which taper to much smaller vessels distally. A large "water-bottle" shaped heart with normal pulmonary vasculature suggests tamponade. Chronic left heart failure is represented by gross cardiomegaly and pulmonary congestion. The left atrium is typically enlarged, demonstrated by a less acute angle between the main stem bronchi. Mitral stenosis has a very distinctive pattern on a chest radiograph, with the triad of a large left atrium, pulmonary congestion, and a *small* left ventricle. Constrictive pericarditis may show calcification of the pericardium, particularly if the etiology is tuberculosis.

II-37.   The answer is B.   *(Ch. 12)*   Patients who have levocardia with situs solitus are entirely normal. It is when patients have levocardia with situs inversus that there is almost a 100 percent incidence of cyanotic congenital cardiac lesions. The majority of patients who have dextroversion have congenitally corrected transposition of the great arteries. Patients having dextrocardia with situs inversus have a 5 percent incidence of congenital heart disease. Patients who have cardiac malpositions with situs ambiguus and have polysplenia tend to be acyanotic and have a milder clinical course than those who have asplenia. Those with asplenia generally die in infancy. The incidence of heart disease of patients with dextroversion is high (98 percent).

II-38.   The answer is C.   *(Ch. 12)*   In straight-back syndrome, the pulmonary trunk cannot be used as an indicator of right ventricular enlargement on chest roentgenogram, as this condition will cause the pulmonary artery to appear more enlarged than it actually is. A "3 sign" on the aorta and an "E sign" on the esophagus indicate the site of coarctation of the aorta. This condition is the most common cause of rib notching. Selective dilation of the ascending aorta is a hallmark sign of valvular aortic stenosis. Generalized dilation of the entire thoracic aorta is seen in aortic regurgitation. When the heart rotates to the left, this is evidenced on roentgenograms by both a smaller aorta and a larger pulmonary trunk.

II-39.   The answer is E.   *(Ch. 12)*   Patients with severe obstructive emphysema demonstrate centralization of blood flow. When the artery-bronchus ratio is less than unity, there is decreased blood flow. Patients with mitral stenosis show cephalization of the pulmonary vasculature. The mechanism responsible for this is intravascular pressure exceeding the oncotic pressure of the blood. When there are equal amounts of blood flow in the base and the apex, this represents an increase in pulmonary blood flow (PBF).

II-40.   The answer is D.   *(Ch. 12)*   Acute left-sided heart failure is characterized by a normal heart and alveolar pulmonary edema in a butterfly pattern. Chronic left-sided heart failure shows gross cardiomegaly, cephalization of the pulmonary vasculature, and interstitial pulmonary edema or fibrosis with multiple, distinct Kerley B lines. Acute right-sided heart failure shows developing centralization of the pulmonary vasculature and dilatation of the right-sided cardiac chambers and venae cavae. The lungs may also show localized or lateralized oligemia. Chronic right-sided heart failure shows diffusely decreased pulmonary vasculature with unusually lucent lungs in patients without pulmonary hypertension. In patients with chronic right-sided heart failure secondary to pulmonary hypertension, a centralized pulmonary blood flow pattern is seen. A cephalized flow with unusually lucent lungs is seen in patients with right-sided heart failure secondary to severe left-sided heart failure.

II-41.   The answer is C.   *(Ch. 13)*   Since sound energy is poorly transmitted through air and bone, a sufficient thoracic window must be present to allow adequate access to cardiac structures. The beam cannot be directed parallel or nearly parallel because little or no sound energy will be reflected to the transducer. A benefit of harmonic energy is that it can transmit energy at one frequency and receive at a higher frequency. When structures reflect such strong signals that they are transmitted again, this leads to reverberations, or the reproduction of anatomic structures in multiple locations within the image. The ultrasound beam diverges with distance from the transducer and has a finite width and will thus display images from the periphery as if they were on the central scan line.

II-42.   The answer is D.   *(Ch. 13)*   The long axis of the heart is best viewed in the parasternal, apical, and occasionally the suprasternal positions. The short axis of the heart is best viewed in the parasternal and subcostal positions. The four-chamber view is best obtained from the apical and subcostal positions.

II-43.   The answer is B.   *(Ch. 13)*   The transducer must be placed (as close to parallel to the flow) as possible to be able to accurately record the velocity. The frequency of sound changes proportional to the velocity and direction of the moving object that it strikes. The Doppler principle is based upon this fact. There is variance between the velocity of blood cells near the wall and near the lumen, which will give a narrowly dispersed signal. When the signal is broad and harsh, this represents turbulent flow. Flow that is shown above baseline represents flow that is moving toward the transducer. Doppler echocardiography can give information about the velocity and direction of blood flow and about the movement of some tissues, but it does not provide structural information. This information is provided by 2D and M-mode echocardiography.

II-44.   The answer is C.   *(Ch. 13)*   Doppler interrogation of the mitral valve diastolic flow velocities has gained widespread use in the diagnosis of diastolic dysfunction. The mitral *e* wave velocity represents passive filling of the left ventricle and, as such, is dependent in large part on the instantaneous pressure difference between the left atrium and the left ventricle. Under conditions where the compliance of the left ventricle is reduced, the left ventricular diastolic pressure is elevated relative to a normal ventricle at any given volume. Thus, the reduction in the peak velocity of the mitral E wave is reflective of decreased passive filling. Under conditions of elevated left atrial pressures, there is augmented early filling of the left ventricle. This can result in an increase in mitral E wave velocity. This becomes problematic when there is concurrent impairment of atrial and ventricular relaxation. Under these conditions, the expected depression of E wave velocity can be partially or completely offset by elevated left atrial pressure resulting in "pseudonormalization" of the mitral inflow pattern. This can be recognized by ancillary Doppler techniques. An impaired systolic filling wave and increased *a* wave flow reversal in the velocity recordings from pulmonary veins, in the setting of a relatively normal transmitral pattern of diastolic filling, suggests elevated left ventricular filling pressures. Restrictive physiology also produces characteristic alterations in the mitral inflow pattern. In restriction, there is an early, rapid filling of the ventricle and subsequent diminished late filling. This results in a very prominent E wave and a diminished or absent *a* wave on the mitral inflow. An E wave velocity that is 2.5 times higher than the *a* wave is considered to be indicative of restrictive physiology. Mitral inflow velocities can be altered by many different factors. The most clinically relevant factor is the effect of changes in preload. As discussed above, elevated left atrial pressure will cause an increase in the mitral E wave velocity, which can obscure the classic finding of impaired relaxation. Conversely, under conditions of relative volume depletion, the mitral E wave velocity can be falsely depressed, thus mimicking impaired relaxation. Other factors such as heart rate, valvular heart disease, and aging also impact the relative magnitudes of the Doppler E and *a* waves.

II-45.   The answer is A.   *(Ch. 13)*   TEE is of great importance for its diagnosis and management of infective endocarditis. The three standard TEE views include posterior to the base of the heart, posterior to the left atrium, and inferior to the heart. The left atrium is particularly well imaged by TEE. With the transducer in the esophagus, posterior structures, particularly the left atrium, appear at the top of the image. TEE is better suited for the Doppler interrogation of the pulmonary veins.

II-46.   The answer is B.   *(Ch. 13)*   Room-air microbubbles that have the diameter of pulmonary capillaries will persist in the blood for less than 1 s. Thus agitated agents injected intravenously will disappear before entering the left heart. The presence of these agents in the left heart indicate a right-to-left shunt. Thus after normal agitated saline solution is injected, a patent foramen ovale could be diagnosed if agitated liquid is present in the left heart.

II-47.   The answer is E.   *(Ch. 13)*   2D and M-mode echocardiography provide indirect evidence of the presence of AR. The important M-mode finding of premature mitral valve closure during diastole does indicate acute, severe AR. To obtain direct evidence of AR, Doppler interrogation is necessary. The AR jet velocity, as measured by CW Doppler, is maximal at the point of valve closure and decreases throughout diastole. The analysis of the size and shape of the flow by CW Doppler, is a semiquantitative measurement of the severity of the regurgitation. Severe, acute AR can cause diastolic mitral regurgitation.

II-48.   The answer is D.   *(Ch. 13)*   2D ultrasound in patients with mitral stenosis shows characteristic findings that are seen in nearly all patients with mitral stenosis. M-mode recordings demonstrate the effects of stenosis on mitral valve motion. A decrease in the E-F slope indicates the severity of the stenosis. Doppler estimates of the mitral valve area are indirect, and they are less accurate than those taken by planimetry of the mitral valve orifice. A score of greater than 9 on the echocardiographic scoring system indicates that percutaneous catheter balloon mitral commissurotomy should not be performed, as the risk of complications is too great.

II-49.   The answer is D.   *(Ch. 13)*   Due to the asymmetrical and crescentic shape of the right ventricle, it is difficult to get accurate calculations of right ventricular volume. With an increased right ventricular pressure load, the interventricular septum remains deformed during both systole and diastole. This can be distinguished from a volume overload, because the interventricular septum flattens during diastole and returns to its normal curvature during systole. In severe pulmonary hypertension, if right atrial pressure is elevated, the inferior vena cava will not decrease in diameter during inspiration as it normally would. Doppler echocardiography showing a high-velocity TR jet, without pulmonic stenosis, indicates pulmonary hypertension. Pulsed-wave Doppler shows a decrease in the velocity-time integral of flow through the pulmonic valve and a shortening of the acceleration time.

II-50.   The answer is B.   *(Ch. 13)*   Vegetations can be visualized with echocardiography. The most reasonable first approach to patients with suspected endocarditis is a screening with TTE. 2D imaging has largely replaced M-mode recordings for description of vegetations. Transesophageal echocardiography provides a more sensitive measurement than TTE in detection of vegetations in infective endocarditis. Echocardiographic evaluations do have limitations. Some of these are that active vegetations cannot be distinguished from healed vegetations, calcifications, myxomatous changes, and rheumatic involvement.

II-51.   The answer is A.   *(Ch. 13)*   Echocardiography is especially valuable in excluding transmural infarctions because these infarcts are usually associated with regional akinesis or dyskinesis. A pseudo-aneurysm is recognized by its localized nature and connection to the ventricle through a narrow neck. Aneurysms are recognized as wide-mouthed, thinned-walled myocardial segments displaying dyskinetic expansion during systole. Calculation of wall motion scores has identified a large cohort of people at increased risk for complications. Echocardiography can detect postinfarction free wall rupture (though most patients die prior to their identification). Echocardiography can likewise detect acquired defects in the interventricular septum. These defects usually present as a latticework of tissue rather than as a discrete orifice.

II-52.   The answer is D.   *(Ch. 13)*   Stress echocardiography has gained wide acceptance in both screening for the presence of significant coronary artery disease and in the preoperative evaluation of patients undergoing non-cardiac surgery. The addition of echocardiography as imaging modality to standard ECG stress testing, markedly increases the sensitivity and specificity of the test. There are two types of stresses that are utilized, exercise (either treadmill or bicycle) or pharmacological (dobutamine.) Many studies have found that the sensitivity and specificity of stress echocardiography is similar to that of exercise and dipyridamole nuclear stress testing. Several outcome studies performed with patients, either after a myocardial infarction or in the setting of preoperative risk stratification for noncardiac surgery, have demonstrated that dobutamine stress echocardiography has a very strong negative predictive value. When ischemia occurs during a stress echo, it is typically identified by a new or worsened regional wall motion abnormality. It is also important to note that the normal response to exercise or dobutamine is a hyperdynamic response. Therefore, the lack of a hyperdynamic response may also be indicative of significant coronary artery disease. In the setting of a preexisting regional wall motion abnormality, a biphasic response consisting of improved contractile function of a previously hypokinetic segment followed by worsening regional function may be observed. This finding is highly predictive of hibernating myocardium. Finally, segments may be severely hypokinetic or akinetic at rest and remain so throughout the stress portion of the test. This finding is indicative of coronary disease. However, it is likely the segment is primarily scar without evidence of a significant amount of hibernating myocardium.

II-53. The answer is C. *(Ch. 13)*   An abnormal "speckled" pattern or "ground-glass" appearance of the myocardium on 2D echocardiography is characteristic of restrictive cardiomyopathy, although the specificity of this finding is not very high because of the great variation in myocardial appearance on echo produced by different gain settings, different brands of equipment, etc. Systolic anterior motion of the mitral valve is seen in hypertrophic cardiomyopathy. Midsystolic closure of the aortic valve is seen in hypertrophic cardiomyopathy, and hypertrophy of some or all of the left ventricular walls is present. Four-chamber dilatation is seen in dilated cardiomyopathy. Infiltration of the myocardium by abnormal material (e.g., amyloid) is seen in restrictive cardiomyopathies.

II-54. The answer is E. *(Ch. 13)*   An ostium primum type ASD is characterized by a lack of interatrial septal tissue between the defect and the base of the interventricular septum. Ostium secundum defects are usually isolated, while ostium primum defects generally are associated with other lesions, such as cleft anterior mitral valve leaflet, mitral regurgitation, and atrioventricular canal ventricular septal defect. Color-flow imaging is the most useful imaging method for detecting a VSD and a patent ductus arteriosus. In the absence of mitral regurgitation, contrast will not enter the left atrium in an isolated VSD with an ASD.

II-55. The answer is D. *(Ch. 13)*   A long, linear, freely mobile structure viewed by echocardiography in the right atrium at the mouth of the inferior vena cava is a persistence of the eustachian valve. The Chiari network is seen as a weblike mobile structure in the posterior right atrium. Aneurysms of the atrial septum are viewed as a protrusion of the interatrial septum of at least 1.5 cm from its longitudinal plane dividing the left and right atriums. Lipomatous hypertrophy appears as a highly reflective thickening of the interatrial septum that typically spares the foramen ovale, creating a dumbbell appearance on an echocardiogram. Right ventricular hypertrophy can result in enlargement of the moderator band coursing along the interventricular septum towards the apex of the right ventricle.

II-56. The answer is B. *(Ch. 13)*   Thrombi that originate in the right atrium tend to be laminar and relatively immobile. Venous thrombo-emboli found in the right atrium tend to be serpentine and mobile. Left atrial thrombi occur in the setting of low cardiac output. Spontaneous echo contrast (or "smoke") is probably produced by transient aggregation of erythrocytes and plasma proteins and indicates stagnant blood flow. This can occur in any of the heart chambers and in the aorta. Left atrial thrombi are of homogenous echo density. Left ventricular thrombi can be either laminar and fixed or protruding and mobile.

II-57. The answer is B. *(Ch. 13)*   Normally, the pericardium is difficult to visualize with echocardiography, as the pericardial cavity is only a potential space. Electrical alternans is created as the heart swinging back and forth in the pericardial space within a moderate or large effusion. An echolucent space seen anterior to the right ventricular should not be the only criteria used to make a diagnosis of pericardial effusion, as this is usually caused by epicardial fat. The subcostal and parasternal views provide the most helpful views to decipher between pleural and pericardial effusions. Constrictive pericarditis is not easily detected with cardiac ultrasound, thus making Doppler flow the best way to diagnose this condition.

II-58.   The answer is B.   *(Ch. 14)*   The adaptation of the cardiovascular system to strenuous exercise is an important part of cardiac physiology. With conditioning induced by chronic bouts of dynamic exercise, a number of cardiovascular adaptations occur leading to a significant increase in maximum oxygen consumption. In addition to increasing the maximal exercise capacity, these adaptations allow sustained submaximal work with an economy of effort. These adaptations affect both the exercising skeletal muscle and the heart. In skeletal muscle, capillary density and the number of mitochondria increases, improving the overall respiratory capacity of the muscle. Oxygen extraction by a conditioned muscle is increased for any given rate of blood flow. The primary cardiac adaptations are hypertrophy and increased dimensions of the cardiac chambers at end diastole leading to an increased stroke volume by the Frank-Starling mechanism. In addition, the rates of systolic contraction and diastolic relaxation are increased, allowing for greater efficient pump function. The resting pulse rate falls as stroke volume increases and thereby allows for greater efficiency and a preserved resting cardiac output. Vagal tone at rest is also increased, decreasing the resting heart rate further. As the workload increases during exercise, even trained muscles need more oxygen. Oxygen consumption is related directly to the amount of work performed. If the capacity to deliver oxygen efficiently to working muscles falls behind, anaerobic metabolism ensues and limits exercise endurance. The maximum ability to deliver oxygen to tissues is the VO_2 max (the maximum consumption of oxygen by the entire body in mL/min). VO_2 max decreases with age and sedentary lifestyle. Local exercise-adaptive changes apply only to those discrete muscles being exercised (e.g., running on a treadmill does not make one fit for upper extremity exercise such as rowing). Each unit of work done requires the same amount of oxygen; trained muscles just deliver that oxygen more efficiently.

II-59.   The answer is E.   *(Ch. 14)*   During exercise, the systolic blood pressure rises as a result of increasing cardiac output while the diastolic pressure stays the same or decreases slightly. Isolated systolic hypertension during vigorous exercise is considered normal. Systolic blood pressure should rise with increasing workload. After a maximal exercise, there is usually a decline in the maximum systolic blood pressure. Systolic blood pressure falls to or below resting levels within 6 min of exercise cessation and often remains below pre-exercise levels for several hours. This fall in blood pressure is primarily due to changes in peripheral vascular resistance due to exercise-induced muscle bed vasodilatation and venous pooling. In some healthy individuals, a sudden and significant drop in blood pressure occurs when exercise is stopped abruptly, leading to pre-syncope or syncope. This is due to venous pooling with loss of the muscle venous pump function. The development of hypotension during exercise is indicative of severe heart disease. Patients with the lowest maximal systolic pressures were often associated with two- or three-vessel disease or reduced ejection fraction or both.

II-60.   The answer is C.   *(Ch. 14)*   The incidence of fatal complications from exercise testing is less than 1 in 10,000. The likelihood of serious arrhythmia or MI is less than 1 in 1000. Therefore, the relative safety of stress testing is well established, especially in view of the fact that many patients with severe cardiac disease safely undergo such tests daily. Unstable angina, endocarditis, and severe aortic stenosis (AS) are absolutely contraindicated. Early reports of sudden death with exercise testing in AS patients has led to a cautious approach in these patients. If there is a high clinical index of suspicion for significant AS (i.e., by history and physical exam), exercise testing should be deferred and echocardiography performed. In adults with mild to moderate AS, exercise testing may be a useful procedure with an acceptable risk when used selectively and with caution.

II-61.   The answer is D.   *(Ch. 15)*   The right femoral vein is recommended to enter the left atrium by transseptal catheterization because the standard technique developed using this approach and potentially drastic complications can occur if performed incorrectly.

II-62. **The answer is A.** *(Ch. 15)* The right ventricular pressure curve is often peaked or triangular in pulmonic stenosis. The LVEDP is recorded where the downslope of the *a* wave meets the upstroke of left ventricular pressure. If this point is not obvious, a standard technique is to use the so-called "Z point," defined by a vertical line drawn from the peak of the R wave down to the left ventricular pressure tracing. The LVEDP is elevated in patients with a dilated failing left ventricle. During diastole, pulmonary artery wedge diastolic mean pressure tends to be higher than left atrial diastolic mean pressure. Although recent advances in technology have improved the accuracy (technically speaking, the frequency response) of fluid-filled systems, true high fidelity pressure recordings require the use of micromanometer-tipped catheters.

II-63. **The answer is B.** *(Ch. 15)* A patient with poor left ventricular reserve would exhibit a decrease in left ventricular stroke work and an increase in LVEDP during the handgrip maneuver.

II-64. **The answer is B.** *(Ch. 15)* Left-to-right and right-to-left shunts may be evaluated by indicator dilution techniques in the cardiac catheterization laboratory. Typically, the indicator substance is injected into the right atrium and sampled in a peripheral arterial site. Flow in a normal heart produces an initial curve with a very large peak and rapid falloff. An early second rise in the curve represents a left to right shunt. A primary curve which occurs very quickly after injection (like the curve in the figure) represents a right to left shunt. Indicator dilution techniques are also used for measuring the volume of flow though various structures, and thus are used in determining cardiac output.

II-65. **The answer is C.** *(Ch. 15)* The right ventricular infundibulum is best seen utilizing a 30° axial right anterior oblique (RAO) and 40° cranial angulation. The four heart chambers and the posterior third of the ventricular septum is viewed in the 40° left anterior oblique (LAO) and 30° cranial position. The anterior two-thirds of the ventricular septum is viewed in the 60° LAO and 30° cranial position. The pulmonary artery and its bifurcation is seen in the frontal position with 30° of cranial angulation.

II-66. **The answer is D.** *(Ch. 15)* The frequency of any complication following cardiac catheterization is low. Arterial complications, such as hematomas, arterial occlusion or stenosis, false aneurysm, and infection, occur more frequently than death, myocardial infarction, thromboembolic events, stroke, or ventricular fibrillation.

II-67. **The answer is E.** *(Ch. 15)* Pressure gradients at rest do not accurately characterize the ischemic potential of a stenosis. The FFR reflects a reduction in myocardial perfusion that results from a stenosis, and is a more accurate prediction of ischemia than just a stenosis pressure gradient. The FFR is independent of hemodynamic and microcirculatory factors. Intravenous injection of adenosine produces similar hyperemia to intracoronary injection, but in a more sustained fashion. Patients with three-vessel coronary disease and no reference vessel provide a major limitation to rCFR.

II-68. **The answer is A.** *(Ch. 16)* ^{99m}Tc-MIBI has relatively stable myocardial concentration with little washout over a 3- to 4-h period. Therefore, it does not demonstrate redistribution phenomenon. To assess the extent of myocardial salvage following thrombolytic therapy, one dose of the tracer is injected prior to the administration of thrombolytic therapy, and imaging is performed several hours later because of the very slow washout. The patient is then reinjected and reimaged 24 h later. The difference between the two defects represents the salvaged myocardium.

II-69. **The answer is D.** *(Ch. 16)* Sestamibi is similar to thallium in that it exhibits high myocardial extraction, and it distributes proportionately to regional myocardial perfusion. ^{99m}Tc-teboroxime clears rapidly from the myocardium and has a half-life for myocardial clearance of about 6 to 10 min. For this reason, images must be acquired rapidly. This limits its use to multidetector systems. ^{99m}Tc-teboroxime is a member of a class that is chemically different from the cationic complexes, which include ^{99m}Tc-MIBI.

II-70. The answer is B. *(Ch. 16)*   The diagnostic value of pharmacologic stress testing is equivalent to that of exercise testing. Dipyridamole blocks the cellular reuptake of adenosine, leading to increased extracellular levels. Caffeine blocks adenosine binding and can thus eliminate the effects of dipyridamole or adenosine on coronary vasodilation. Dobutamine more commonly has side effects and thus it is not the agent of first choice for myocardial perfusion scintigraphy. It is used in patients with asthma or who have recently ingested caffeine.

II-71. The answer is A. *(Ch. 16)*   Changes in MIBG uptake has shown a loss of effective sympathetic innervation in heart failure patients. MIBG uptake is decreased in denervated myocardium. Myocardial necrosis occurs before denervation. ^{123}I compounds are very useful, but cannot currently be obtained in the United States. IPPA washes out of normal myocardium faster than out of ischemic myocardium.

II-72. The answer is C. *(Ch. 16)*   Patients who have a low probability (< 15%) of CAD should not have an exercise ECG for the purpose of making a diagnosis of CAD, but may be useful in risk stratification of patients with known CAD. Patients who have an intermediate probability of 15 to 50% should have a standard ETT. If the test yields positive results, the patient might need a stress SPECT if abnormalities of the resting ECG decrease the specificity of a standard ETT. A patient with a high risk of CAD (>85 percent) does not need an exercise SPECT to make a diagnosis of CAD, but perhaps to localize an area of ischemia to a particular area of myocardium or define the extent of jeopardized myocardium. Sensitivity is the probability that a patient with disease is identified by the test to be abnormal. The referral bias seen in SPECT testing leads to an overestimation of the sensitivity and a lowering in test specificity.

II-73. The answer is C. *(Ch. 16)*   Diabetics with mildly to moderately abnormal scans have a lower rate of event-free survival than those without diabetes. Myocardial perfusion SPECT is a good predictor of cardiac events in patients with LBBB. Nondiabetic women who are under the age of 45 may show false-positive results on ^{201}Tl imaging. This is thought to be related to soft tissue (breast) attenuation in the anterior and anterolateral segments. Abnormalities in exercise thallium imaging are accurate in predicting a high-risk population in people over age 65. Nuclear testing in noncardiac surgery patients has been recommended in those patients with an intermediate risk for a cardiac event at the time of the procedure.

II-74. The answer is B. *(Ch. 16)*   Patients with LBBB and patients presenting late after chest pain are both candidates for myocardial perfusion scintigraphy to determine whether they should have thrombolytic therapy or PCI. Myocardial perfusion SPECT combined with resting LV function provides information on myocardial stunning. Myocardial perfusion scintigraphy provides an efficient and less expensive before and after test to determine the efficacy of therapy. There is evidence that a relationship exists between the size of a very early myocardial perfusion defect and subsequent mortality from an acute MI.

II-75. The answer is E. *(Ch. 17)*   Ultrafast computed tomography (ultrafast CT) has primarily been a research tool; however, recent technical advances have vaulted this technology into greater importance in cardiac diagnoses for several disease entities. Ultrafast CT is an excellent diagnostic tool for visualizing the heart and great vessels. Because the scan times are in the millisecond range, cardiac motion can be stopped, allowing for good resolution of cardiac structures. Ultrafast CT has been shown to predict accurately the patency of coronary artery bypass grafts when compared to conventional angiography. It is also one of the diagnostic modalities of choice for evaluating the pericardium. One of the most promising applications for ultrafast CT may be the early diagnosis of CAD in asymptomatic patients. Diagnosis of coronary artery disease by ultrafast CT is made by visualizing calcification in the coronary arteries. The amount of calcium (Ca^{2+}) in the coronary arteries can be graded and correlated with the severity of disease. This may be very useful to clinicians who can diagnose coronary artery disease in asymptomatic patients and then focus on risk-factor modification. Currently, a number of studies are designed to evaluate the long-term incidence and prevalence of asymptomatic coronary disease as well as the effects of risk-factor modifications on the long-term prognosis of these patients. It should be mentioned, however, that the routine use of ultrafast CT as a screening test for CAD in asymptomatic patients is controversial and awaits the outcome of the major trials. Ultrafast CT is also useful in evaluating patients with suspected dissecting aortic aneurysms. Relative to MRI, the ultrafast CT has a much more open architecture that allows continued medical treatment of patients with suspected dissecting aortic aneurysms. Thus ultrafast CT and TEE are useful diagnostic tests for making the diagnosis of dissecting aneurysms. Echocardiography continues to be the diagnostic standard for evaluating native leaflet structure and motion.

II-76. **The answer is B.** *(Ch. 17)* Ultrafast CT has a very high resolution and scanning frequency. This technology is seen as a potential tool for evaluating and diagnosing CAD. Ultrafast CT can be used to determine regional left ventricular function and volumes and to detect coronary calcification. In general, the higher the amount of calcification present, the more severe the coronary disease; however, coronary calcification is an age-related phenomenon. Even normal elderly patients without angiographically significant coronary disease have a higher level of coronary calcification than younger patients (as determined by ultrafast CT). There is a relatively high sensitivity for predicting obstructive CAD in patients older than fifty. Younger patients with acute myocardial infarction frequently do not have significant calcification on ultrafast CT scanning. The presumed reason is that the acute infarction is caused by the rupture of a soft plaque, platelet aggregation, and thrombosis and not by a chronic high-grade stenosis within the coronary artery. One small study has actually shown a decrease in the severity of coronary calcification in patients who are aggressively treated with risk-factor modification. The current generation of scanners is not adequate to permit clinically diagnostic coronary angiography, although future developments in spatial resolution may make it feasible to perform diagnostic coronary angiography with this device. Studies have shown that most (~85 percent) patients with obstructive CAD also have coronary calcification. At the present time, ACC/AHA guidelines do not recommend selective coronary arteriography if the CT is positive for calcium.

II-77. **The answer is D.** *(Ch. 17)* CT scanning is useful in detecting myxomas, as well as the presence and extent of intracardiac tumors. CT scanning can also delineate metastatic tumors within the myocardial wall. Although CT scanning detects all of the other conditions, other modalities are better suited than CT. Congenital heart diseases, such as tetralogy of Fallot, are best detected by MRI, because it does not require x-ray exposure or the need for intravenous contrast material for both structural and functional delineation. Intracardiac tumors are easily detected by noninvasive two-dimensional echocardiography. Echocardiography is the best method for assessing pericardial abnormalities, such as pericardial effusion and pericardial cysts.

II-78. **The answer is E.** *(Ch. 18A)* As nuclei return to the B_0 axis following a radio frequency (RF) pulse, they lose the energy that they gained from the RF. Each type of tissue in the body has different T1 and T2 relaxation properties. To obtain general cardiovascular imaging, special magnetic resonance (MR) systems are not necessary. Specialized software can make most clinical MR systems able to obtain cardiovascular images. To obtain optimal cardiovascular MR, however, a specialized system dedicated to cardiovascular imaging is needed. The magnetic field must vary over the field of interest in order to obtain an image. In the presence of rapidly flowing blood, no signal is produced because the blood does not experience the refocusing pulse.

II-79. **The answer is A.** *(Ch. 18A)* In Chapter 18, the author states that there has never been a report of an incident with a heart valve prosthesis in an MRI with the possible exception of the pre-6000 series Starr-Edwards valve. Magnetic resonance techniques are contraindicated if (1) there is the potential to move or dislodge the device; (2) the RF field will heat a conductor such as a pacemaker electrode; (3) there is the potential for inducing current in a pacing electrode; or (4) there is the generation of artifacts which can confound diagnosis.

II-80.   **The answer is C.**   *(Ch. 18A)*   The fibrous tissue of the pericardium yields a lower signal intensity. MR can both show valvular regurgitation and assess the volume of the regurgitant flow. MR measures the amount of regurgitant flow by comparing right ventricular and left ventricular stroke volumes. Echocardiography provides an estimate of the valve leaflets with both high spatial and temporal resolution. Magnetic resonance is not able to accurately assess and reproduce the valve leaflets. Both echocardiography and MRI detect pericardial effusions, but MRI can detect small fluid accumulations that echocardiography could not. MRI has the ability to view hypertrophy at the apex, an area where hypertrophy is difficult to visualize with echocardiography.

II-81.   **The answer is D.**   *(Ch. 18B)*   An ECG-gated fast spin echo used in black blood imaging requires only 32 heartbeats. In a conventional gradient echo in white blood imaging, 128 heartbeats are needed to get an adequate image. With this long scan time, the patient cannot hold his/her breath for the full image, subjecting this method to respiratory motion artifacts. The signal-to-noise ratio of segmented k-space techniques is lower that that of conventional gradient echo cine acquisitions, due to shorter TRs required for smaller flip angles. The total scan time in segmented k-space scans, is inversely proportional to the number of views per segment. The long scan times in conventional single-phase, multiple-slice ECG-gated spin-echo (SE) make them extremely sensitive to respiratory motion.

II-82.   **The answer is B.**   *(Ch. 18B)*   The small diameter of the coronary arteries presents a challenge to magnetic imaging. There is often an overestimation of the flow velocity. MRA can sometimes be superior to coronary angiography in the identification of anomalous coronary arteries. An MRI should not be performed for several weeks following a coronary stent placement. A saphenous vein graft is easily visualized with MRA due to its stationary position and straight path. Research shows that magnetic resonance makes it possible to distinguish between normal vessel wall components and atherosclerotic plaque.

II-83.   **The answer is A.**   *(Ch. 19)*   A PTI of .75 indicates damage to the myocardium, whether through scar tissue formation or interstitial fibrosis. A low PTI has a negative predictive valve, but a near normal PTI does not accurately predict viability. Women demonstrate higher MBF than men. This is thought to be related to their higher HDL levels and lower plasma triglyceride levels. One of the benefits of using ^{82}Rb to measure MBF is its short half-life, which allows repeat studies in 10-min intervals. [^{13}N]ammonia has a longer half-life, which produces higher diagnostic quality images, but they must be obtained at 40- to 50-min time intervals. When the slope and size of the rapid clearance phase of [^{11}C]palmitate declines, this indicates ingestion of carbohydrates and thus a switch from FFA use by the myocardium to glucose use.

II-84.   **The answer is E.**   *(Ch. 19)*   PET has been used mainly in cardiology for the identification and characterization of CAD and detection of myocardial viability.

II-85.   **The answer is C.**   *(Ch. 19)*   Reversible and irreversible impairment of contractile function of the myocardium share several common features. Among these features are reduced myocardial blood flow, abnormal systolic wall function, and electrocardiographic abnormalities. Persistence of metabolic function and recruitable contractile reserve are seen in only reversible impairment of contractile function.

PART III
HEART FAILURE

III. HEART FAILURE

QUESTIONS

DIRECTIONS: Each question listed below contains five suggested responses. Select the **one best** response to each question.

III-1. Circulatory congestion refers specifically to which of the following?

(A) inadequacy of the cardiovascular system due to inadequate blood volume

(B) inadequacy of the cardiovascular system due to decreased venous return

(C) congestion due to either heart failure or noncardiac circulatory overload

(D) congestion due to inadequate oxyhemoglobin

(E) edema from any cause

(page 656)

III-2. Which of the following statements regarding the staging of heart failure (HF) is true?

(A) a patient in stage D heart failure is at risk of developing HF due to comorbid conditions associated with developing HF

(B) a patient with current or prior symptoms of HF associated with underlying structural disease is in stage B heart failure

(C) a person with coronary artery disease is in stage B heart failure

(D) a stage A heart failure patient has symptoms of heart failure at rest despite maximal medical therapy

(E) a patient with left ventricular hypertrophy is in stage C heart failure

(page 657–658)

III-3. Which of the following statements regarding systolic and diastolic ventricular dysfunction is true?

(A) an S_4 gallop is heard in systolic heart failure

(B) myocardial ischemia is common in diastolic dysfunction

(C) there is a well-established treatment for diastolic heart failure

(D) systolic heart failure is the primary feature of hypertensive heart disease

(E) elderly women more commonly have systolic dysfunction

(page 658)

III-4. Which of the following statements regarding the mechanism of heart failure is true?

(A) salt and water retention leads to the long-term maladaptive response of cell death

(B) hyperplasia and apoptosis play a large role in myocardial remodeling

(C) a systemic compensatory mechanism for heart failure is decreased oxygen extraction by tissues

(D) maladaptive remodeling of myocytes occurs long before clinical heart failure begins

(E) the role of neurohormones in heart failure is to protect perfusion pressure

(pages 662–665)

III-5. Which of the following statements regarding molecular, physiologic, and biochemical alterations seen with progression to heart failure is true?

(A) the switch from β-MHC to α-MHC, when translated into protein expression, results in decreased myosin ATPase enzyme velocity

(B) there is impaired sarcoplasmic reticulum (SR) uptake of Ca^{2+} in heart failure, but sarcolemmal uptake remains intact

(C) a widening of the coronary arteriovenous oxygen difference occurs in heart failure

(D) it has been shown that mitochondrial mass increases relative to the mass of the myofibrils

(E) with heart failure, there may be a downregulation of $β_2$ receptors, leaving $β_1$ receptors to mediate chronotropic and inotropic responses

(pages 665–667)

III-6. Which of the following diagnostic tests should be performed only in patients with symptoms of heart failure and angina?

(A) metabolic exercise testing

(B) blood work

(C) coronary angiography

(D) echocardiography

(E) electrocardiography

(page 678)

III-7. Which of the following statements regarding the mechanical and hemodynamic features of heart failure is true?

(A) a dilated, failing heart becomes less sensitive to preload and more sensitive to afterload

(B) an increase in the wall thickness of the ventricle results in an increase in wall tension

(C) no hyperplasia occurs in the heart

(D) hibernation is the mechanical dysfunction that persists after reperfusion, despite absence of irreversible damage

(E) it is important to recognize myocardial stunning because reperfusion can lower cardiovascular event rate

(pages 668–671)

III-8. Which of the following statements regarding non-cardiac adaptations to heart failure is true?

(A) increased quantities of the natriuretic peptides found in the blood in heart failure are regulatory in function

(B) AT_1 receptor-blocking (ARB) drugs enhance AT_2 receptor activity

(C) plasma norepinephrine levels are decreased in patients with heart failure

(D) decreased activation of V_1 receptors in vascular tissue contributes to both heightened vascular resistance and myocardial dysfunction in heart failure

(E) atrial natriuretic peptide (ANP) works cooperatively with endothelin

(pages 672–674)

III-9. A 43-year-old man complains of dyspnea on exertion and exertional chest pain. An echocardiographic demonstrates an aortic valve orifice area of less than 0.70 cm², making it most appropriate to schedule the patient for which of the following?

(A) cardiothoracic surgical consultation for possible aortic valve replacement

(B) coronary angiography

(C) follow-up evaluation with echocardiography in 6 months

(D) follow-up evaluation with echocardiography in 2 years

(E) an exercise test to rule out concomitant coronary disease

(pages 1675–1677)

III-10. A 45-year-old woman with a history of mitral valve prolapse presents with the acute onset of shortness of breath and fever. Physical examination reveals an early systolic murmur at the apex and bilateral pulmonary rales. Chest x-ray demonstrates bilateral pulmonary edema but not car-

diomegaly. In addition to blood cultures, the next test that should be performed is which of the following?

(A) left and right cardiac catheterization

(B) bronchoscopy

(C) ventilation-perfusion lung scan

(D) echocardiography

(E) myocardial biopsy

(page 399)

III-11. Which of the following statements regarding the pathophysiology and diagnosis of heart failure is true?

(A) myocyte slippage occurs during the first stage of chronic heart failure (HF)

(B) activation of the sympathetic nervous system and the renin-angiotensin system can result in myocyte loss

(C) symptoms of heart failure present when ventricular remodeling occurs

(D) as patients pass from New York Heart Association (NYHA) class I to class IV, there is a greater reduction in ejection fraction than in exercise capacity

(E) the left ventricular ejection fraction (LVEF) provides a good measure of systolic ventricular performance in a patient with mitral regurgitation and heart failure

(689–691)

III-12. Which of the following statements regarding angiotensin-converting enzyme (ACE) inhibitors is true?

(A) initial hemodynamic changes accurately predict the long-term clinical response to ACE inhibitors

(B) ACE inhibitors provide relief from vasoconstriction, but not a long-term change in vasculature structure or function

(C) structural alterations in the heart by ACE inhibitors lead to the initial decrease in left ventricular end diastolic volume

(D) captopril has been shown to reduce systemic arterial pressures and lower ventricular filling pressures

(E) long-term ACE inhibition also reliably lowers plasma aldosterone levels

(pages 693–694)

III-13. Which of the following patients should not be treated with ACE inhibitors?

(A) a patient receiving aspirin

(B) a patient with aortic regurgitation with no signs of heart failure

(C) a patient with progressive heart failure

(D) a diabetic patient

(E) a patient with bilateral renal artery stenosis

(pages 694–695)

III-14. Which of the following statements regarding alternatives to ACE inhibitors is true?

(A) angiotensin-converting enzyme (ACE) escape can be attenuated by the addition of AT_1 receptor-blocking (ARB) drugs

(B) ARB drugs are widely used for treatment of patients with heart failure

(C) daily doses of hydralazine and isosorbide dinitrate may reduce hospitalization, but not mortality, for patients with chronic heart failure

(D) prostacyclin has shown some benefits in patients with heart failure

(E) calcium channel antagonists are recommended for the treatment of heart failure

(pages 696–697)

III-15. Which of the following patients with heart failure should be treated with β-adrenergic blockade?

(A) a patient with reversible airway obstructive disease

(B) a patient with NYHA class III heart failure

(C) a patient with advanced heart block

(D) a patient with sinus rhythm and a resting heart rate of 40

(E) a patient with depression

(page 700)

III-16. Which of the following statements regarding β-adrenergic blockade is true?

(A) recent studies have shown that metoprolol does not further lower mortality in patients treated with ACE inhibitors and diuretics

(B) $β_1$ receptors are upregulated in the failing myocardium

(C) trials with carvedilol have demonstrated both mortality reduction and a dose-dependent improvement in LVEF

(D) the β-adrenergic blockade causes almost immediate improvement, with positive results seen several days following onset of therapy

(E) patients with class IV heart failure are the best candidates for β-adrenergic blockade

(page 698)

III-17. Which of the following statements regarding the use of diuretics in heart failure patients is true?

(A) the most potent diuretics act on the renal collecting ducts

(B) loop diuretics compete with potassium for binding to the $Na^+/K^+/2Cl$ cotransporter

(C) the newer loop diuretic torsemide has an 80 to 90 percent bioavailability and is excreted primarily by the kidneys

(D) the braking phenomenon, seen with long-term loop diuretic administration, refers to an increase in tubular sodium resorption by the distal tubule

(E) diuretics given orally rather than intravenously are more effective in decompensated heart failure

(pages 700–701)

III-18. Which of the following is a feature of spironolactone?

(A) an intravenous route of administration is preferred

(B) it increases both sodium and potassium reabsorption

(C) it is an endogenous hormone

(D) it is a water-soluble potassium-sparing diuretic

(E) it has been associated with reduced mortality in CHF, possibly by reducing arrhythmic death

(page 702)

III-19. Which of the following statements regarding digoxin is true?

(A) digoxin is of limited value for right-sided heart failure

(B) the benefits of reduced hospitalization are seen in patients with ejection fractions greater than 50 percent

(C) digoxin sensitizes the baroreflexes to increase efferent sympathetic activity

(D) digoxin has been shown to prolong survival in heart failure

(E) digitalis glycosides act on the cyclic AMP system

(pages 703–705)

III-20. Which of the following statements regarding catecholamines is true?

(A) dobutamine is indicated in the treatment of severe left ventricular failure with profound hypotension

(B) $α_2$ receptors are presynaptic and their stimulation causes a decrease in norepinephrine release

(C) $β_1$ receptors are located in vascular smooth muscle tissue

(D) catecholamines act by inhibiting the Na^+-K^+-ATPase

(E) dopamine administered in high doses causes peripheral vasodilation

(pages 705–707)

III-21. Which of the following activities is not safe for a patient with chronic heart failure to perform?

(A) limiting salt intake

(B) moderate walking

(C) limiting alcohol intake

(D) receiving an influenza vaccine

(E) performing isometric exercises

(pages 712–713)

III-22. Which of the following patients with heart failure would be the best candidate for a heart transplant?

(A) a 57-year-old man with an estimated survival of 1 year

(B) a 55-year-old woman with ongoing substance abuse

(C) a 60-year-old man with an estimated survival of 8 months

(D) a 75-year-old woman with an estimated survival of 1 year

(E) a 50-year-old man with lung cancer

(page 727–728)

III-23. Which of the following statements regarding the postoperative management of heart transplant patients is true?

(A) immune reactivity and the risk of graft rejection increase over time

(B) the preferable management strategy in the use of immunosuppressants is to give higher doses of a smaller number of drugs

(C) physical signs of graft rejection are few until the rejection is far advanced

(D) surveillance biopsies should be performed every month for a year following the transplant

(E) severe rejection episodes are treated with an increase in oral steroid dose

(pages 730–732)

III-24. Which of the following statements regarding allograft vasculopathy is true?

(A) this condition results in early death following transplantation

(B) it is characterized by asymmetric and calcified plaques

(C) patients first present with angina

(D) a calcium channel blocker given early following transplant may reduce the incidence of vasculopathy

(E) revascularization procedures are highly effective for long-term treatment of this condition

(pages 733–734)

III-25. Which of the following statements regarding alternatives to heart transplantation is true?

(A) a percutaneous intraaortic balloon pump (IABP) can be used as a long-term alternative to a heart transplant

(B) wound infection is the most common complication seen with IABPs

(C) ventricular assist devices (VADs) have been approved as a bridge to transplantation

(D) permanent VADs, implantable devices with rechargeable batteries, are being used in a wide variety of patient populations

(E) primate hearts are the most useful to use for xenotransplantation due to their appropriate size, anatomic structure, and available numbers for human transplantation

(pages 735–736)

III-26. Which of the following statements regarding endomyocardial biopsy is true?

(A) an endomyocardial biopsy is usually performed in the left ventricle

(B) an inflammatory infiltrate of eosinophils with nonischemic damage or necrosis of adjacent myocytes seen on biopsy is characteristic of sarcoidosis

(C) the appearance on biopsy of interstitial, subendocardial, or vascular deposits of finely fibrillar, eosinophilic material characterizes idiopathic cardiomyopathy

(D) hypertrophic cardiomyopathy is not readily distinguished on endomyocardial biopsy

(E) biopsy-shown changes of myofibrillar loss with Z-band remnants and sarcotubular dilatation within myocytes is seen with cardiac amyloidosis

(pages 738–740)

III-27. The presence of atypical lymphocytes, immunoblastic cell infiltrates, abundant tissue necrosis, and frequent mitotic figures on endomyocardial biopsy suggest

(A) acute rejection of transplant

(B) posttransplant lymphoproliferative disorder

(C) previous biopsy site

(D) Quilty effect

(E) infectious myocarditis

(page 743)

III. HEART FAILURE

ANSWERS

III-1. **The answer is C.** *(Ch. 20)* Circulatory failure is inadequacy of the cardiovascular system in providing nutrition to the cells of the body and inadequate retrieval of breakdown by-products of metabolism. The causes may be either cardiac (pump failure) or noncardiac. Noncardiac causes include inadequate oxyhemoglobin, inadequate blood volume, increased capacity of the vascular system, and peripheral vascular abnormalities. Circulatory congestion is excess blood volume from either cardiac or noncardiac causes. Noncardiac causes include conditions in which there is an increase in blood volume (salt-retaining steroids, excess fluid administration, and renal insufficiency) and then conditions in which there is increased venous return or decreased peripheral resistance (atrioventricular fistulae, beriberi, severe anemia, and end-stage cirrhosis).

III-2. **The answer is B.** *(Ch. 20)* There are four stages of (HF) Stage A is a patient with a strong risk of developing HF due to comorbid conditions. This patient has no structural or functional abnormalities of the valves or ventricles. A patient with coronary artery disease would be in stage A. Stage B is a patient who has developed structural heart disease that is strongly associated with HF development, but has no symptoms nor has ever manifested signs or symptoms. A patient with left ventricular hypertrophy is in stage B. Stage C is a patient with current or prior symptoms of HF associated with underlying structural heart disease. Stage D is a patient with marked symptoms of HF at rest, despite maximal therapy.

III-3. **The answer is B.** *(Ch. 20)* An S_3 gallop is frequently present in systolic heart failure. Systolic dysfunction usually occurs in the setting of normal or low blood pressure. The treatment of systolic dysfunction is much better established than the treatment of isolated diastolic dysfunction. Diastolic heart failure more commonly affects elderly women. An S_4 gallop is common in hypertensive heart disease. Hypertensive heart disease is characterized by increasing left ventricular hypertrophy, which causes diastolic relaxation abnormalities. Systolic function in hypertensive heart disease is usually normal or hyperdynamic for a prolonged period of time. Eventually, systolic function deteriorates as well.

III-4. **The answer is D.** *(Ch. 20)* There are four compensatory mechanisms of the body in response to low cardiac output. These mechanisms are salt and water retention, vasoconstriction, increased cardiac adrenergic drive, and transcription factor activation. Of these, salt and water retention is the only mechanism that does not lead to the long-term maladaptive response of cell death. Hyperplasia and apoptosis involve less than 1 percent of the cardiac myocytes. Myocyte hypertrophy plays the largest role in myocardial remodeling. Tissues extract increased oxygen from the blood as a compensatory response to heart failure. The maladaptive response of cardiac myocytes occurs long before the onset of clinical heart failure. Neurohormones play a role in both protecting perfusion pressures as well as in facilitating the left ventricular remodeling process.

III-5. **The answer is C.** *(Ch. 20)* Mechanical stress causes the shift from α- to β-MHC expression. The β-MHC isoform is less active. This shift leads to a decreased myosin ATPase enzyme velocity and thus a slower speed of contraction. Sarcolemmal Ca^{2+} uptake may be defective in heart failure as well as in SR release. SR uptake, however, remains intact. The total amount of oxygen consumed by the heart increases with the myocardial changes, thus a greater amount of oxygen is extracted from the coronary blood, leading to a widening of the coronary arteriovenous oxygen difference. The decrease or lack of change in mitochondrial mass in the presence of myocyte hypertrophy may be one of the limitations of severe hypertrophy. In heart failure, β_1 receptors are selectively downregulated, leaving a high percentage of β_2 receptors to mediate chronotropic and inotropic responses.

III-6. **The answer is C.** *(Ch. 20)*   The use of coronary angiography in patients with heart failure is controversial. It is a usually indicated if there is evidence of ischemic viable myocardium because revascularization may improve left ventricular systolic function. The presence of angina strongly suggests viability in at least some portion of the myocardium.

III-7. **The answer is A.** *(Ch. 20)*   A dilated, failing heart becomes less sensitive to preload and has increased sensitivity to afterload. According to the law of Laplace, an increase in wall thickness results in a decrease in wall tension. There is significant hyperplasia of fibroblasts in the heart. Fibroblasts outnumber myocytes by 3:1 to 4:1. When myocytes are lost, it is the fibroblasts that are the major source of collagen in the heart. *Myocardial stunning* is the mechanical dysfunction of viable myocardium that may persists for up to several weeks after reperfusion. *Hibernation* is the term given to myocardium which is viable but chronically ischemic. This myocardium has little or no mechanical activity but may improve substantially with revascularization. Recognition of which nonmoving heart muscle retains viability is one of the important challenges in the management of coronary artery disease and ischemic cardiomyopathy.

III-8. **The answer is B.** *(Ch. 20)*   The increased natriuretic peptides found in the circulation in heart failure are considered to be counterregulatory. They reduce right atrial pressure, systemic vascular resistance, aldosterone secretion, sympathetic nerve stimulation and hypertrophy of cells, and enhanced sodium excretion. ARBs increase angiotensin II levels and thus enhance the activity of unoccupied AT_2 receptors. Plasma norepinephrine levels are increased in patients with heart failure. Activation of V_1 receptors in vascular tissue contributes to both increased vascular resistance and myocardial dysfunction present in heart failure. ANP is the antagonist of vasopressin.

III-9. **The answer is B.** *(Ch. 20)*   Valvular heart disease is an important, potentially reversible, cause of heart failure. An adult with symptoms of significant aortic stenosis (i.e., dyspnea, angina pectoris, or syncope) in whom echocardiographic features suggest critical aortic stenosis should have coronary angiography performed promptly. It may or may not be appropriate, depending on the clinical situation, to cross the aortic valve during catheterization to confirm the transvalvular pressure gradient. The principal reason for performing coronary angiography is to assess the status of the coronary arteries, since the prevalence of coronary artery disease is greatly increased in patients with aortic stenosis. Exercise testing in patients with severe aortic stenosis may be hazardous, and exercise-induced ST changes are usually unreliable in detecting ischemia since these changes could be to due to the omnipresent left ventricular hypertrophy.

III-10. **The answer is D.** *(Ch. 20)*   The patient presents with a classic history of acute mitral regurgitation from endocarditis on a previously abnormal valve. In acute heart failure consequent to infective endocarditis of the aortic or mitral valves, ruptured chordae tendinae, papillary muscle infarction, or ruptured interventricular septum, echocardiography should be performed immediately to assess the mechanical cause of the heart failure and to evaluate left ventricular function. Vegetations may not be detected in the acute stage of endocarditis. Transesophageal echocardiography may also be necessary to assess the extent of the infection and to determine if mitral valve repair is possible or if valve replacement is necessary. Prior to surgical intervention, cardiac catheterization should be performed to determine the status of the coronary arteries.

III-11. **The answer is B.** *(Ch. 21)*   *Myocyte slippage* is the displacement of myocytes or groups of myocytes which occurs with sustained diastolic loads. This occurs during the second phase of heart failure. Activation of the sympathetic nervous system as well as the renin-angiotensin system causes further vasoconstriction and salt accumulation. These factors, combined with myocyte hypertrophy, can lead to myocyte loss. As patients pass from NYHA class I to class IV, the reduction in the exercise capacity is greater than the decrease in the ejection fraction. In a patient with chronic severe mitral regurgitation, the LVEF represents the fraction of blood ejected into the left atrium as well as the systemic circulation. Since a dilated left atrium is a low resistance structure, much of left ventricular ejection is spent in filling the atrium. Therefore the LVEF does not provide an true measure of the patient's systolic ventricular function.

III-12. **The answer is D.** *(Ch. 21)* The initial hemodynamic changes seen with ACE inhibitor therapy do not predict the long-term clinical response. The principal benefit of ACE inhibitors is from a structural or functional change in the peripheral vasculature or from effects on myocardial cellular alterations. The initial reduction in left ventricular end diastolic volume is related to the decreased loading of the failing ventricle, not structural changes in the heart. Captopril has been shown to both reduce systemic arterial pressure and lower ventricular filling pressures. Aldosterone levels are regulated by factors other than the rennin-angiotensin system. Aldosterone is also regulated by potassium levels, corticotropin, and endothelin. Thus, long-term ACE inhibition does not provide a reliable means for lowering plasma aldosterone levels.

III-13. **The answer is E.** *(Ch. 21)* A patient with bilateral renal artery stenosis should not be treated with ACE inhibitors. There is a potential drug-drug interaction with ACE inhibitors and aspirin, but the finding has not been substantiated in recent analyses. ACE inhibition therapy would be appropriate in the other conditions.

III-14. **The answer is A.** *(Ch. 21)* The addition of ARB drugs to ACE inhibitors negates the detrimental effects of elevated levels of tissue and circulating angiotensin. The use of ARB drugs for treatment of heart failure is currently recommended for patients who experience cough or angioedema while receiving ACE inhibitors. Treatment with the combination of the two agents has not been shown to be superior to their individual use. Treatment with the combination of hydralazine and isosorbide dinitrate has been shown to reduce mortality, but not hospitalization, for heart failure. Prostacyclin has not been shown to have any benefits for patients with heart failure. Multiple studies have failed to show any benefit in the treatment of heart failure with calcium channel antagonists, and some studies have shown a worse outcome compared to placebo.

III-15. **The answer is B.** *(Ch. 21)* Patients with reactive airway disease may have worsening of bronchospasm if treated with β-adrenergic blockade. Patients with class III heart failure have been shown to benefit from β-adrenergic blockade therapy with improvement in symptoms and prolongation of survival. Advanced heart block or resting bradycardia are contraindications for β-adrenergic blockade therapy, unless permanent pacemaker implantation is contemplated. Clinically significant depression is a relative contraindication for β-adrenergic blockade therapy, although treatment with an antidepressant may ameliorate this side effect.

III-16. **The answer is C.** *(Ch. 21)* In a recent study, metoprolol lowered mortality by 34 percent in patients with heart failure who had already treated with ACE inhibitors and diuretics. There is a predominance of β_2 receptors in the failing myocardium, due to a downregulation of β_1 receptors. Carvedilol trials have shown a reduction in mortality and a dose-dependent improvement in LVEF. The β-adrenergic blockade takes weeks to months to show benefits. Frequently, there is an initial decrease in LVEF, then a return to normal, and finally an improvement of about 10 percent. Selected patients with class IV heart failure may be candidates for β-adrenergic blockade, but treatment with ACE inhibitors, digoxin, loop diuretics, and spironolactone should be instituted first.

III-17. **The answer is D.** *(Ch. 21)* The most potent diuretics act on the ascending limb of Henle. Loop diuretics compete with chloride for binding the $Na^+/K^+/2Cl$ cotransporter. Torsemide is primarily (80 percent) metabolized by the liver. The *braking phenomenon* refers to an increase in sodium reabsorption by the distal tubules after long-term administration of loop diuretics. In decompensated heart failure, absorption of orally administered diuretics may be compromised, and the intravenous route of administration is preferred.

III-18. **The answer is E.** *(Ch. 21)* Spironolactone is administered orally. It increases sodium reabsorption, but the exchange of sodium for potassium is reduced. Aldosterone, but not spironolactone, is an endogenous hormone. Spironolactone is a lipid-soluble, potassium-sparing diuretic. It has been associated with reduced mortality in heart failure, possibly by maintaining potassium levels and therefore reducing arrhythmic death.

III-19. **The answer is A.** *(Ch. 21)* Digoxin is of limited value for patients with right-sided heart failure and ejection fractions of greater than 40 percent. Digitalis glycosides act to sensitize the baroreflexes and decrease efferent sympathetic activity. Digoxin has been shown to decrease hospitalization and improve symptoms in patients with ejection fractions of less than 40 percent. It has no effect on mortality. Digitalis glycosides act on the Na^+-K^+-ATPase on the surface membrane of myocardial cells.

III-20. **The answer is B.** *(Ch. 21)* Dobutamine is indicated in selected patients with severe refractory heart failure. It does not cause peripheral vasoconstriction and therefore does not raise blood pressure. α_2 receptors are presynaptic; their stimulation causes a decrease in the amount of norepinephrine released. β_1 receptors are located in the myocardium, while β_2 receptors are located in vascular smooth muscle. Catecholamines increase intracellular Ca^{2+} levels by acting on β-adrenergic receptors and the adenyl cyclase system. Dopamine, a naturally occurring substance, causes renal vasodilation when administered at low doses and vasoconstriction at higher doses.

III-21. **The answer is E.** *(Ch. 21)* A patient with chronic heart failure should be encouraged to obtain physical exercise such as moderate walking. Exercise improves symptoms and quality of life in patients with heart failure, but has not been shown to prolong survival. Isometric exercises, however, may be harmful. Patient should be advised to limit salt and alcohol intake. Vaccines for pneumococcal pneumonia and influenza should be administered.

III-22. **The answer is A.** *(Ch. 22)* The upper limit on the age of candidates for heart transplantation has traditionally been 60 years old, but there have been many individual exceptions. They should have an estimated survival time of 1 to 2 years. They cannot have other diseases that would limit their long-term survival. Candidates must also not have behavior patterns that suggest limited compliance with post-transplant treatment regimens.

III-23. **The answer is C.** *(Ch. 22)* Immune reactivity and the chance of graft rejection are highest during the months following the transplant and decrease with time. The preferable strategy with immunosuppressive agents is to use several drugs simultaneously at lower doses. The physical signs of a graft rejection are few until the rejection is advanced. Surveillance biopsies are performed every week for the first 4 to 6 weeks following the transplant, and then at a minimum of every 3 months for a year. Most centers continue to do biopsies every 4 to 6 months. An increase in oral steroids is usually sufficient for mild rejection, but more serious rejection requires intravenous steroids.

III-24. **The answer is D.** *(Ch. 22)* Allograft vasculopathy is currently the principal factor limiting long-term survival in heart transplant patients. The asymmetric and calcified plaques that are seen in conventional atherosclerosis are not present in the lesions of transplant vasculopathy. Patients usually do not have angina, as most patients usually have a persistent state of both afferent and efferent denervation. One study has shown that a calcium channel blocker given early following surgery reduces the incidence of vasculopathy. Revascularization procedures have a 94 percent success rate and an acceptable complication rate; however, restenosis eventually occurs in a high number of cases.

III-25. **The answer is C.** *(Ch. 22)* IABPs can only be used for a short period of time in patients awaiting transplant or for patients in acute situations, such as cardiogenic shock. The most common complication seen with IABPs is ischemia of the extremity distal to the femoral insertion site. VADs are approved as a bridge to patients awaiting a transplant. Permanent VADs are undergoing trials in a patient population not eligible for a heart transplant. Primates are the most obvious choice for supplying hearts for human transplants, due to their homology to humans for both hormones and cell surface receptors. However, the supply of primates is much too limited to fill the demand and ethical considerations play a major role. Swine hearts are the next most likely candidates, due to their appropriate size, anatomic structure, and available numbers for transplants.

III-26. **The answer is D.** *(Ch. 22)* Endomyocardial biopsy is usually performed in the right ventricle, although some conditions require a left ventricular biopsy. Sarcoidosis is usually characterized by a lymphocytic infiltration associated with nonischemic damage or necrosis of adjacent myocytes. Interstitial, subendocardial, or vascular deposits of finely fibrillar, eosinophilic material seen on biopsy characterizes cardiac amyloidosis. Hypertrophic cardiomyopathy is not readily distinguished by endomyocardial biopsy. Anthracycline toxicity can be determined by myofibrillar loss with Z-band remnants and sarcotubular dilatation within myocytes.

III-27. **The answer is B.** *(Ch. 22)* The presence of atypical lymphocytes, plasmacytoid or immunoblastic cell infiltrates, abundant tissue necrosis, and frequent mitotic figures suggest posttransplant lymphoproliferative disorder. All conditions mentioned may be confused with acute rejection on endomyocardial biopsy.

PART IV
RHYTHM AND
CONDUCTION DISORDERS

IV. RHYTHM AND CONDUCTION DISORDERS

QUESTIONS

DIRECTIONS: Each question listed below contains five suggested responses. Select the **one best** response to each question.

IV-1. Which of the following is the dominant pacemaker rate of the heart?

(A) atrial pacemaker rate of 20 to 40 beats per minute
(B) ventricular pacemaker rate of 60 beats per minute
(C) sinus node rate of 60 to 100 beats per minute
(D) atrioventricular nodal rate of 20 beats per minute
(E) His-Purkinje rate of 20 beats per minute

(page 751)

IV-2. Which one of the following arrhythmogenic mechanisms is correctly matched with the electrical stimulation that identifies it?

(A) automaticity and termination by overdrive pacing
(B) reentry and initiation by electrical stimulation
(C) delayed afterdepolarization and triggered activity and entrainment during overdrive pacing
(D) early afterdepolarization and triggered activity and entrainment during overdrive pacing
(E) automaticity and initiation by overdrive pacing

(pages 751–778)

IV-3. Which of the following statements regarding exercise stress testing for cardiac arrhythmias is true?

(A) the stress test should usually be accompanied by thallium or sestamibi scintigraphy
(B) the test is particularly useful for detecting atrial arrhythmias
(C) the test is useful in distinguishing autonomic from structural disease mechanisms
(D) the test is not helpful in evaluating the proarrhythmic effects of antiarrhythmic agents
(E) the test should not be used in patients with the Wolff-Parkinson-White syndrome

(page 799)

IV-4. Identify the abnormality illustrated in the rhythm strip below and choose the correct first-line therapy.

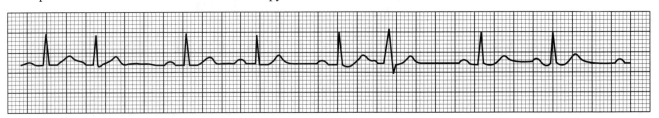

(A) premature atrial depolarization and a beta blocker
(B) premature atrial depolarization and amiodarone
(C) premature atrial depolarization and reassurance
(D) premature ventricular depolarization and sotalol
(E) premature ventricular depolarization and procainamide

(page 805)

IV-5. What does the ECG below illustrate?

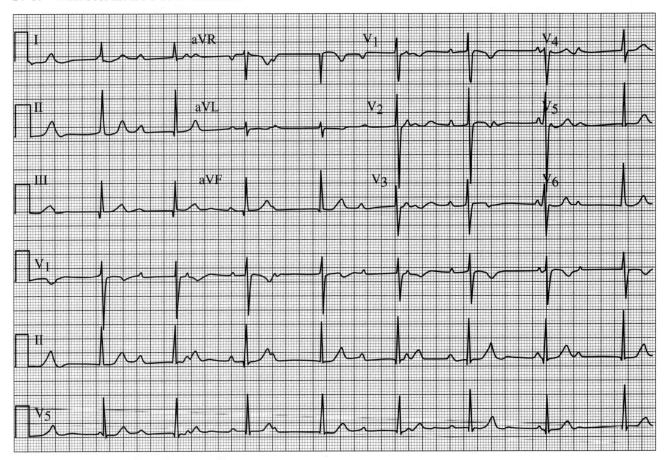

(A) first-degree atrioventricular (AV) block
(B) type I second-degree AV block
(C) type II second-degree AV block
(D) third-degree AV block
(E) accelerated junctional rhythm

(page 860)

IV-6. Which of the following statements regarding the ECG below is true?

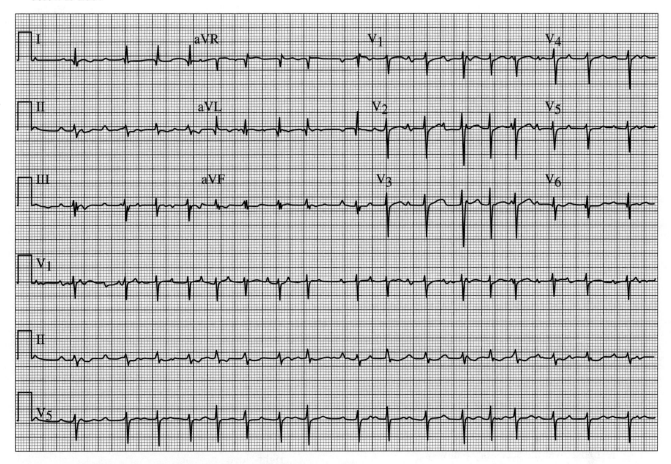

(A) it may be seen in a patient with chronic lung disease
(B) it is unlikely to be seen in a patient with aminophylline toxicity
(C) it illustrates a triggered mechanism
(D) it illustrates a reentrant mechanism
(E) the PR intervals are constant

(page 819)

IV-7. Which of the following statements regarding a premature atrial contraction (PAC) is true?

(A) a PAC is characterized by a P wave which occurs before the next expected sinus impulse and a normal P wave axis
(B) an negative P wave in II, III, and aV_F suggests an origin in the upper part of the left atrium
(C) a P wave which is positive in I and negative in V_1 suggests a right atrial origin
(D) a P wave which is negative in I and V_6 but is positive in V_1 suggests a right atrial origin
(E) a P wave which is negative in I and V_6 but is positive in the inferior leads suggests a left atrial origin

(page 805)

IV-8. The rhythm strip shown below has which of the following characteristics?

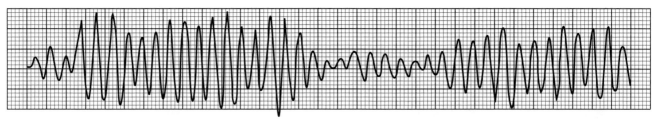

(A) its mechanism is due to triggered activity
(B) it is seen as a complication in patients with Romano-Ward syndrome
(C) it is seen as a complication in patients with Lown-Ganong-Levine syndrome
(D) it is seen as a complication in patients who have an intracranial lesion
(E) it is seen as a complication in phenothiazine therapy

(page 762)

IV-9. Which of the following statements regarding iatrogenic complications of electrophysiological studies is true?

(A) complete heart block in patients with preexisting left bundle branch block (LBBB) is a rare complication of right ventricular catheterization
(B) in a patient with Wolff-Parkinson-White syndrome and paroxysmal supraventricular tachycardia (PSVT), atrial fibrillation should be initiated at the end of the study to assess ventricular response over the accessory pathway
(C) patients with a prior history of atrial fibrillation are more prone to developing sustained ventricular tachycardia in the laboratory
(D) the overall complication rate is very low with an almost negligible mortality when left heart catheterization is done for electrophysiological studies
(E) catheter damage to the cardiac valves is an uncommon but well reported complication

(page 896)

IV-10. The only antiarrhythmic agent which has not been associated with excess mortality after myocardial infarction is which of the following?

(A) encainide
(B) flecainide
(C) moricizine
(D) amiodarone
(E) quinidine

IV-11. Which of the following statements regarding side effects of antiarrhythmic agents is true?

(A) disopyramide has significant negative inotropic properties

(B) quinidine has significant negative dromotropic (atrioventricular nodal blocking) properties
(C) flecainide rarely demonstrates proarrhythmic effects when used to treat supraventricular arrhythmias
(D) more than 25 percent of patients treated with amiodarone will demonstrate some evidence of pulmonary toxicity during the course of therapy
(E) sotalol does not prolong the QT interval

(page 815)

IV-12. Which of the following statements regarding the ECG in the Wolff-Parkinson-White (WPW) syndrome is true?

(A) during sinus rhythm with WPW, the P to J interval is shortened (the J point is where the ST segment begins)
(B) if the delta wave is positive in lead I and negative in V_1, the accessory pathway (AP) is probably right-sided
(C) if the delta wave is positive in the inferior leads, the AP is probably posterior
(D) if the delta wave is negative in aV_L, a right lateral AP is likely
(E) most episodes of PSVT are wide complex arrhythmias with a rate of 120 to 180

(page 816)

IV-13. Which of the following statements regarding atrial tachycardia is true?

(A) digoxin toxicity is an unlikely cause
(B) the most common mechanism is reentry
(C) most patients with atrial tachycardia have no obvious underlying cause
(D) primary therapy is radiofrequency catheter ablation
(E) atrial tachycardias may originate from atrial suture lines after surgical treatment of congenital heart disease

(page 819)

IV-14. Which of the following statements regarding atrial flutter is true?

(A) type I flutter is utilizes a macroreentrant pathway located in the left atrium

(B) type I flutter usually has a clockwise direction of propagation

(C) type I flutter usually has a distinct slowing in the subeustachian isthmus

(D) one of the differences between type I and type II flutter is the ability to entrain the latter with overdrive pacing

(E) the rate of type II flutter is usually very close to 300

(page 820)

IV-15. Which of the following statements regarding the treatment of atrial flutter is true?

(A) ibutelide, a newer class III agent, is quite effective without significant risk of torsades de pointes

(B) overdrive pacing is seldom effective in the treatment of recent onset atrial flutter

(C) a linear radiofrequency ablation between the tricuspid annulus and the inferior vena cava (IVC) has an 85 percent long-term success rate

(D) atrial flutter is relatively common in normal patients

(E) patients with chronic atrial flutter do not need long-term warfarin anticoagulation

(page 823)

IV-16. Which of the following statements regarding atrial fibrillation is true?

(A) the most common mechanism of atrial fibrillation is focal atrial tachycardia in the muscle fibers of the distal pulmonary veins

(B) the presence of PACs has no relation to the likelihood of developing atrial fibrillation

(C) the morphology of PACs has no relation to the mechanism of atrial fibrillation

(D) the hemodynamic consequences of atrial fibrillation are due to a loss of atrial systole and shortening of the diastolic filling period

(E) mitral stenosis is still the most common cause of atrial fibrillation

(page 824)

IV-17. Which of the following statements regarding anti-coagulation in atrial fibrillation is true?

(A) an acceptable alternative to three weeks of warfarin anticoagulation prior to direct current (DC) cardioversion is the lack of left atrial thrombi on transesophageal echocardiography

(B) recent studies have shown that fixed-dose warfarin plus aspirin was as effective in preventing stroke as conventional dose-adjusted warfarin

(C) anticoagulation for atrial fibrillation associated with thyrotoxicosis has not been shown to be beneficial

(D) an international normalized ratio (INR) of 3.5 to 4.5 has been shown to have the best risk/benefit ratio

(E) one recent large trial reported that the risk of a major hemorrhagic event was three times more likely with warfarin than with aspirin or placebo

(pages 826–829)

IV-18. Which of the following statements regarding the treatment of atrial fibrillation is true?

(A) recent studies suggest there is a favorable risk/benefit ratio in attempting to maintain sinus rhythm in patients with chronic atrial fibrillation

(B) among patients with advanced underlying heart disease, only about 20 percent who are taking a newer antiarrhythmic agent will revert to atrial fibrillation in one year

(C) surgical approaches for the prevention of atrial fibrillation have proven to be effective in less than 25 percent of cases

(D) dofetilide and azemilide are newer class III agents which may be useful in maintaining sinus rhythm

(E) an atrial implantable cardiac defibrillator (ICD) has proven to be very useful in the maintenance of sinus rhythm

(page 828)

IV-19. Which of the following statements regarding the treatment of premature ventricular contractions (PVCs) is true?

(A) There are no data supporting the theory that PVC suppression itself improves mortality rates, despite the connotation of risk in specific clinical settings

(B) it is still recommended to administer lidocaine to all patients having an acute MI who have any number of PVCs

(C) recent large trials have shown that amiodarone improved total mortality post MI

(D) class IC agents should be considered in patients with symptomatic PVCs

(E) ICDs have been shown to prolong life in patients with frequent PVCs and ejection fractions less than 30 percent

(page 832–837)

IV-20. Which of the following statements regarding the treatment of sustained ventricular tachycardia (VT) is true?

(A) intravenous amiodarone is third-line therapy (after lidocaine and procainamide) in the treatment of sustained VT

(B) invasive electrophysiological (EP) studies should be used to guide the choice of antiarrhythmic agents in the treatment of sustained VT

(C) invasive EP studies are most useful in predicting which patients are candidates for ICDs

(D) a recent trial showed that patients who had inducible VT on a baseline EP study and did not respond to antiarrhythmic therapy had no improvement in survival with an ICD

(E) surgical therapy is superior to an ICD for left ventricular aneurysms that are sources of sustained VT

(pages 843–845)

IV-21. Which of the following statements regarding the use of ICDs in the treatment of sustained VT is true?

(A) ICDs should not be implanted until at least three EP-guided antiarrhythmic agents have been unsuccessful

(B) ICDs suffer from lack of backup pacing for bradyarrhythmic episodes

(C) ICDs should rarely be used in patients with ejection fractions greater than 40 percent

(D) a recent study showed a favorable survival trend in patients undergoing coronary artery bypass graft (CABG) surgery who had abnormal signal-averaged ECGs but no history of VT

(E) a significant limitation in the use of ICDs is in the patient who has many runs of sustained VT

(page 845)

IV-22. Which of the following statements regarding the arrhythmogenic right ventricular dysplasia (ARVD) syndrome is true?

(A) there is no familial association with right ventricular dysplasia

(B) the surface ECG is not useful in the diagnosis of right ventricular dysplasia

(C) sustained VT from ARVD has a LBBB morphology

(D) amiodarone is effective therapy in most patients with ARVD

(E) patients with ARVD without a history of syncope are at minimal risk for sudden death

(pages 847–848)

IV-23. Which of the following statements regarding the congenital long QT syndromes is true?

(A) congenital long QT syndromes have been shown to be due to mutations on one of five different genes

(B) there is an abnormality of cardiac autonomic neural innervation

(C) the Romano-Ward syndrome has an autosomal recessive pattern of inheritance

(D) the Jervell and Lange-Nielsen syndrome is much more common than the Romano-Ward syndrome

(E) the preferred treatment is the use of an ICD

(pages 847–852)

IV-24. Which of the following statements regarding the congenital long QT syndromes is true?

(A) congenital long QT syndromes have been shown to be due to mutations on one of five different genes

(B) there is an abnormality of cardiac autonomic neural innervation

(C) the Romano-Ward syndrome has an autosomal recessive pattern of inheritance

(D) the Jervell and Lange-Nielsen syndrome is much more common than the Romano-Ward syndrome

(E) the preferred treatment is the use of an ICD

(pages 847–852)

IV-25. Which of the following statements regarding atrioventricular block is true?

(A) second-degree AV block type I usually demonstrates prolongation of the H-V interval on an EP study

(B) patients who develop high-grade AV block after an acute inferior MI require permanent pacing and have a high mortality

(C) asymptomatic patients with congenital third-degree AV block should have permanent pacing

(D) frequently there is a slight variation in the P-P interval in patients in sinus rhythm and third-degree block

(E) pacing is never indicated in patients with sinus bradycardia and first-degree AV block

(pages 857–859)

IV-26. Which of the following statements about ambulatory electrocardiography (AECG) is true?

(A) AECG has a high sensitivity but low specificity for predicting risk in post myocardial infarction (MI) patients

(B) a standard 24-h AECG (Holter monitor) is useful for detecting ischemic ST segment changes

(C) a "pre-event" recording device is appropriate for patients who have frank syncopal episodes

(D) a 30-day event monitor is useful for the determining heart rate variability

(E) a subcutaneous implantable recorder is appropriate for events which occur weekly

(pages 879–880)

IV-27. Which of the following statements regarding recent advances in EP mapping techniques is true?

(A) the main value of endocardial mapping is to determine the utility of various antiarrhythmic drugs

(B) the CARTO endocardial mapping system (manufactured by Cordis Webster) utilizes a magnetic field generator pad under the patient table coupled with an endocardial reference catheter to produce a color-coded 3D image of the direction of impulse propagation

(C) the EnSite 3000 endocardial mapping system (manufactured by Endocardial Solutions) uses a balloon with an array of 64 sensors on its surface coupled with an external high-frequency transmitter to produce a 3D image of the direction of impulse propagation

(D) the CARTO device is not applicable to the mapping of atrial flutter

(E) the EnSite 3000 is useful for mapping the site of left-sided accessory pathways

(pages 887–888)

IV-28. Which of the following statements regarding radiofrequency catheter ablation is true?

(A) ablation of unifocal atrial tachycardias, atrioventricular nodal reentry, and accessory pathways results in a cure from 70 to 80 percent of the time

(B) patients with VT associated with ischemic myocardial scarring are poor candidates for ablation

(C) ablation may be an important adjunct to ICD therapy for VT

(D) patients should be tried on at least two different medications prior to being considered for to ablation for any arrhythmia

(E) serious complications, including deep venous thrombosis, pulmonary embolism, infection at catheter sites, systemic infection, pneumothorax, and perforation of a cardiac chamber occur in up to 10 percent of patients undergoing ablation

(pages 895–896)

IV-29. Which of the following statements regarding amiodarone is true?

(A) the only current FDA indication for amiodarone is life-threatening ventricular arrhythmias

(B) the CHF STAT trial showed that amiodarone reduced all cause mortality when used prophylactically in patients with ejection fractions of less than 40 percent and at least 10 PVCs per hour

(C) the CAMIAT and EMIAT trials demonstrated a lower all cause mortality rate in post MI patients treated with amiodarone

(D) the AVID trial showed that patients resuscitated after sudden death or with sustained VT did equally well with amiodarone or an ICD

(E) a recent study reported intravenous amiodarone had no effect when used for the prevention of postoperative atrial fibrillation

(pages 912–913)

IV-30. Which of the following statements regarding ibutilide and dofetilide is true?

(A) ibutilide is a potent class III antiarrhythmic agent which has been shown to be effective in converting about 25 percent of patients from atrial fibrillation or flutter to sinus rhythm when given intravenously

(B) almost 10 percent of patients in controlled trials developed either torsades de pointes or sustained monomorphic VT, even after excluding patients with hypokalemia or QT_c intervals greater than 400 ms

(C) dofetilide is a very potent class III antiarrhythmic agent which has been shown to be equivalent to sotalol in converting patients to sinus rhythm from atrial fibrillation

(D) in the DIAMOND trial, dofetilide was shown to improve all cause mortality in patients with reduced ejection fractions and heart failure symptoms

(E) dofetilide therapy can be safely initiated in outpatients

(pages 915–917)

IV-31. Which of the following statements regarding radiofrequency catheter ablation is true?

(A) recent studies have shown that catheter ablation may be effective therapy for a subset of patients with atrial fibrillation initiated by abnormal automaticity of muscle cells located along the medial side of the inferior vena cava as it enters the right atrium

(B) few complications have been reported after catheter ablation in patients with inappropriate sinus tachycardia

(C) atrioventricular junctional ablation for control of refractory rapid ventricular response in patients with atrial fibrillation has a success rate of 85 percent

(D) successful ablation of accessory pathways has been shown to be more likely in left-sided rather than right-sided locations

(E) ablation for atrioventricular nodal re-entrant tachycardia has a 95 percent success rate and a risk of developing complete heart block in less than 0.5 percent of patients

(pages 927–929)

IV-32. Which of the following statements regarding external cardioversion is true?

(A) cardioversion may be particularly beneficial in patients with "giant" scarred atria or previous mitral valve replacement

(B) current-based defibrillation, rather than delivery of a predetermined amount of energy, has been advocated in the treatment of ventricular fibrillation

(C) optimal electrode size for adults appears to be from 15 to 22 cm

(D) chest impedance increases after each successive shock delivery

(E) a sternotomy increases impedance for at least one month following cardiothoracic surgery

(pages 934–938)

IV-33. Which of the following statements regarding external defibrillator waveforms is true?

(A) original defibrillators used direct current

(B) most modern direct-current defibrillators use an undamped capacitor discharge with a long time constant that is then truncated, so the waveform resembles a trapezoid

(C) a biphasic (alternating-current) defibrillator requires more energy to achieve successful cardioversion than a direct-current defibrillator

(D) an alternating-current defibrillator has been developed which automatically adjusts the duration of the waveform for transthoracic impedance

(E) direct-current defibrillators are lighter, cheaper, and easier to maintain

(pages 934–938)

IV-34. Which of the following statements regarding VT detection by an ICD is true?

(A) up to 50 percent of ICD discharges are inappropriate when rate is employed as the sole criterion for VT therapy

(B) algorithms which utilize onset criteria and sustained-rate criteria increase specificity of VT detection and result in fewer inappropriate shocks

(C) dual-chamber pacemaker-defibrillators have no VT detection advantages, but are useful as back-up atrioventricular sequential pacemakers for bradyarrhythmias

(D) the programmable options for VT detection also function in the VF detection zone

(E) the addition of morphology criteria to VT detection algorithms does not improve specificity

(pages 947)

IV-35. Which of the following statements regarding the benefits of an ICD is true?

(A) a meta analysis of the three large trials which compared ICDs to antiarrhythmic drug therapy (mostly amiodarone) in patients who had survived life-threatening ventricular arrhythmias demonstrated a decrease in mortality of 15 percent with an ICD versus conventional medical therapy

(B) the MADIT trial showed that patients with a prior MI, poor LV function [left ventricular ejection fraction (LVEF) of 35 percent], nonsustained VT, and nonsuppressible VT/VF on EP had no survival benefit with either an ICD or EP guided antiarrhythmic therapy versus no antiarrhythmic therapy

(C) the MUSTT trial showed that patients with known coronary artery disease (CAD), decreased left ventricular function (LVEF of 40 percent), nonsustained VT, and inducible VT/VF on EP had no difference in the risk of cardiac arrest or arrhythmic death with an ICD or EP-guided antiarrhythmic therapy compared to no anti-arrhythmic therapy

(D) the CABG-Patch trial showed that patients who were post CABG, had poor left ventricular function (LVEF < 36 percent), and a positive signal-averaged ECG showed no survival benefit with an ICD versus a control group with no ICD

(E) the CAT trial showed that patients who had dilated cardiomyopathies (LVEF < 30 percent) and no symptomatic ventricular arrhythmias had no survival benefit with an ICD versus a control group with no ICD

(pages 954–957)

IV-36. Which of the following statements regarding the indications for permanent pacemaker implantation is true?

(A) permanent pacing is indicated in all symptomatic patients with congenital third-degree block

(B) permanent pacing is not indicated in the treatment of the tachycardia-bradycardia syndrome

(C) studies have shown that patients with neurocardiogenic syncope do not benefit from permanent pacing

(D) recent studies have shown a substantial benefit from permanent DDD pacing in patients with hypertrophic cardiomyopathy and left ventricular outflow gradients

(E) DDD pacing dramatically improves the symptoms of heart failure in patients with severely decreased left ventricular function

(pages 967–968)

IV. RHYTHM AND CONDUCTION DISORDERS

ANSWERS

IV-1. **The answer is C.** *(Ch. 23)* The dominant pacemaker of the heart is in the sinus node, which fires at a rate of 60 to 100 beats per minute. The typical rate of atrial tissue, the atrioventricular (AV) node, and the His-Purkinje system is 40 to 60 beats per minute. Ventricular myocardial cells are capable of an intrinsic rhythm of approximately 20 to 40 beats per minute.

IV-2. **The answer is B.** *(Ch. 23)* Electrical stimulation of arrhythmias is frequently useful in identifying the underlying physiological mechanism. Stimulation of an arrhythmia by electrical pacing indicates that the arrhythmia is caused by either reentry or delayed afterdepolarization/triggered activity. Termination of an arrhythmia by overdrive pacing is indicative of reentry or delayed afterdepolarization/triggered activity. Entrainment is seen with reentry mechanisms and is not expected in other arrhythmias. An automatic rhythm is neither terminated nor induced by overdrive pacing.

IV-3. **The answer is C.** *(Ch. 24)* Exercise stress testing may be very useful in evaluation of arrhythmias, especially if the rhythm disturbances are exercise-related. Nuclear studies are not needed unless ischemia is the suspected inciting factor of the arrhythmia. Exercise testing is more useful for detecting ventricular arrhythmias. The test is useful in distinguishing autonomic from structural disease mechanisms, particularly for sinus or atrioventricular nodal dysfunction. Exercise testing may be very helpful in evaluating the rate-related proarrhythmic effects of antiarrhythmic agents such as flecainide. The test may be useful in obtaining general information about the refractory period of the accessory pathway in the Wolff-Parkinson-White syndrome.

IV-4. **The answer is C.** *(Ch. 24)* The rhythm strip and the ladder diagram beneath it demonstrate a premature atrial depolarization with aberrant intraventricular conduction. Correct identification of the premature beat as originating from the atria is essential. The P wave is "buried" in the preceding T wave, and the compensatory pause is less than complete. Even if the event is symptomatic, the best treatment is reassurance. If intervention is needed, a beta blocker should be tried first. Membrane-active agents such as class IA or III antiarrhythmic agents should be avoided.

IV-5. **The answer is D.** *(Ch. 27)* In first-degree atrioventricular (AV) block, AV conduction is prolonged (i.e., the PR interval is greater than 200 ms), but all impulses are conducted to the ventricle. Type I second-degree AV block is characterized by progressive AV block until a P wave fails to elicit a QRS complex. The cycle then recurs, producing group beating of the QRS complexes. In type II second-degree AV block, conduction usually proceeds from the sinus node to the ventricles; however, occasionally, P waves are not followed by QRS complexes. The block is infranodal (i.e., a manifestation of bilateral bundle branch block), permanent, and usually progresses to complete AV block. In complete third-degree AV block, there is a either a junctional escape mechanism with a rate of 40 to 60 beats per minute or a ventricular escape mechanism with a wide QRS with a rate less than 45 beats per minute. This ECG shows sinus rhythm with AV disassociation consistent with third-degree AV block. The escape rhythm rate is 58 beats per minute and the QRS complexes are narrow, indicating a junctional origin. Most cases of acquired third-degree AV block require permanent pacing, but this ECG is from a 23-year-old female with congenital third-degree block. See Answer IV-25 for further information on this situation.

IV-6.   **The answer is D.**   *(Ch. 24)*   The rhythm strip demonstrates multifocal atrial tachycardia. This arrhythmia is frequently encountered in patients with chronic lung disease, in patients with aminophylline or digoxin toxicity, and in patients with metabolic or electrolyte abnormalities. The ECG requirements are: at least three P wave morphologies, varying PR intervals, and a rate greater than 100. The mechanism of this rhythm is automatic. Treatment with beta or calcium channel blockers has been tried but is frequently unrewarding. The most effective treatment is correction of the underlying abnormality.

IV-7.   **The answer is C.**   *(Ch. 24)*   A PAC is characterized by an early P wave which has an abnormal axis. The location of the P wave can be ascertained by examining its axis in various leads. A P wave which is negative in II, III, and aVF suggests an origin in the lower part of the atrium. A P wave which is positive in I and negative in V_1 suggests a right atrial origin. A P wave which is negative in I and V_6 but is positive in V_1 suggests a left atrial origin. A P wave which is narrower than a nearby sinus P wave and is positive in aVR and aVL suggests a septal origin. Finally, a P wave which is negative in I and V_6 but is positive in the inferior leads suggests a right superior pulmonary vein origin. In recent years, repetitive PACs or atrial tachycardia have been identified as sources of paroxysmal atrial fibrillation and have responded to radiofrequency ablation.

IV-8.   **The answer is C.**   *(Ch. 24)*   The rhythm strip demonstrates a particular form of polymorphic ventricular tachycardia called *torsades de pointes* (twisting of the points). The ECG features include varying polarity of the QRS axis back and forth around the baseline. Additionally, the QT interval is prolonged. Although still debated, the current mechanism is thought to be triggered activity. Any pharmacological intervention or condition associated with prolongation of the QT interval may result in this abnormality. These include congenital prolongation of the QT interval seen in Romano-Ward or Jervell and Lange-Nielson syndromes or as a complication of increased intracranial pressure. Lown-Ganong-Levine syndrome is a form of accelerated atrioventricular conduction with a normal QRS configuration.

IV-9.   **The answer is B.**   *(Ch. 29)*   Atrial fibrillation will obviously not permit study of other forms of supraventricular tachycardia (SVT); however, in patients with the Wolff-Parkinson-White syndrome and SVT, if atrial fibrillation must be initiated for diagnostic purposes, it should be performed at the end of the study. This allows complete diagnostic EP testing of the bypass tracts and supraventricular arrhythmias first. Frequently, atrial fibrillation develops during the initial placement of the catheters; therefore, excessive manipulation of catheters in the atria should be avoided. The mechanical irritation from the catheters can cause a variety of arrhythmias and conduction disturbances. In patients with underlying LBBB, complete atrioventricular block can occur as the catheter disturbs the right ventricular septum. In general, EP testing has a low complication rate but complications such as deep venous thrombosis, pulmonary embolism, infection, pneumothorax, and perforation of cardiac chambers have been reported. Valvular damage has not been reported. Development of electromechanical dissociation in the laboratory should prompt a thorough search for pneumothorax or perforation of a cardiac chamber or coronary sinus.

IV-10.   **The answer is D.**   *(Ch. 30)*   The Cardiac Arrhythmia Suppression Trial (CAST) was designed to test the hypothesis that suppression of asymptomatic ventricular arrhythmias in patients with recent myocardial infarction would reduce mortality from cardiac arrest or arrhythmic sudden death. Encainide and flecainide were removed because of a two- to three-fold increase in mortality compared with placebo in CAST I. CAST II was terminated prematurely because moricizine was producing a similar trend with no chance for a beneficial effect. Because of poor results with sodium channel blocking drugs, a class III drug that prolongs the action potential (amiodarone) was studied and found to have somewhat favorable results. Amiodarone does not appear to decrease overall mortality, but there is a reduced incidence of ventricular fibrillation or arrhythmic death among survivors of myocardial infarction. The D isomer of sotalol (not the racemic mixture commonly prescribed), a drug which prolongs action potential but has less serious side effects than amiodarone, has unfortunately also been found to increase mortality after myocardial infarction. Quinidine has long been known to have substantial side effects and proarrhythmic effects and has not been included in any recent trials.

IV-11. **The answer is A.** *(Ch. 24)* Disopyramide, a 1A agent, has a substantial negative inotropic effect, making it useful therapy in some patients with hypertrophic obstructive cardiomyopathy. It is generally contraindicated in patients with systolic heart failure. Quinidine enhances atrioventricular nodal conduction and can be accelerate the ventricular rate in atrial fibrillation or flutter. Unfortunately, flecainide has been shown to have proarrhythmic effects in patients with underlying CAD, even when used to treat atrial fibrillation or flutter. Pulmonary toxicity is a serious complication of therapy with amiodarone, but it occurs in only about 2 percent of patients. Pulmonary toxicity can occur shortly after therapy, but usually occurs after months or years. The effect may be total-dose related and may also be more likely to occur in patients with underlying pulmonary disease. Pulmonary toxicity is usually reversible after stopping amiodarone, but about 10 percent of affected patients will die. Sotalol can cause sinus bradycardia and prolongation of the PR, QRS, and QT intervals.

IV-12. **The answer is B.** *(Ch. 24)* In the Wolff-Parkinson-White (WPW) syndrome, the PR interval is shortened because the delta wave occurs earlier than the QRS complex would normally begin. The distance from the P wave to the J point is normal. In the Lown-Ganong-Levine syndrome, the PR interval is actually short, and the P to J interval is also shorter than normal. In general, the following rules for localizing the AP on the surface ECG are accurate: (1) if the delta wave is positive in lead I and negative in V_1, the AP is probably right-sided; the vectors are generally opposite for left-sided tracts; (2) if the delta wave is positive in the inferior leads, the AP is probably anterior, and if it is negative in these leads, probably posterior; and (3) if the delta wave is negative in aVL, a left lateral AP is likely. The most common pattern recorded during PSVT using the AP is a narrow-complex rhythm with rates from 160 to 240 per minute.

IV-13. **The answer is E.** *(Ch. 24)* Ectopic atrial tachycardias rarely occur in normal individuals. The most common mechanism is automatic, although reentry and triggered activity have occasionally been implicated. Digoxin, with its property of enhancing automaticity, should be suspected as the most likely cause in any patient taking that medication, particularly if significant atrioventricular block is present on the ECG. Other causes include decompensated chronic lung disease, metabolic abnormalities, acute alcohol abuse, electrolyte disturbances, hypoxia, recent MI, and previous atrial surgery in patients with congenital heart disease. Treatment of the underlying cause is the primary therapy. Catheter ablation for persistent atrial tachycardia after the underlying cause has been eliminated has a success rate of up to 80 percent.

IV-14. **The answer is C.** *(Ch. 24)* Atrial flutter has been separated into two types: classic, or type I, and type II. The former utilizes an obligate reentrant circuit in a counterclockwise pathway up the interatrial septum, down the right atrial free wall, and along the crista terminalis. The other boundaries of the circuit include the tricuspid valve ring and an area of probable anatomic block extending from the venae cavae to the eustachian valve and ridge on the other side. Type I flutter type usually has a distinct slowing in the subeustachian isthmus The distinction between the two types is based on (1) the ability to entrain interrupt type I flutter with atrial pacing and (2) the faster rate in type II. Untreated type I has atrial rates between 280 and 320 per minute, with limits of 240 to 340. Type II has rates of 340 to 350 per minute and occasionally as fast as 450.

IV-15. **The answer is C.** *(Ch. 24)* Atrial flutter can be treated with medications, overdrive pacing, DC cardioversion, and radiofrequency ablation. Newer type III antiarrhythmic agents such as ibutelide are very effective in restoring sinus rhythm, but patients require observation during its initiation because of the small but significant risk of *torsades de pointes.* Overdrive pacing is usually effective in restoring sinus rhythm is patients with type I atrial flutter. Radiofrequency ablation across the subeustachian isthmus between the tricuspid annulus and the IVC has an 85 percent long-term success rate. Atrial flutter is very uncommon in normal patients. Recent retrospective studies have suggested that the risk of stroke in patients with atrial flutter may be as high as that in patients with atrial fibrillation. Warfarin anticoagulation is currently recommended for chronic atrial flutter.

IV-16.   **The answer is D.**   *(Ch. 24)*   The most common mechanism of atrial fibrillation by far is multiple reentrant atrial wavelet circuits. An important alternate mechanism in some patients is focal atrial tachycardia in the muscle fibers of the distal pulmonary veins in the left atrium or other right atrial locations. The latter mechanism may lend itself to catheter ablation. The presence of frequent PACs is associated with the likelihood of developing atrial fibrillation, and the morphology of repetitive PACs may be evidence of an atrial tachycardia focus. Regardless of the mechanism, the hemodynamic consequences of atrial fibrillation are due to a loss of atrial systole and shortening of the diastolic filling period. Mitral stenosis is no longer the most common cause of atrial fibrillation in industrialized countries. Hypertensive and ischemic cardiomyopathies are now responsible for the majority of atrial fibrillation.

IV-17.   **The answer is A.**   *(Ch. 24)*   The stroke risk of various strategies prior to elective DC cardioversion has not been studied as thoroughly as chronic anticoagulation, but it seems reasonable to use warfarin 3 to 6 weeks prior to elective cardioversion. A recent alternative has been to use transesophageal echocardiography to detect the presence of left atrial appendigeal thrombi and to proceed with cardioversion if none are present. The effectiveness of this technique in avoiding stroke is still subject to considerable debate, however. Atrial fibrillation in any setting except lone atrial fibrillation in otherwise healthy individuals requires anticoagulation. Traditional dose-adjusted warfarin therapy has been shown in prospective trials to be superior to fixed-dose warfarin plus aspirin. One such study reported the risk of serious hemorrhage to be as low as 1.5 percent per treatment year, similar to aspirin or placebo. The risk of hemorrhage clearly increases with INR, and is quite substantial with INRs over 5.0. The current recommendation is an INR between 2.0 and 3.0. There are obviously patients who are not candidates for anticoagulation (see Table 24-9 in *Hurst's The Heart,* 9th edition).

IV-18.   **The answer is D.**   *(Ch. 24)*   There is considerable controversy regarding the extent of effort to maintain sinus rhythm in patients with chronic atrial fibrillation. The obvious advantages of sinus rhythm include physiological rate control, better filling of the ventricles, decreased risk of stroke, less risk of hemorrhage by avoiding warfarin therapy, and, usually, improvement in symptoms. Disadvantages include exposure to the risks of antiarrhythmic drugs, increased bleeding risk, complications of various procedures and devices, and the enormous expense of the effort. Studies are ongoing to compare aggressive strategies to maintain sinus rhythm versus rate control and chronic anticoagulation. In spite of current medical therapy, some two-thirds of patients with advanced heart disease will revert to atrial fibrillation within a year after DC cardioversion. Surgical approaches, including the "corridor" procedure and the MAZE procedure, have a success rate of over 50 percent. They are most appropriate if cardiothoracic surgery is indicated for another reason. Several new class III antiarrhythmic agents are awaiting approval by the FDA as therapy for atrial fibrillation. The extent of their usefulness in clinical practice remains to be determined. Current models of implantable atrial defibrillators have had only limited applicability in clinical practice.

IV-19.   **The answer is D.**   *(Ch. 24)*   One of the greatest shifts in thinking among cardiologists in the past 15 years is the movement away from the concept that most patients with PVCs need anti-arrhythmic therapy. In spite of the well-demonstrated association between the density of PVCs and the risk of cardiac events, there are no data to support that suppression of PVCs proffers any survival advantage. The treatment in the setting of acute MI has also changed in that routine administration of lidocaine is no longer indicated. Large trials with amiodarone in post MI patients and in patients with chronic heart failure showed no benefit in survival. β-adrenergic blocking agents, however, have been shown to decrease the risk of sudden death post MI and should be part of the post MI treatment regimen unless contraindicated. Class IC agents were shown to increase mortality in the CAST trial. If patients require therapy for symptomatic PVCs, a class III agent, such as sotalol, should be considered. Studies are ongoing to determine the role of implantable defibrillators in patients with low ejection fractions and PVCs post MI.

IV-20.   The answer is C.   *(Ch. 24)*   A recent study showed that intravenous amiodarone was slightly superior to lidocaine in patients with sustained VT surviving to reach the hospital after a cardiac arrest. Reliance on invasive electrophysiology studies to guide the selection of an appropriate antiarrhythmic agent for the treatment of sustained VT has largely yielded to empiric therapy, ablative procedures, and ICDs. EP studies may still be useful for risk stratification and indicating which patients should have ICDs. ICDs have been shown to be superior to antiarrhythmic agents and surgical procedures in a variety of patients with serious underlying cardiac disease.

IV-21.   The answer is D.   *(Ch. 24)*   The technology of ICDs has improved dramatically in the last few years, and these devices frequently have antitachycardia pacing, backup atrioventricular sequential pacing for bradyarrhythmias, and ECG storage for retrieving and analyzing events. The practice of requiring multiple EP guided trials of anti-arrhythmic agents prior to using an ICD has been abandoned. Even patients with ejection fractions greater than 40 percent who have failed even one antiarrhythmic agent are considered candidates for an ICD. The CABG-Patch trial showed a favorable trend in the use of ICDs in patients undergoing CABG who have an abnormal signal-averaged ECG but no history of VT. ICDs with antitachycardia pacing may terminate many episodes of sustained VT without having to use a DC shock. Some patients, however, may still require concomitant antiarrhythmic therapy, usually with amiodarone.

IV-22.   The answer is C.   *(Ch. 24)*   ARVD may occur spontaneously but may have a familial association in 40 to 50 percent of patients. The surface ECG may reveal inverted T waves across the precordial leads and a curious notching in the early part of the ST segment in V_1 and V_2 (the so-called "epsilon" wave). VT from this lesion has a LBBB morphology because of its origin in the right ventricle. No antiarrhythmic agent has been shown to protect these patients entirely from sudden death, and most receive an ICD. Patients with a history of syncope do appear to be at greater risk for sudden death than those without, but the first evidence of ARVD may be a VF arrest.

IV-23.   The answer is A.   *(Ch. 24)*   The congenital long QT syndromes were previously thought to be due to abnormalities of autonomic cardiac innervation, but there is now conclusive evidence that these disorders represent mutations which can occur on at least five different chromosomes. The defects produce abnormalities in membrane ion-channel molecular function. The two most recognized forms are the Romano-Ward syndrome and the Jervell and Lange-Nielsen syndrome. The former has an autosomal dominant inheritance pattern, and the latter is autosomal recessive, associated with congenital deafness, and is much less common. Most patients respond to beta-blocker therapy and left sympathetic ganglion ablation, but some require ICDs for recurrent arrhythmias.

IV-25.   The answer is D.   *(Ch. 24)*   Abnormalities of atrioventricular (AV) conduction can usually be localized to the AV node or the His bundle. A His bundle electrogram, obtained during an EP study, can determine the location of the conduction defect. First-degree AV block and second degree AV block type I (AV Wenckebach) have prolongation of the atrial to His (A-H) interval and represents block at the level of the AV node. Second-degree AV block and third-degree (or complete) heart block usually involve failure of the His to ventricular (H-V) interval. A-H block is usually clinically benign and does not need treatment unless the patient has symptomatic bradycardia. Prolongation of the H-V interval to more than 100 msec is a serious situation and usually requires permanent pacing, even in asymptomatic patients. Significant AV block accompanies about 15 percent of inferior MIs and is due to AV nodal ischemia. The block is usually transient, requires temporary pacing only for symptomatic bradycardia, and does not increase the long-term need for permanent pacing. AV block accompanying an anterior MI signifies a very high mortality, since the mechanism of AV block is damage to both bundle branches in the septum. The size of an infarct required to damage both bundles is large and has a 40 to 60 percent in-hospital mortality. Congenital third-degree AV block occurs because of complete separation of the AV ring at the level of the AV node. Patients usually have an adequate junctional escape mechanism and do not require pacing, but pacing is indicated if the escape rhythm has chronotropic incompetence and limits the ability to exercise. The slight variation in the P-P interval in patients in sinus rhythm and third-degree block is called ventriculophasic sinus arrhythmia and is a common feature of AV dissociation. Pacing may be indicated in sinus bradycardia with or without AV block if the patient is symptomatic.

IV-26. **The answer is C.** *(Ch. 25)* A variety of AECG devices are available, and each is particularly appropriate for a specific circumstance. A 24-h AECG (Holter monitor) is useful for evaluating heart rate variability, QT dispersion, numbers of abnormal beats, and arrhythmias which occur on a daily basis. Specialized 24-h AECGs and scanning techniques are required for ST segment analysis to detect ischemia. Event monitors, usually worn for periods of 30 days or more, are useful for recording symptomatic arrhythmias which occur less frequently. "Post-event" monitors are patient-activated and record from the point of activation forward. The information can be stored by the device and transferred transtelephonically for analysis. Patients who have frank syncope require a "pre-event" monitor which loops continuously and can be activated after the patient regains consciousness. A subcutaneous pre-event monitor, which also requires patient activation, is available for symptoms which occur with even less frequency than 30 days. It has the advantage of not requiring the patient to apply electrodes and deal with leads and a recording device.

IV-27. **The answer is B.** *(Ch. 26)* Substantial progress has occurred recently in the techniques for mapping the origin and direction of flow of electrical activity in the cardiac chambers. This information is extremely useful in elucidating the nature of arrhythmias, assessing the feasibility of radiofrequency ablation, and guiding ablation therapy. Two manufacturers have recently developed products which use different approaches to endocardial mapping. The CARTO system (by Cordis Webster) utilizes a magnetic field generator pad under the patient table coupled with an endocardial reference catheter to produce a color-coded 3D image of the direction of impulse propagation. The EnSite 3000 system (by Endocardial Solutions) uses an intracardiac balloon with an array of 64 sensors on its surface coupled with an internal roving catheter to collect geometric information. Both systems obviously utilize sophisticated computer software to aid in the acquisition, analysis, and 3D reconstruction of data and images. Both devices are useful in a wide variety of reentrant and automatic arrhythmias, including atrial flutter. The EnSite 3000 system is currently only approved for use in the right atrium, but this restriction is likely to be removed as more experience and safety information is acquired.

IV-28. **The answer is C.** *(Ch. 26)* Radiofrequency catheter ablation has become increasingly useful in the treatment of supraventricular and ventricular arrhythmias. Ablation of unifocal atrial tachycardias, atrioventricular nodal reentry, and accessory pathways results in a cure 90 percent of the time. Because of the success of the aforementioned mapping techniques, ablation has been applicable to more cases of VT. Ablation may be an important adjunct to ICD therapy by decreasing the frequency of sustained ventricular arrhythmias which require use of the defibrillator. Ablation is the treatment of choice for several arrhythmias, particularly those using an accessory pathway. Serious complications are less likely to occur with right heart ablation procedures, and the mortality is negligible. Left heart procedures are slightly riskier.

IV-29.   The answer is A.   *(Ch. 27)*   Amiodarone currently is only indicated by the FDA for life-threatening ventricular arrhythmias because of (1) the documented potentially lethal complications of chronic therapy; (2) the complications associated with its variable onset of action; and (3) its multiple dangerous drug interactions. CHF STAT showed that amiodarone offered no long-term survival benefit in heart failure patients with frequent PVCs. CAMIAT and EMIAT trials demonstrated similar all cause mortality rates in post MI patients treated with amiodarone, although CAMIAT showed a decrease in VF and arrhythmic death in amiodarone patients. The AVID trial showed ICDs to be superior to amiodarone in reducing mortality rates in high-risk patients. Although not yet approved for this use, a recent study showed that intravenous amiodarone decreased the risk of postoperative atrial fibrillation. It is encouraging to note that none of the long-term trials showed an increase in mortality in the amiodarone groups, as had been the case with several drugs in the CAST trial.

IV-30.   The answer is B.   *(Ch. 27)*   Ibutilide is approved only in the intravenous form for the rapid conversion of atrial fibrillation and flutter to sinus rhythm. In one study, 44 percent of patients with atrial fibrillation converted to sinus rhythm after one or two doses of ibutilide compared to 2 percent for placebo. The response time ranged from 5 to 88 min after infusion. Other studies showed that rates of conversion were similar between atrial fibrillation and flutter. Almost 10 percent of patients in controlled trials developed either *torsades de pointes* or sustained monomorphic VT, even after excluding patients with hypokalemia or QT_c intervals greater than 400 m. In one study, 30 percent of patients given oral dofetilide converted to sinus rhythm versus 6 percent given sotalol and 1 percent given placebo. In the DIAMOND trial, there was a lower incidence of atrial fibrillation and admission for heart failure in patients with reduced ejection fractions, but no difference in mortality. In spite of excluding patients with hypokalemia or a prolonged QT_c interval, the incidence of *torsades de pointes* was 3.3 percent. The manufacturer is requiring practitioners to have additional training prior to using dofetilide, and all therapy must be initiated on an inpatient basis.

IV-31.   The answer is E.   *(Ch. 28)*   Recent sophisticated mapping studies have shown there is a subset of patients with atrial fibrillation initiated by abnormal automaticity of muscle cells in one of the pulmonary veins, and that ablation of these sites is highly effective in eliminating recurrence of the arrhythmia. The procedure requires transseptal catheterization, however, and there are no long-term studies on effectiveness or the incidence of complications like pulmonary venous stenosis. There have been small numbers of patients with persistent sinus tachycardia who have responded to ablation of the fastest focus in the sinoatrial nodal area. However, cases of narrowing of the superior vena cava-right atrium junction have been reported, and more experience is needed before the use of this procedure can be recommended. Atrioventricular junctional ablation for control of refractory rapid ventricular response in patients with atrial fibrillation has a success rate of 98 percent. Ablation of APs is successful (according to data from the NASPE registry) in 96 percent of right free wall pathways, 94 percent of left free wall pathways, and 84 percent of septal pathways. Ablation for atrioventricular nodal reentrant tachycardia has been very rewarding with a 95 percent success rate and a risk of developing complete heart block of less than 0.5 percent of patients.

IV-32.   The answer is B.   *(Ch. 29a and 29b)*   Patients with "giant" scarred atria, previous mitral valve replacement, or recurrent paroxysmal atrial fibrillation may not benefit from cardioversion. Since the amount of current delivered to the heart varies considerably with changes in chest impedance, some have advocated using current-based defibrillation rather than a predetermined amount of energy (e.g., 360 J) in the treatment of ventricular fibrillation. Optimal electrode size for adults appears to be from 8 to 12 cm. Chest impedance decreases after each successive shock delivery and is also decreased for at least a month following sternotomy.

IV-33.   **The answer is D.**   *(Ch. 29b)*   The original defibrillators used alternating current but have since been replaced by direct current models which deliver a monophasic damped sinusoidal waveform. Recently, biphasic alternating current defibrillators have been developed which are lighter, cheaper, and easier to maintain. In several studies they appear to require less energy for cardioversion than direct current models. An alternating current defibrillator has been developed which automatically adjusts the duration of the waveform for transthoracic impedance, but it has not been studied sufficiently to determine if it has any clinical advantages.

IV-34.   **The answer is B.**   *(Ch. 30)*   Up to 50 percent of ICD discharges are inappropriate when rate is employed as the sole criterion for VT therapy. Specificity for detecting VT is increased by the use of onset criteria (VT is usually paroxysmal), sustained rate criteria (all the VT beats are greater than a certain rate), and morphology criteria (VT has wider and more bizarre QRS complexes). The increased specificity, however, comes at the cost of decreasing sensitivity of detection, so most of these devices are used with a sustained-rate criterion programmed "on." Dual chamber pacemakers do offer a theoretical advantage in the specificity of VT detection, since they can detect atrioventricular dissociation and V to A conduction. One study, however, failed to demonstrate a decrease in inappropriate therapies for atrial fibrillation over single-chamber devices.

IV-35.   **The answer is D.**   *(Ch. 30)*   There is a substantial amount of information available recently which sheds light on the subsets of patients who are likely to benefit from an ICD. A meta-analysis of the three large trials (AVID, CIDS, and CASH) which compared ICDs to antiarrhythmic drug therapy (mostly amiodarone) in patients who had survived life-threatening ventricular arrhythmias demonstrated a decrease in mortality of 27 percent with an ICD versus conventional medical therapy. It is now accepted practice that these patients should have an implantable device unless there are good reasons not to. In patients who are at high risk for increased arrhythmic death but have not had a life-threatening episode, the data is less clear: The MADIT trial showed that patients with a prior MI, poor left ventricular function (LVEF ≤ 35 percent), nonsustained VT, and nonsuppressible VT/VF on EP had a 16 percent 6-year mortality compared to 39 percent in the group with no antiarrhythmic therapy. The MUSTT trial showed that patients with known CAD, decreased left ventricular function (LVEF ≤ 40 percent), nonsustained VT, and inducible VT/VF on EP had a 25 percent 6-year risk of cardiac arrest or arrhythmic death with an ICD or EP-guided antiarrhythmic therapy compared to a 32 percent risk with no antiarrhythmic therapy. The CABG-Patch trial showed that patients who were post CABG, had poor left ventricular function (LVEF ≤ 36 percent), and a positive signal-averaged ECG showed no survival benefit with an ICD versus a control group with no ICD. The ongoing CAT trial showed that patients who had dilated cardiomyopathies (LVEF ≤ 30 percent) and no symptomatic ventricular arrhythmias had no survival benefit at a 6-year interim analysis with an ICD versus a control group with no ICD. All of the studies demonstrated the substantial mortality associated with heart failure in spite of any form of antiarrhythmic therapy, in the range of 5 to 15 percent annually in mild heart failure and 20 to 50 percent in patients with severe heart failure. The results of the negative trials (CABG-Patch and CAT) emphasize the fact that ICDs prolong survival in a population of patients only if that population has a sufficiently high incidence of life-threatening ventricular arrhythmias and a sufficiently low incidence of death from all other causes. For the current ACC/AHA guidelines for ICD implantation, see the ACC website at http://www.acc.org/ or the National Guideline Clearinghouse at http://www.guideline.gov/.

IV-36.   **The answer is A.**   *(Ch. 31)*   A permanent pacemaker is indicated in any patient with symptomatic bradycardia which is not due to a correctible cause (e.g. medications, electrolyte abnormalities, hypoxia, ischemia, etc.). There is an increased mortality in patients who have congenital third-degree block, particularly if they have resting bradycardia, prolonged QT interval, cardiomegaly, atrial enlargement, decreased left ventricular function, periods of junctional exit block, or mitral regurgitation. Permanent pacemaker implantation is indicated if patients have symptomatic bradycardia when a supraventricular tachycardia terminates suddenly. Some patients with neurocardiogenic syncope do benefit symptomatically from a permanent pacemaker, particularly if bradycardia is a prominent part of their presentation. There are conflicting reports concerning the utility of permanent DDD pacing in patients with hypertrophic cardiomyopathy and left ventricular outflow gradients. Hemodynamic benefits should be demonstrated in the laboratory with temporary transvenous DDD pacing a permanent device is implanted. Subsequent studies have not shown a discernable benefit from DDD pacing in patients with severe heart failure.

PART V
SYNCOPE, SUDDEN DEATH, AND CARDIOPULMONARY RESUSCITATION

V. SYNCOPE, SUDDEN DEATH, AND CARDIOPULMONARY RESUSCITATION

QUESTIONS

DIRECTIONS: Each question listed below contains five suggested responses.
Select the **one best** response to each question.

V-1. A 30-year-old female in her third trimester of pregnancy has a witnessed syncopal episode while lying supine on a couch. Physical examination reveals a systolic flow murmur and third heart sound. What is the most likely diagnosis?

  (A) peripartum cardiomyopathy
  (B) postprandial syncope
  (C) neurocardiogenic syncope
  (D) hyperventilation syndrome
  (E) mitral valve prolapse

(page 2280)

V-2. Which of the following situations may bring on a neurocardiogenic syncopal episode?

  (A) increased sodium intake
  (B) exertion in a cool environment
  (C) prolonged time in a supine position
  (D) being in an upright position for an extended period of time during pregnancy
  (E) a stressful or emotional situation

(page 996)

V-3. Which of the following statements regarding orthostatic hypotension is true?

  (A) it is most common in short, overweight individuals
  (B) slowly rising from a recumbent position may prevent orthostatic hypotension in some individuals
  (C) venous pooling occurs in individuals taking fludrocortisone acetate to augment salt retention
  (D) a large decrease in heart rate is associated with the idiopathic form of orthostatic hypotension
  (E) orthostatic hypotension lasts for several seconds and then returns to normal

(pages 998–999)

V-4. A 70-year-old man with a history of coronary artery disease has a witnessed syncopal episode while playing table tennis. Physical examination reveals a right supraclavicular bruit and a diminished right brachial pulse. What is the most likely diagnosis?

  (A) sick sinus syndrome
  (B) vertebrobasilar insufficiency
  (C) carotid sinus syndrome
  (D) subclavian steal syndrome
  (E) idiopathic subaortic stenosis

(page 1000)

V-5. A 20-year-old female presents with syncope following exertion. Physical examination reveals no murmurs. What is the most likely diagnosis?

  (A) aortic stenosis
  (B) cardiac tamponade
  (C) hypertrophic cardiomyopathy
  (D) mitral stenosis
  (E) primary pulmonary hypertension

(page 1003)

V-6. Which of the following statements regarding the epidemiology of sudden cardiac death (SCD) is true?

  (A) the incidence of SCD is higher in whites than in blacks
  (B) there is no defined set of risk factors for SCD
  (C) the incidence of SCD without evidence of coronary heart disease is higher in men than women
  (D) the majority of SCD in the pediatric population occur in those with surgically treated congenital cardiac abnormalities
  (E) there is a higher incidence of SCDs following myocardial infarctions in highly educated men

(pages 1016–1019)

V-7. Which of the following is the strongest independent predictor of sudden cardiac death?

- (A) left ventricular hypertrophy
- (B) frequent ventricular extrasystoles and nonsustained ventricular tachycardia
- (C) left ventricular dysfunction
- (D) heart rate variability
- (E) ventricular couplets

(pages 1018–1019)

V-8. Of the various congenital coronary anomalies, which of the following is most frequently identified in patients with sudden cardiac death?

- (A) origin of the left main artery from the right coronary sinus
- (B) single coronary artery
- (C) origin of the left circumflex from the right coronary artery
- (D) coronary artery fistula
- (E) coronary artery from the pulmonary artery

(page 1024)

V-9. Which of the following is associated with the worst prognosis for sudden death in patients with hypertrophic cardiomyopathies?

- (A) increased left ventricular wall thickness
- (B) onset of spontaneous, sustained monomorphic ventricular tachycardia in childhood
- (C) outflow tract obstruction
- (D) asymptomatic nonsustained ventricular tachycardia
- (E) mutations of β-myosin heavy chain

(page 1025)

V-10. In patients with idiopathic dilated cardiomyopathy, the best clinical predictor of sudden cardiac death is which of the following?

- (A) left ventricular ejection fraction less than 25 percent
- (B) nonsustained ventricular tachycardia
- (C) late potentials on signal average electrocardiogram
- (D) interventricular conduction defect on electrocardiogram
- (E) syncope

(page 1025)

V-11. Which of the following statements regarding electrical abnormalities in the heart and sudden cardiac death is true?

- (A) arrhythmic events in patients with long-QT syndrome 1 are often triggered by auditory stimuli
- (B) the risk of sudden death in Wolff-Parkinson-White syndrome is high and often occurs in otherwise healthy individuals

- (C) patients with idiopathic polymorphic ventricular tachycardia have a good prognosis
- (D) younger patients who have survived SCD have a higher incidence of idiopathic ventricular fibrillation
- (E) most cases of idiopathic ventricular tachycardias originate from the left ventricular outflow tract

(page 1028)

V-12. Which of the following statements regarding patients who have had an out-of-hospital cardiac arrest is true?

- (A) the most important determinant of successful resuscitation is the mechanism that caused the cardiac arrest
- (B) bystander performed cardiopulmonary resuscitation (CPR) is not associated with an increase in survival rate following cardiac arrest
- (C) patients who required four or more shocks for defibrillation have a higher risk of in-hospital mortality
- (D) when CPR is performed early following the cardiac arrest, there is a greater chance of the patient being admitted with bradycardia
- (E) patients admitted with bradycardia as the presenting rhythm have a good prognosis for being discharged alive

(pages 1030–1031)

V-13. Which of the following patients has the lowest risk for sudden cardiac death following a myocardial infarction (MI)?

- (A) a 48-year-old man who suffered cardiac arrest at the first documented episode of arrhythmia
- (B) a 58-year-old man who has ventricular fibrillation 2 weeks following the MI
- (C) a 50-year-old woman with class III heart failure
- (D) a 63-year-old woman who has ventricular tachycardia 3 months following an MI
- (E) a 56-year-old man with a history of previous MIs

(page 1032)

V-14. Which of the following pharmacologic agents demonstrate a proarrhythmic effect and a low incidence of sudden cardiac death, but a high recurrence rate of ventricular arrhythmias?

- (A) angiotensin-converting enzyme (ACE) inhibitors
- (B) metoprolol
- (C) diltiazem
- (D) class I antiarrhythmic drugs
- (E) amiodarone

(pages 1034–1035)

V-15. Which of the following statements regarding the mechanisms of blood flow during CPR is true?

(A) during chest compression (the systolic phase of CPR), the heart acts as a pump that directly increases blood flow to the brain

(B) intrathoracic pressure increases during chest compression as a direct result of the compression of lung tissue

(C) transesophageal electrocardiography in humans during CPR shows that the mitral valve closes during chest compressions, thereby directing forward blood flow through the aortic valve

(D) greater sternal force during CPR augments myocardial and cerebral perfusion

(E) the recommended rate for chest compression in adults is 60 beats per minute

(page 1050)

V-16. Which of the following statements regarding alternative techniques of cardiopulmonary resuscitation is true?

(A) interposed abdominal compression (IAC) is beneficial because it can be performed by one bystander, using no special equipment

(B) active compression-decompression CPR (ACD CPR) slightly improves vascular pressures and air exchange

(C) "high-impulse" CPR requires a special suction-cup plunger-type device

(D) aortic infusion of fluids in humans has been shown to improve both coronary flow and survival

(E) perithoracic high-pressure vest inflation is a widely used technique to increase vascular pressure

(page 1051)

V-17. Which of the following statements regarding ventilation and chest compression during CPR is true?

(A) clearing the airway is the most important step in CPR

(B) ventilation with the bag-valve mask technique is superior to simple mouth-to-mouth or mouth-to-nose ventilation

(C) an esophageal obturator airway is a safe and effective alternative to endotracheal intubation

(D) endotracheal intubation has been shown to be much more effective than the bag-valve mask technique

(E) the purpose of a barrier device is to provide constant pressure during ventilation

(page 1054)

V-18. Which of the following statements regarding ventricular tachycardia (VT) and ventricular fibrillation (VF) is true?

(A) high-energy defibrillation (≥ 400 J) results in a higher successful resuscitation rate

(B) there is no data supporting the use of lidocaine in patients with refractory (VF/VT)

(C) attempts at defibrillation are often more successful if the ECG shows fine ventricular fibrillation waves

(D) early epinephrine use makes the heart less responsive to defibrillation

(E) patients given intravenous amiodarone in shock-refractory VF/VT have a higher survival to hospital discharge

(page 1055)

V. SYNCOPE, SUDDEN DEATH, AND CARDIOPULMONARY RESUSCITATION

ANSWERS

V-1. **The answer is C.** *(Ch. 32)* Neurocardiogenic syncope of an unusual type may be seen in pregnancy. The syncope may, in part, may be related to inferior vena caval compression by the gravid uterus when the patient is supine and is usually relieved by moving to the lateral decubitus position. Peripartum cardiomyopathy is a very uncommon disorder of unknown etiology. It would most likely present with symptoms of heart failure, although syncope from ventricular arrhythmias is possible. The physical examination findings are related to the normal physiology of pregnancy. Syncope from cardiac arrhythmias in patients with mitral valve prolapse is rare.

V-2. **The answer is E.** *(Ch. 32)* Exertion in a warm environment, prolonged upright posture, sodium restriction, and stressful situations are important triggers for a neurocardiogenic syncopal episode. In pregnancy, the postural relationships are reversed, in that syncope is more likely to occur in the supine position than with upright posture.

V-3. **The answer is B.** *(Ch. 32)* Orthostatic hypotension is most common in tall, asthenic individuals with poorly developed musculature. Some patients may prevent orthostatic hypotension by rising slowly from a recumbent position. Venous pooling occurs in many situations, some of which are dehydration, prolonged bed rest, and blood loss. Patients with the idiopathic form of orthostatic hypotension also have a relatively fixed heart rate, anhidrosis, nocturnal polyuria, urinary and anal sphincter dysfunction, and impotency. The hypotension is progressive over a period of seconds to minutes, depending on the degree of loss of adaptation in that patient.

V-4. **The answer is D.** *(Ch. 32)* Syncope in the subclavian steal syndrome is caused by significant arterial stenosis proximal to the origin of the vertebral artery. Upper extremity activity initiates retrograde shunting of blood flow from the circle of Willis to the distal subclavian. The exam findings in this patient are typical of this entity. Carotid sinus hypersensitivity is more often associated with brisk rotation of the neck, whereas syncope related to vertebrobasilar insufficiency is nearly always preceded by vertigo, diplopia, and ataxia. Sick sinus syndrome is the most common manifestation of sinoatrial disease and is related mostly to increasing age. Episodes of paroxysmal atrial fibrillation or flutter, common in the elderly with hypertension and/or coronary artery disease, overdrive the sinus node. When these arrhythmias terminate abruptly, the sinus node may not depolarize or may not capture the atrium [sinoatrial (SA) exit block] within in the normal 1000 ms [sinus node recovery time (SNRT)], and syncope may ensue.

V-5. **The answer is E.** *(Ch. 32)* All patients with a history of syncope should have a careful history and physical examination. The history should emphasize the description of the event (to determine a cardiac or neurologic source) and the presence of symptoms which might indicate the presence of structural heart disease. The examination should include postural blood pressure and heart rate measurements and should concentrate on signs of structural heart disease. A resting ECG and basic laboratory tests are indicated. Echocardiography should be performed if there is any suggestion of structural heart disease. Exercise testing may be indicated in some patients, to assess for inducible arrhythmias or ischemia. Prolonged ambulatory ECG monitoring and/or tilt table testing may be necessary. A young female patient who presents with syncope during or shortly following exertion and has no cardiac murmurs should be considered to have primary pulmonary hypertension until proven otherwise. Physical examination would almost certainly have revealed some of the many findings of pulmonary hypertension.

V-6.   The answer is B.   *(Ch. 33)*   The incidence of sudden cardiac death is higher in blacks than in whites. Sudden cardiac death (SCD) without evidence of coronary heart disease is more likely in women than in men. About 40 percent of cardiac deaths in the pediatric population occur in patients who have been surgically treated for congenital cardiac abnormalities. The majority of SCDs are the first manifestation of underlying cardiac disease. The incidence of SCD following myocardial infarctions is higher in men with lower levels of education than in men with higher levels and the same arrhythmias. There is not, as of yet, a defined set of risk factors for SCD, excepting, of course, a previous episode of SCD.

V-7.   The answer is C.   *(Ch. 33)*   The exact mechanisms by which left ventricular dysfunction precipitates SCD are not completely understood but involve mechano-electric feedback and, usually, the precipitation of sustained ventricular tachycardia or ventricular fibrillation. Increases in left ventricular preload and contractility shorten the action potential duration, probably mediated by intracellular calcium fluxes. Left ventricular systolic function (commonly represented by the ejection fraction) is one of the most powerful predictors of prognosis in any cardiac condition.

V-8.   The answer is A.   *(Ch. 33)*   Origin of the left main artery from the right coronary sinus and origin of the right coronary artery from the left coronary sinus are the most common anomalies associated with SCD. The deaths are often exercise-induced and occur in patients from 25 to 45 years of age. The etiology of sudden death is presumably ventricular arrhythmias caused by myocardial ischemia. The latter arises when the aorta and pulmonary artery enlarge during exercise and compress the anomalous coronary artery running between them. Anomalous coronaries which course behind the aorta are very unlikely to be associated with SCD. Another explanation of the induction of ischemia is the acute angle of take-off of the coronary artery from the aorta and the associated slit-like origin of the artery.

V-9.   The answer is B.   *(Ch. 33)*   A clinical history of spontaneous, sustained monomorphic VT, sudden death in family members, or onset of symptoms in childhood indicates the worst prognosis. Left ventricular wall thickness and outflow tract obstruction are not useful in identifying patients at high risk for SCD. The predictive value of asymptomatic nonsustained ventricular tachycardia is limited. Mutation in β-myosin heavy chain is not a good predictor of SCD either, as some mutations can be benign. As seen in most genetic disorders, phenotypic expression of a genetic abnormality varies from person to person. The majority of autopsies in young persons who have SCD during exercise are normal, but hypertrophic cardiomyopathy is the commonest cardiac abnormality encountered.

V-10.   The answer is E.   *(Ch. 33)*   Advanced congestive heart failure increases total mortality but does not predict SCD. The predictive values of nonsustained ventricular arrhythmias and intraventricular conduction defects are poor, due to their low specificity. An abnormal signal averaged electrocardiogram is useful but is found in only a minority of patients. Although the etiology may include severe orthostasis or arrhythmias, syncope in the setting of idiopathic dilated cardiomyopathy is the best clinical predictor of sudden cardiac death.

V-11.   The answer is D.   *(Ch. 33)*   Exercise-related events are the most common in patients with long-QT syndrome 1. Patients with long-QT syndrome 2 suffer from arrhythmias in response to auditory stimuli. The risk of sudden death in patients with Wolff-Parkinson-White syndrome is low. However, it is important to consider because sudden death can occur with this condition in otherwise healthy patients. Patients with idiopathic polymorphic ventricular tachycardias have a high incidence of SCD. The majority of idiopathic ventricular tachycardias originate from the right ventricular outflow tract. Younger patients who have had SCD and female survivors of SCDs unrelated to MI have a higher incidence of idiopathic ventricular fibrillation.

V-12.   **The answer is C.**   *(Ch. 33)*   The time between cardiovascular collapse and initial intervention is the most important determinant of successful resuscitation. Bystander CPR has been associated with a greater than twofold odds ratio of survival. The risk for in-hospital mortality increases following an out-of-hospital arrest in patients 60 or older, cardiogenic shock after defibrillation, requirement of four or more shocks for defibrillation, absence of an acute MI, and coma on admission to the hospital. The earlier CPR is performed, the greater the likelihood that the patient will be in ventricular fibrillation. Patients who are admitted with bradycardias or electromechanical dissociation as the presenting rhythm have a poor prognosis for being discharged alive.

V-13.   **The answer is D.**   *(Ch. 33)*   There are four variables that indicate a worse prognosis for sudden cardiac death following an MI. These variables are: (1) cardiac arrest at the first documented episode of arrhythmia; (2) NYHA class III or class IV heart failure; (3) ventricular fibrillation or ventricular tachycardia occurring 3 days to 2 months following the MI; and (4) a history of previous MIs. A patient who has ventricular fibrillation or ventricular tachycardia more than 2 months following an MI has a very low incidence of sudden cardiac death at 26 months.

V-14.   **The answer is E.**   *(Ch. 33)*   Amiodarone has been shown to reduce SCD in selected patients, although there is a relatively high recurrence rate of arrhythmias. One large trial (CHF STAT), however, showed no difference in 5-year mortality in patients with heart failure who received amiodarone or placebo. The effect of ACE inhibitors on SCD has not been clarified. Metoprolol and other β-adrenergic antagonists have been shown to decrease sudden cardiac death. Calcium channel antagonists have not been shown to have an effect on SCD. Certain class I antiarrhythmic drugs have been shown to increase the risk of SCD.

V-15.   **The answer is D.**   *(Ch. 34)*   The exact hemodynamic mechanisms that move blood out of the thorax to the vital organs during CPR are not entirely clear, but some facts are known. The relationship between aortic pressure, jugular venous pressure, and intrathoracic pressure is complex. In order for cerebral blood flow to occur during CPR, the carotid pressure must be greater than the venous pressure in the jugular veins. During the systolic phase of chest compression, the same pressure is transmitted to the carotid arteries and the greater veins. However, at the thoracic outlet, the veins collapse, preventing complete transmission of this pressure to the jugular veins and creating a pressure differential that promotes cerebral blood flow. Therefore, the heart itself acts as a passive conduit, not an active pump during CPR. Transesophageal echocardiography during CPR has shown that the mitral valve both closes and stays open with chest compression. Thus, mitral valve closure, in itself, cannot be used to identify a primary mechanism of blood flow during CPR. Despite the uncertainties of the mechanism of blood flow during CPR, it is clear that more vigorous chest compression results in increased myocardial and cerebral perfusion. The current recommendations of the American Heart Association for CPR in adults is a compression rate of 80 to 100 beats per minute. These higher compression rates (i.e., 80 to 100 instead of 60 beats per minute) result in an overall chest compression duration of 50 percent of the cycle or more. The rise in thoracic pressure that occurs during chest compression is probably the result of small airway collapse with resultant air trapping. The air trapping in the small airways occupies volume in the lung that forces blood through the lungs during chest compression. This increase in thoracic pressure during chest compression is an important part of the CPR pumping mechanism. Thus, pulmonary blood flow occurs via an indirect mechanism during chest compression. A similar mechanism operates during coughing. Indeed patients who can initiate repetitive coughs during an episode of ventricular tachycardia can maintain a blood pressure as long as they can sustain the coughing efforts.

V-16. **The answer is B.** *(Ch. 34)*   Three health care providers are necessary to perform interposed abdominal compression CPR, although no special equipment is required. Active compression-decompression CPR slightly improves vascular pressures and air exchange. A special suction-cup-plunger type device is necessary for this procedure. High-impulse CPR, which needs no special equipment, refers to the increased sternal pressure and increased frequency of compressions currently recommended by the American Heart Association. Aortic infusion of fluid in animals has been shown to increase both coronary flow and survival, but studies in humans are limited. Perithoracic high-pressure vest inflation may be of value, but currently there is limited data.

V-17. **The answer is A.** *(Ch. 34)*   Clearing the airway of the patient is the most important step in CPR. It requires considerable training and practice to obtain adequate ventilation using the bag-valve mask technique, but is certainly preferable from an infectious disease standpoint than direct contact with the patient's oral-nasal area. Esophageal obturator airways have been associated with life-threatening complications. Safe and effective alternatives to endotracheal intubation are the Combitube and the laryngeal tracheal mask airway. The value of endotracheal intubation over an appropriately performed bag-valve mask technique has not been demonstrated, perhaps due to the delay that occurs during patient intubation. The use of a barrier device is to prevent the spread of infectious disease.

V-18. **The answer is B.** *(Ch. 34)*   High-energy defibrillation likely causes more cardiac injury and increases postshock myocardial dysfunction, and there is no clear evidence that it results in an increased rate of successful resuscitations. Although lidocaine is often given to patients with shock refractory VF/VT, there are no data that support its use. When the ECG shows fine fibrillation waves, attempts at defibrillation are often unsuccessful. The early administration of epinephrine makes the heart more responsive to defibrillation. Its use, however, is not supported by improved survival in clinical trials in patients who have fine fibrillation waves. Patients who are given intravenous amiodarone in shock-refractory VF/VT have an improved survival on the way to and in the early phase of hospitalization, but not an increased survival to discharge.

PART VI
CORONARY HEART DISEASE

VI. CORONARY HEART DISEASE

QUESTIONS

DIRECTIONS: Each question listed below contains five suggested responses. Select the **one best** response to each question.

VI-1. Which of the following statements regarding the study of atherogenesis in susceptible mice is true?

(A) deoxy low-density lipoprotein (LDL) present in the subendothelial space is responsible for making the vessel more atherogenic
(B) the recruitment of B cells into the arterial intima is one of the earliest detectable signs of atherogenesis
(C) low shear stress has an atheroprotective effect
(D) minimally oxidized LDL is a prime candidate for the upregulation of monocyte chemoattractant protein 1 (MCP-1) in the vessel wall
(E) MCP-1 is a potent attractor of granulocytes and B cells

(pages 1066–1067)

VI-2. Which of the following statements regarding human atherosclerosis is true?

(A) evidence has suggested that flow patterns determine the degree of adaptive intimal thickening
(B) the presence of fatty streaks in the aorta is a sign of atherosclerosis
(C) risk of plaque disruption depends on the plaque size
(D) the atheromatous core of a plaque is collagen rich
(E) proteins like albumin can be found in atherosclerotic plaques

(pages 1071–1072)

VI-3. Which of the following atherosclerosis-related features is true?

(A) coronary angiography is an excellent technique for determining the likelihood of plaque rupture
(B) vasospasm is localized to a discrete area in an acute coronary syndrome
(C) the degree of stenosis is a good predictor of acute coronary events
(D) dystrophic calcification occurs in lipid-rich atherosclerotic plaques

(E) the extent of the calcification of a plaque correlates closely with its risk of sudden occlusion

(pages 1074–1076)

VI-4. Which of the following statements regarding risk factors for atherogenesis is true?

(A) very low-density lipoproteins (VLDLs) are responsible for a large proportion of atherosclerosis in arteries
(B) smoking causes increased atherogenesis without the presence of other risk factors
(C) there is no correlation between serum total cholesterol and the extent of atherosclerosis
(D) hypertension in a cholesterol-independent risk factor
(E) atherosclerotic plaques in smokers with high cholesterol levels progress faster than those in nonsmokers with high cholesterol levels

(pages 1077–1078)

VI-5. Which of the following statements regarding risk factors for atherogenesis is true?

(A) diabetes is a powerful cholesterol-dependent, sex-independent risk factor
(B) the presence of C-reactive protein, serum amyloid A, and fibrinogen in the blood are specific markers of coronary events
(C) elevated homocysteine levels are more closely linked with thrombus-mediated coronary events than with coronary atherosclerosis
(D) plaque rupture is the primary mechanism of thrombosis in diabetic patients
(E) the health benefits of regular versus irregular intake of alcoholic beverages are similar

(pages 1079–1082)

VI-6. Which of the following statements regarding clinical symptoms and plaque types is true?

(A) the majority of advanced plaques are not angiographically visible

(B) clinical symptoms develop with plaques of types III to Va

(C) the majority of major coronary thrombi are the result of endothelial erosion

(D) reduction of blood flow (i.e., vasospasm) to an area following a plaque disruption will decrease the likelihood of major thrombosis within the core

(E) increase in lipid-filled macrophages in plaques raise the amount of stress needed to cause plaque disruption

(pages 1098–1101)

VI-7. Which of the following statements regarding the pathology of clinical syndromes in ischemic heart disease is true?

(A) thrombus was recovered from the majority of plaques retrieved by atherectomy in patients with stable angina

(B) there is no difference in the vasospastic component of acute ischemic events in men and women

(C) the majority of occlusive coronary thrombi are due to plaque rupture that contains only an intraluminal component

(D) non-ST-segment elevation infarcts more often have previously established collateral flow or anterograde flow restoration over the plaque

(E) in radiolabeling studies, the intraplaque component of the thrombus is labeled

(pages 1102–1103)

VI-8. Which of the following statements regarding the regression and progression of plaques is true?

(A) high-grade lesions occur at sites where lower-grade lesions were initially present

(B) high-grade stenoses more frequently cause total occlusion

(C) it is possible to predict the sites that are more likely to cause infarction

(D) lipid lowering trials reduce the degree of narrowing in arteries

(E) lesions usually progress in areas of the artery that have an irregular outline

(pages 1104–1105)

VI-9. Which of the following statements regarding the physiologic control of myocardial perfusion is true?

(A) myogenic control of vasomotor tone keeps vessel wall tension constant in response to changing vascular distending pressures

(B) perfusion pressure and flow-mediated vasodilation determines vasomotor tone in arterioles

(C) there is a greater density of nerve endings in epicardial coronary arteries than in prearterioles or arterioles

(D) abolition of α-adrenergic tone causes a decrease in resting coronary blood flow

(E) the purinergic receptor, P_2, is most sensitive to adenosine

(pages 1111–1112)

VI-10. Which of the following statements regarding flow-limiting stenosis is true?

(A) a greater basal transstenotic pressure results in increased coronary flow reserve

(B) the subepicardium is most vulnerable to ischemia in the presence of a decreased poststenotic pressure

(C) coronary angiography provides the best assessment of the degree of coronary stenoses

(D) dynamic stenoses are usually eccentric

(E) all patients with flow-limiting stenosis develop collateral circulation

(pages 1115–1116)

VI-11. Which of the following statements regarding acute thrombosis is true?

(A) strong thrombogenic stimuli cause the growth of white thrombi

(B) a local inflammatory activation by infectious or noninfectious stimuli represents a strong thrombogenic stimuli

(C) thrombus formation is the first physiologic self-limiting step of vascular injury repair

(D) occlusive thrombosis can be caused by weak, nonpersistent thrombogenic stimuli with a normal circulatory state

(E) plaque vulnerability usually lasts for only a few days

(pages 1119–1120)

VI-12. Which of the following is a metabolic consequence of myocardial ischemia?

(A) there is a loss of intracellular sodium

(B) there is no change in protein synthesis

(C) potassium binds to calcium binding sites on contractile proteins

(D) there is a loss of intracellular potassium
(E) water moves out of the cell

(page 1120)

VI-13. Which of the following cellular changes contributes to myocardial stunning?

(A) loss of sarcomeres
(B) extracellular matrix alterations
(C) increased calcium sensitivity of myofilaments
(D) loss of T tubules
(E) tropomyosin degradation

(page 1122)

VI-14. Which of the following statements regarding variant angina is true?

(A) episodes have a poor response to sublingual nitrates
(B) angina occurs primarily on exertion
(C) angina usually persists, sometimes lasting up to $\frac{1}{2}$ h
(D) episodes may occur in clusters of two to three in the early morning hours
(E) β-adrenergic blocking agents are an effective treatment

(pages 1124–1125)

VI-15. Which of the following statements regarding LDL as a risk for coronary artery disease (CAD) is true?

(A) cholesterol lowering in hypercholesterolemic male CAD patients, ages 45 to 54, has not been shown to be cost-effective
(B) marked reductions of LDL will stop progression of coronary lesions, but will not cause them to regress
(C) patients who are at intermediate risk for CAD should always be treated with cholesterol-lowering drugs
(D) patients at low risk for CAD should have an LDL-cholesterol level of less than or equal to 130 mg/dL
(E) LDL lowering causes coronary lesion stabilization

(pages 1136–1138)

VI-16. Which of the following statements regarding CAD risk factors is true?

(A) pipe smoke and cigar smoke, when not inhaled, carry a low risk
(B) first-line treatment for atherogenic dyslipidemia is fibric acids or nicotinic acid
(C) the individualized approach to dietary intervention is more cost-effective than a population-wide approach
(D) the benefits reported from abstaining from an atherogenic diet were not as good as those seen from lipid-lowering drugs

(E) a reduction in smoking is an acceptable goal in patients with cardiovascular disease

(pages 1139–1141)

VI-17. Which of the following statements regarding CAD risk factors is true?

(A) insulin resistance has an indirect effect on CAD
(B) the majority of insulin resistance is due to genetic factors
(C) high-intensity physical activity is needed to achieve a mortality benefit
(D) obesity is generally considered an independent risk factor for CAD
(E) it is currently not recommended that postmenopausal women with CAD be treated with estrogen replacement therapy to prevent CAD events

(pages 1142–1145)

VI-18. Which of the following is an unmodifiable risk factor?

(A) plasma homocysteine level
(B) hypertension
(C) socioeconomic status
(D) insulin resistance
(E) obesity

(page 1147)

VI-19. Which of the following statements regarding pharmacologic therapy for CAD is true?

(A) fibrinogen levels correlate closely with dyslipidemia
(B) the risk-to-benefit ratio for aspirin use to prevent myocardial infarction (MI) in women differs from that of men
(C) evidence shows that a reduction in fibrinogen levels may be helpful in preventing CAD
(D) angiotensin-converting enzyme (ACE) inhibitors are an effective treatment due to their ability to bring about a reduction in the incidence and complexity of ventricular arrhythmias
(E) ACE inhibitors should be used for primary prevention due to their cost-effectiveness

(pages 1148–1150)

VI-20. Which of the following coronary artery anomalies is characterized by a slit-like ostium?

(A) single coronary artery
(B) ostial fibrous ridges
(C) high-takeoff coronary ostia
(D) coronary artery fistula
(E) origin of both right and left coronary artery from the same sinus of Valsalva

(pages 1164–1168)

VI-21. Which of the following statements regarding causes of nonatherosclerotic CAD is true?

(A) aneurysm formation of the coronary arteries is always an acquired condition

(B) the most common location for a coronary artery emboli is the left main coronary artery

(C) primary coronary artery dissections are more common than secondary dissections

(D) spiral dissection is a serious condition which may occur as a complication of coronary angioplasty

(E) coronary arteries with smooth muscle depletion, seen in atherosclerotic plaques with advanced degrees of luminal narrowing, have increased vasospastic potential

(pages 1169–1171)

VI-22. Which of the following statements regarding coronary artery arteritis is true?

(A) in a direct extension route of entry, the coronary intimal layer is usually involved

(B) tuberculous arteritis is characterized by a chronic inflammation with adventitial fibrosis and patchy destruction of media with a lymphoplasmacytic infiltrate

(C) temporal arteritis has its highest incidence in young to middle-aged Asian females

(D) Buerger's disease can result from the placement of a saphenous vein bypass graft

(E) patients with infantile polyarteritis nodosa have infarction or hemorrhage in various organs from necrotizing vasculitis

(pages 1172–1176)

VI-23. Which of the following statements regarding non-atherosclerotic causes of CAD is true?

(A) disorders of metabolism such as primary oxalosis and Fabry's disease affect major epicardial coronary arteries

(B) accelerated intimal fibrous hyperplasia involving coronary arteries is believed to be a result of intimal damage from immunologic rejection

(C) metastatic myocardial lesions from various tumors are usually surrounded by areas of necrotic myocardium

(D) the intimal lesions seen in radiation-induced CAD consist of fibrous tissue with extracellular lipid deposits

(E) cocaine use has been associated with a myocardial oxygen demand-supply disproportion

(pages 1180–1184)

VI-24. Which of the following statements regarding the diagnosis of CAD is true?

(A) Baye's theorem states that the pretest prevalence of disease influences the posttest likelihood of significant CAD

(B) a resting 12-lead ECG will be abnormal in most patients with chronic stable angina

(C) simple clinical observations such as pain type, age, and sex do not have a powerful predictive value for the probability of CAD

(D) chest roentgenograms usually appear abnormal in patients with stable angina pectoris

(E) exercise stress testing is valuable because of its relatively high sensitivity for detecting CAD

(pages 1210–1212)

VI-25. Which of the following statements regarding the diagnosis of CAD is true?

(A) exercise stress testing is most valuable when the pretest probability of CAD is high

(B) most patients undergoing a diagnostic evaluation for angina should have a resting echocardiogram

(C) patients with left bundle branch block (LBBB) should undergo cardiac stress imaging in addition to ECG

(D) planar imaging is more sensitive than ^{201}thallium single photon emission computed tomography (SPECT) for diagnosing CAD

(E) coronary angiography is most appropriate for a patient with an intermediate-risk exercise stress test outcome

(pages 1212–1214)

VI-26. Which of the following statements regarding the pathophysiology of ischemic heart disease is true?

(A) myocardial contractility is often a primary factor for therapeutic intervention

(B) nitrate therapy acts by decreasing preload

(C) the vasodilator response is especially important when coronary perfusion pressure drops below 60 mm Hg

(D) the vasodilator mechanism remains intact until an artery is almost occluded

(E) normal and atherosclerotic arteries react in the same way to the α-adrenergic agonist, phenylephrine

(pages 1215–1216)

VI-27. Which of the following statements regarding the pathophysiology of ischemic heart disease is true?

(A) the larger, epicardial vessels are most important in the pathogenesis of angina pectoris
(B) patients with capillary narrowing exhibit a different response than controls to nonendothelial-dependent vasodilators
(C) the phenomenon of mixed angina involves vasoconstriction in the microvasculature
(D) the threshold for precipitating anginal attacks in patients with stable angina is highest in the morning
(E) anginal pain travels through unmyelinated and small myelinated fibers to the spinothalamic tract

(pages 1217–1218)

VI-28. Which of the following patients with ischemic heart disease would be at high risk for an MI?

(A) a man with normal stress echocardiographic wall motion
(B) a woman with a Duke treadmill score of –6
(C) a man with a stress-induced moderate perfusion defect without left ventricular dilatation or increased lung intake (^{201}thallium)
(D) a woman who had stress-induced multiple perfusion defects of moderate size
(E) a man with a resting left ventricular ejection fraction (LVEF) of 45 percent and known CAD

(page 1222)

VI-29. In which of the following conditions is there a relative contraindication for beta-blocker therapy?

(A) mild peripheral vascular disease
(B) migraine of vascular headaches
(C) depression
(D) mitral regurgitation
(E) hyperthyroidism

(page 1226)

VI-30. Which of the following statements regarding treatments for chronic stable angina is true?

(A) ticlopidine, a thienopyridine derivative that inhibits platelet aggregation, has been shown to decrease adverse cardiovascular events
(B) lipid-lowering therapy should be used for patients with moderate to high elevations of LDL-cholesterol
(C) β-adrenergic blocking agents act mainly through cyclic AMP formation
(D) a combination of β-adrenergic blocking agents and nitrates is more effective than treatment with β-adrenergic blocking agents alone

(E) when pharmacologic treatment for hypertension is necessary, short-acting calcium channel antagonists should be used

(pages 1223–1225)

VI-31. Which of the following statements regarding the pathophysiology of unstable angina is true?

(A) plaque erosion tends to be more common than plaque rupture in hyperlipidemic men
(B) interferon-gamma, produced by T lymphocytes, inhibits collagen production in regions surrounding the plaque
(C) nuclear factor-κB (NF-κB) is elevated in patients with stable angina, but not in those with unstable angina
(D) antibodies to cytomegalovirus or *Helicobacter* are used as predictors of future cardiovascular events
(E) most lesions that progress to cause acute coronary events are usually greater than 50 percent stenotic

(pages 1239–1241)

VI-32. Which of the following statements regarding the diagnosis of patients with unstable angina is true?

(A) unstable angina often occurs during exertion
(B) unstable angina is relieved by nitroglycerin
(C) the duration of chest discomfort is usually longer in stable angina than in unstable angina
(D) patients who describe their pain as sharp, jabbing, or knifelike are likely to have unstable angina
(E) when unstable angina is suspected in patients under age 50, it is important to ask about cocaine use

(pages 1241–1242)

VI-33. Which of the following statements regarding the diagnosis of patients with unstable angina is true?

(A) at coronary angiography, women presenting with unstable angina are more likely to have significant coronary lesions than men
(B) when ST depression is a persistent feature of ECGs recorded in a patient with or without chest pain, this is highly specific for unstable angina
(C) myocardial stunning distal to the culprit lesion is probably responsible for a persistently negative T wave pattern over the involved territory
(D) the majority of patients with unstable angina will have elevated troponin levels on admission
(E) The MB isoenzyme of creatine kinase (CK-MB) levels are useful in making a diagnosis when a patient presents late after a coronary event

(pages 1242–1244)

VI-34. Which of the following statements regarding treatment of unstable angina is true?

(A) nitroglycerin reduces thrombin-induced platelet aggregation, but this effect disappears when nitroglycerin tolerance occurs

(B) administration of captopril or *N*-acetylcysteine may reduce nitrate tolerance

(C) β-adrenergic blocking agents reduce the risk of myocardial infarction

(D) dihydropyridine calcium channel blockers slow heart rate and reduce afterload

(E) nifedipine is helpful in controlling angina in patients who are not receiving β-adrenergic blocking agents

(pages 1248–1250)

VI-35. Which of the following statements regarding treatments for unstable angina is true?

(A) platelet GP IIb/IIIa inhibition at the time of angioplasty reduces ischemic complications

(B) symptoms are easier to control in a patient who has previously taken antianginal drugs

(C) the effect of aspirin in reducing cardiac events, particularly death, is relatively small

(D) due to the negative interactions between aspirin and ACE inhibitors, aspirin should be withheld in patients who are receiving ACE inhibitors in the absence of severe heart failure

(E) ticlopidine is the drug of choice to use with aspirin to prevent thrombotic complications in the weeks following coronary stenting

(pages 1251–1255)

VI-36. Which of the following statements regarding treatments for unstable angina is true?

(A) low-molecular-weight heparins (LMWHs) have equivalent activity against factor Xa and thrombin

(B) a disadvantage of LMWHs is that they have a greater inhibition of activation of the protein C anticoagulant pathway than regular heparin

(C) thrombolytic therapy reduces cardiovascular events in unstable angina

(D) hirudin is not recommended for use in patients with unstable angina

(E) LMWHs are the most effective treatment for prevention of venous thrombosis in patients undergoing total hip replacement

(pages 1257–1260)

VI-37. Which of the following statements regarding variant angina is true?

(A) the underlying coronary lesions, as demonstrated by coronary angiography, usually have subtotal occlusion

(B) surgery almost invariably eliminates variant angina and has an excellent long-term outcome

(C) it is likely that either parasympathetic nervous system overactivity or reduced sympathetic activity cause variant angina

(D) coronary angiography is usually not necessary in patients with variant angina

(E) β-adrenergic blockers are very effective in preventing attacks of variant angina

(pages 1263–1265)

VI-38. Which of the following statements regarding the clinical aspects of acute myocardial infarction is true?

(A) the risk for myocardial infarction is highest in the late afternoon

(B) pulmonary emboli can precipitate a myocardial infarction by increasing catecholamine levels

(C) it is not unusual for an MI to go unnoticed by the patient

(D) sinus tachycardia that is present 24 h following a myocardial infarction shows that the patient is not experiencing significant hemodynamic compromise

(E) an inspiratory rise in jugular venous pressure is normal in a patient with an acute inferior MI

(pages 1278–1279)

VI-39. Which of the following statements regarding plasma diagnostic markers of acute myocardial infarction is true?

(A) the use of total creatine kinase (CK) alone to diagnose MI has a high specificity

(B) cardiac troponin I is upregulated in injured skeletal muscle

(C) myoglobin is a very sensitive test in the first few hours following myocardial infarction

(D) if CK-MB accounts for less than 5 percent of total CK, a skeletal muscle source should be considered for elevated plasma CK-MB activity

(E) the LDH level is the best indicator of myocardial infarction 48 to 72 h following an MI

(pages 1283–1288)

VI-40. Which of the following modalities is most useful in diagnosing acute myocardial infarction (AMI)?

(A) roentgenogram
(B) magnetic resonance imaging
(C) echocardiography
(D) computed tomography
(E) radionuclide scintigraphy

(page 1290)

VI-41. Which of the following statements regarding the management of patients with chest pain in the emergency department is true?

(A) with increasingly specific tests now available, the missed diagnosis rate has dropped

(B) the administration of nitroglycerin upon admission with chest pain is useful to distinguish between MI and gastrointestinal disturbances

(C) oxygen should be administered to all patients with an acute MI

(D) evidence shows benefits of routine, long-term use of nitrates in uncomplicated acute MI

(E) all patients with ST-segment elevation should be considered for rapid reperfusion

(pages 1294–1299)

VI-42. For which of the following patients should primary percutaneous coronary intervention (PCI) be considered over thrombolytic therapy?

(A) a 78-year-old patient with ST elevation

(B) a 55-year-old patient with new left bundle branch block

(C) a 60-year-old patient with ST-segment depression

(D) a 58-year-old patient with blood pressure on presentation of 190/110 mmHg

(E) a 70-year-old patient with ST elevation and a time to therapy of 12 h or less

(page 1301)

VI-43. Which of the following statements regarding management of patients with ST-segment elevation is true?

(A) primary angioplasty is superior to thrombolytic therapy in nearly every way

(B) patients with atrial fibrillation should receive subcutaneous unfractionated heparin

(C) rescue angioplasty is recommended as a routine strategy for failed thrombolysis

(D) atropine should administered to patients with asymptomatic sinus bradycardia and a heart rate greater than 40 beats per minute

(E) heart block with an inferior MI may have a more favorable prognosis than heart block with an anterior MI

(page 1305–1309)

VI-44. Which of the following statements regarding patients who present with ischemic-type chest pain without ST-segment elevation is true?

(A) enoxiparin is superior to unfractionated heparin in treating patients with unstable angina and non-ST-segment elevation myocardial infarctions

(B) non-ST-segment elevation myocardial infarctions involve loss of a larger amount of myocardium than Q-wave infarctions

(C) patients with non-ST-segment elevation infarctions do not usually benefit from secondary prevention

(D) diltiazem and verapamil are used to treat acute MI with associated left ventricular dysfunction

(E) β-adrenergic blocking agents have a positive effect on reducing reinfarction rates in patients following non-ST-segment elevation myocardial infarctions

(pages 1311–1314)

VI-45. Which of the following statements regarding management of the high-risk patient with acute myocardial infarction is true?

(A) the recurrence of chest pain following non-ST-segment elevation infarction is not associated with a greater mortality rate

(B) indomethacin is the best treatment to give a patient with early postinfarction pericarditis

(C) systolic dysfunction usually precedes diastolic dysfunction in acute MI

(D) abnormal right ventricular function following an inferior MI is most often due to stunning rather than massive infarction

(E) a patient with right ventricular infarction should be treated with diuretics

(pages 1318–1321)

VI-46. Which of the following statements regarding the management of heart failure in acute MI is true?

(A) digoxin is the drug of choice in acute heart failure in myocardial infarction

(B) invasive monitoring is not necessary in uncomplicated acute MI as long as there is careful clinical observation

(C) the primary use of dobutamine in heart failure in MI is to raise blood pressure

(D) the most common cause of in-hospital death following MI is sudden death due to ventricular fibrillation

(E) diuretics should be used initially in the treatment of pulmonary congestion in acute MI

(pages 1322–1325)

VI-47. Which of the following statements regarding other complications of acute MI is true?

(A) prophylactic anticoagulant therapy should be given to all patients following a myocardial infarction

(B) a pseudoaneurysm has a narrow base

(C) ventricular thrombi are commonly found in patients with inferior infarction

(D) the location of the aneurysm is usually apical, posterior, or anteroapical

(E) the prognosis for patients with aneurysms is related to the risk of aneurysm rupture

(pages 1327–1328)

VI-48. Which of the following arrhythmias or conduction disturbances complicating acute MI is common and usually has a bad prognosis?

(A) paroxysmal supraventricular tachycardia
(B) atrial flutter
(C) second-degree atrioventricular (AV) block in an inferior MI
(D) escape AV junctional rhythm with right coronary occlusion
(E) sinus tachycardia

(pages 1328–1329)

VI-49. Which of the following statements regarding thrombosis in acute coronary syndromes is true?

(A) the late phase of saphenous vein graft disease is characterized by intimal hyperplasia
(B) macrophages and T lymphocytes found at the site of plaque disruption are generally in a deactivated state
(C) the first component of thrombus formation is a platelet monolayer
(D) the large calcified plaque has the highest thrombogenicity of all types of plaques
(E) the intrinsic pathway of the coagulation cascade is the predominant mechanism for initiating hemostasis

(pages 1374–1379)

VI-50. Which of the following statements regarding the role of blood coagulation in thrombosis is true?

(A) tissue factor X requires activation by minor proteolysis
(B) a congenital deficiency of factor XII results in bleeding problems
(C) factor VII is activated only by the phospholipids of the platelet membrane
(D) to be fully active, factor Xa has to form a complex with factor Va
(E) factor X contributes to the stability of the fibrin network

(pages 1381–1383)

VI-51. Which of the following statements regarding the fibrinolytic system is true?

(A) physical exercise causes an increase in the level of tissue-type plasminogen activator (t-PA) in the blood
(B) the presence of thrombin directly enhances the plasminogen-activating property of t-PA
(C) t-PA is synthesized and secreted by vascular smooth muscle cells
(D) only platelets produce the plasminogen activator inhibitor 1 (PAI-1)
(E) PAI-1 binds to its target in an irreversible complex

(pages 1385–1388)

VI-52. Which of the following statements regarding anti-thrombotic drugs is true?

(A) aspirin inhibits adherence of the initial layer of platelets to both the subendothelium and to atherosclerotic plaques
(B) there is a dose related response in the efficacy of aspirin
(C) thienopyridines (e.g., clopidogrel) do not appear to have a permanent effect on platelets
(D) ticlopidine is more potent than clopidogrel in the inhibition of ADP-induced aggregation of human platelets
(E) ticlopidine combined with aspirin is effective in reducing thrombosis in patients undergoing coronary stent implantation

(pages 1388–1394)

VI-53. Which of the following statements regarding platelet glycoprotein (GP) IIb/IIIa receptor blockers is true?

(A) because abciximab has a short half-life, antiplatelet activity reverses after a few hours when drug infusion is discontinued
(B) GP IIb/IIIa inhibitors may reduce the development of myocardial necrosis
(C) eptifibatide and tirofiban bind tightly to the GP IIb/IIIa receptor, and thus their effects last much longer than the infusion period
(D) the 6-month endpoint of death, MI, or any target vessel revascularization was significantly reduced when abciximab was used in primary coronary intervention
(E) there is no evidence that increased benefit can be gained from the use of GP IIb/IIIa inhibitors combined with heparin

(pages 1394–1398)

VI-54. Which of the following statements regarding oral GP IIb/IIIa inhibition is true?

(A) sibrafan has a relatively low incidence of bleeding at levels needed to achieve effective chronic platelet inhibition
(B) a recent study showed that sibrafan had double the rate of minor bleeding when given twice rather than once per day
(C) there is a suggested benefit from combining aspirin with oral GP IIb/IIIa inhibitors
(D) thrombocytopenia generally occurs during long-term follow-up of patients taking GP IIb/IIIa inhibitors
(E) there has been little interpatient variability seen in drug level and degree of platelet inhibition with oral GP IIb/IIIa inhibitors

(pages 1401–1402)

VI-55. Which of the following statements regarding unfractionated heparin is true?

(A) more heparin is needed to prevent the formation of the initial thrombus than is needed to prevent the extension of venous thrombosis

(B) the bioavailability of unfractionated heparin after subcutaneous injection is >90 percent

(C) the risk of bleeding is higher when unfractionated heparin is given by continuous infusion

(D) unfractionated heparin does not increase vascular permeability

(E) lower initial doses of heparin in the setting of thrombolytic therapy reduce the rates of intracranial and other major hemorrhages

(pages 1404–1406)

VI-56. Which of the following statements regarding LMWHs is true?

(A) factor Xa bound to the platelet membrane in the prothrombinase complex is resistant to inactivation by LMWHs

(B) LMWHs have a shorter half-life than unfractionated heparins

(C) higher doses (1.25 mg/kg twice per day) of enoxaparin have been found to be most effective in lowering the rate of recurrent ischemic events without increasing bleeding complications

(D) danaparoid sodium may be associated with fewer bleeding episodes than heparin

(E) LMWHs exhibit greater interpatient variability of the anticoagulant response than unfractionated heparin

(pages 1407–1408)

VI-57. Which of the following would NOT be inhibited by warfarin?

(A) factor VII

(B) protein C

(C) factor XII

(D) factor II

(E) protein S

(page 1411)

VI-58. Which of the following statements regarding thrombolytic drugs is true?

(A) all thrombolytic drugs, whether they are natural activators endogenous to humans or not, are fibrinogen activators

(B) the plasmin-staphylokinase complex is rapidly inhibited by α_2-antiplasmin

(C) renewed treatment with streptokinase within 4 to 6 months of the first treatment is highly effective

(D) plasmin formed on the fibrin surface is rapidly inhibited by α_2-antiplasmin

(E) anistreplase is not affected by streptokinase antibodies

(pages 1413–1421)

VI-59. Which of the following statements regarding new devices and strategies for coronary intervention is true?

(A) aspirin combined with warfarin gives the lowest rate of stent thrombosis

(B) Gianturco-Roubin flex stent is the stent that revolutionized interventional cardiology

(C) intermediate data available from studies involving stents versus coronary artery bypass graft (CABG) in multivessel disease show increased 1-year survival free of death, MI, and reintervention in the stent group

(D) patients treated with IIb/IIIa platelet receptor inhibitors have shown decreased composite endpoints of death or nonfatal MI in the setting of coronary intervention

(E) diabetics treated with abciximab while undergoing stent placement have had a higher repeat target vessel revascularization than without abciximab treatment

(pages 1443–1446)

VI-60. Which of the following statements regarding indications for coronary intervention is true?

(A) the favorable cost-effectiveness of percutaneous intervention is seen in both single-vessel and multivessel diseases

(B) complete revascularization is achieved in a majority of patients with multivessel disease who undergo coronary intervention

(C) the risks of percutaneous coronary intervention increase in the presence of female gender

(D) diabetics and nondiabetics with stents have roughly the same mortality rates

(E) patients with stable and unstable angina have the same risk for abrupt closure following coronary intervention

(pages 1447–1448)

VI-61. Which of the following statements regarding the selection of lesions for PCI is true?

(A) a lesion with heavy calcification has a 60 to 85 percent success rate

(B) a type C lesion has a high success rate following coronary intervention

(C) eccentric lesions have a low success rate

(D) a lesion that is diffuse (>2 cm in length) carries a moderate risk

(E) in-stent restenosis occurs through a combination of negative remodeling and intimal proliferation

(pages 1449–1450)

VI-62.   Which of the following statements regarding the results of coronary intervention is true?

(A)   complication rates of coronary intervention have increased as increasingly difficult cases are attempted

(B)   the strongest predictor of major complications is ventricular arrhythmia requiring emergent cardioversion

(C)   the risk of perforation in laser angioplasty is highest in small, tortuous lesions

(D)   the hydrophilic coronary guidewire carries a significant risk of perforation

(E)   patients at increased risk for microparticulate embolization from rotational atherectomy are those who have tortuous lesions

(pages 1459–1461)

VI-63.   Which of the following statements regarding primary angioplasty is true?

(A)   low-risk patients do not benefit from primary angioplasty

(B)   most patients are eligible for both thrombolytic therapy and primary angioplasty

(C)   primary angioplasty is not useful in any patient who presents more than 12 h after the onset of symptoms

(D)   reperfusion rates in patients with acute MI due to saphenous vein graft occlusion are similar to those in patients with acute MI due to native vessel occlusion

(E)   the total cost for primary angioplasty is less than for thrombolytic therapy

(pages 1475–1478)

VI-64.   Which of the following patients would have the least benefit from primary angioplasty?

(A)   a man with an acute MI and cardiogenic shock

(B)   an elderly woman with an acute MI

(C)   a woman with nonanterior wall myocardial infarction

(D)   a man with anterior wall myocardial infarction

(E)   a woman with an acute MI and cardiogenic shock

(page 1474)

VI-65.   Which of the following statements regarding primary angioplasty is true?

(A)   TIMI 3 flow is achieved most often in primary angioplasty if treatment occurs within 2 h of the onset of symptoms

(B)   there is little role for intraaortic balloon counterpulsation after primary angioplasty in hemodynamically stable patients

(C)   if reperfusion is not established when a guidewire is passed through an occlusion, the balloon should be inflated to establish reperfusion

(D)   noninfarct arteries can be dilated in addition to the infarct artery when primary angioplasty is performed

(E)   intraaortic balloon counterpulsation has great benefit when used alone in high-risk patients

(pages 1480–1483)

VI-66.   Which of the following statements regarding the characterization of atherosclerosis with coronary intravascular ultrasound imaging is true?

(A)   current ultrasound devices make it possible to view fatty streaks

(B)   fibromuscular lesions are usually hypoechoic

(C)   a zone of reduced echogenicity is diagnostic of a thrombus

(D)   if no calcification is visualized on an angiogram, there is a low chance of detecting a large superficial arc of calcium by ultrasound

(E)   intravascular ultrasound can reliably diagnose thrombi

(pages 1492–1493)

VI-67.   Which of the following statements regarding diagnostic clinical applications of coronary intravascular ultrasound imaging is true?

(A)   there is good correlation between ultrasonic and angiographic dimensions in atherosclerotic arteries

(B)   trailing-edge measurements accurately describe the locations of boundaries

(C)   studies have shown good correlation between the apparent circumferential pattern of a plaque seen by angiography and the actual plaque distribution shown by ultrasound

(D)   intravascular ultrasound and angiography are similar in their ability to quantify left main coronary artery lesions

(E)   the prognosis has not been worse in patients with atherosclerosis demonstrated only by ultrasound

(pages 1494–1496)

VI-68.   Which of the following statements regarding interventional clinical applications and coronary intravascular ultrasound imaging is true?

(A)   superficial calcium detected by ultrasound predicts poor tissue retrieval in directional atherectomy

(B)   a larger postprocedure lumen using ultrasound guidance for directional atherectomy results in a lower restenosis rate without an increase in complications

(C) demonstration of a heavily calcified vessel by angiography or ultrasound is an indication for directional atherectomy

(D) additional procedures rarely result after ultrasound imaging of high-pressure coronary stenting

(E) interventions designed to prevent intimal hyperplasia may be more important in preventing recoil than interventions to prevent chronic recoil

(pages 1498–1500)

VI-69. Which of the following statements regarding types of bypass grafts and their outcomes is true?

(A) grafts occluded within 1 to 2 months of surgery exhibit a hypercellular, proliferative hyperplasia involving the intima

(B) vein graft atherosclerosis is a proximal, eccentric, and intermittent lesion that is often covered by a fibrous cap

(C) the strategy of bilateral internal mammary artery grafting has become widespread in use

(D) the gastroepiploic artery has been shown to function well as a graft to the posterior descending branch of the right coronary artery

(E) radial artery grafts are superior to left internal mammary grafts

(pages 1511–1515)

VI-70. Which of the following statements has the greatest predictive value of in-hospital death following bypass surgery?

(A) female gender

(B) acuteness of operation

(C) reduced left ventricular ejection fraction

(D) number of coronary systems with more than 50 percent stenosis

(E) left main coronary artery with 50 percent stenosis

(page 1515)

VI-71. Which of the following statements regarding current operative strategies and risk of coronary bypass surgery is true?

(A) there is no decrease in hospital mortality when internal mammary grafts are used

(B) obesity and diabetes are associated with a greater risk of sternal complications following surgery

(C) patients undergoing operation in the face of acute ischemia require asanguineous, cold, high-in-potassium cardioplegic solutions

(D) the most important predictor for type II neurologic abnormalities is proximal aortic atherosclerosis

(E) patients with a history of unstable angina and stroke are at increased risk of type II deficits

(pages 1516–1517)

VI-72. Which of the following statements regarding coronary bypass surgery is true?

(A) young patients have an increased survival rate following bypass surgery

(B) patients need not have any graft failure to be a candidates for reoperation

(C) emergency bypass operation is associated with a large increase in risk

(D) late stenoses in vein grafts are no more dangerous than those in native coronary lesions

(E) patients who have early vein graft stenoses have an improved late survival rate with surgery

(pages 1518–1519)

VI-73. Which of the following statements regarding the postoperative management of a patient following bypass surgery is true?

(A) the transient myocardial depression that is present following bypass surgery is attributed to the effects of cardiopulmonary bypass (CPB)

(B) depressed myocardial function is directly related to CPB time

(C) hypothermia may result in postoperative hypotension

(D) generally a localized bleeding site, such as an internal mammary pedicle, is responsible for severe, postoperative bleeding

(E) if vasodilation with increased venous capacitance is considered responsible for hypotension, the patient should be given colloids

(pages 1526–1527)

VI-74. Which of the following statements regarding the approach to postoperative cardiovascular problems after bypass surgery is true?

(A) pain can cause sinus tachycardia following surgery

(B) the most common cause of low cardiac output postoperatively is increased systemic vascular resistance

(C) hydralazine, which acts mainly through venous dilatation, is generally given to patients with high filling pressures and active myocardial ischemia

(D) ventricular ectopy is the most common rhythm disturbance following bypass surgery

(E) ventricular fibrillation following surgery is seen only in the presence of acute myocardial ischemia

(pages 1528–1530)

VI-75. Which of the following statements regarding respiratory management following bypass surgery is true?

(A) pulmonary problems infrequently cause morbidity following cardiac surgery

(B) there is usually an increase in lung water, unrelated to cardiac filling pressures, following routine CPB

(C) patients should not be given opioids during bypass surgery or postoperatively due to the risk of respiratory depression

(D) atelectasis is the most common pulmonary complication

(E) inhaled forms of bronchodilators given to patients with bronchospasm following cardiac surgery can have detrimental cardiovascular effects

(pages 1530–1532)

VI-76. Which of the following statements regarding the approach to postoperative cardiovascular complications after bypass surgery is true?

(A) the appearance of jaundice following bypass surgery can be normal

(B) hypomagnesemia is a bad prognostic sign following cardiac surgery

(C) a fever seen after surgery is generally a result of phlebitis

(D) the risk of developing postbypass renal failure is related to the patient's underlying renal function

(E) encephalopathy seen following bypass surgery is not generally reversible

(pages 1532–1534)

VI-77. Which of the following statements regarding exercise training in the rehabilitation of patients with coronary heart disease is true?

(A) an increase in stroke volume during aerobic exercise generally does not occur in elderly patients

(B) a clinical benefit of exercise training is improved resting ejection fraction

(C) activity-related symptoms, such as claudication or angina, are not generally reduced with exercise training

(D) patients should exercise at a heart rate between 70 to 85 percent of the highest level safely achieved at exercise testing

(E) beta-blocking drugs attenuate the improvement in physical work capacity gained in exercise training

(pages 1538–1540)

VI-78. Which of the following statements regarding the rehabilitation of patients with CAD is true?

(A) continuous ECG monitoring has been shown to provide added safety to low-risk patients during supervised exercise

(B) there are a number of complications and adverse outcomes associated with exercise testing in the elderly

(C) the mortality rate in patients with coronary heart disease living alone is greater than in those who live with others

(D) the ventricular ejection fraction is a good predictor of the exercise capacity and potential for improvement of a patient with heart failure

(E) the return-to-work rate following bypass surgery is quite high

(pages 1541–1545)

VI. CORONARY HEART DISEASE

ANSWERS

VI-1. **The answer is D.** *(Ch. 35)* The presence of minimally oxidized LDL in the subendothelial space makes the vessel more atherogenic. T-cell recruitment into the arterial intima is one of the earliest signs of atherogenesis. High shear stress has an atheroprotective effect. Minimally oxidized LDL may upregulate MCP-1 in the vessel wall. MCP-1 is a potent attractor of monocytes and T cells. It does not attract neutrophils, eosinophils, or B cells.

VI-2. **The answer is E.** *(Ch. 35)* Evidence has shown that the shape of a vessel, not flow patterns, may determine the degree of adaptive intimal thickening. The presence of fatty streaks and its implications remains controversial. Fatty streaks are present in the arteries of human fetuses. Fatty streak comparisons between different racial groups and sexes do not parallel the risk of atherosclerosis associated with each race and sex. The risk of plaque disruption depends on the type of plaque, rather than on the size. Soft, lipid-rich plaques are more vulnerable and prone to rupture than hard, collagen-rich plaques. The atheromatous core of a plaque is lipid rich and has no collagen present. As the endothelium becomes denuded during atherogenesis, blood-derived components like albumin and fibrinogen can be present in the lesions.

VI-3. **The answer is B.** *(Ch. 35)* Coronary angiography demonstrates flow limiting lesions, but there is poor, if any, correlation between plaque size and propensity for rupture. The vulnerability and thrombogenicity of atherosclerotic plaques, rather than the degree of stenosis, are the main determinants of the occurrence of an acute coronary event. Vasospasm is usually localized to the culprit lesion in acute coronary syndromes. Calcification of both lipid-rich and collagen-rich plaques occurs in an active and controlled manner, similar to that seen in bone. The extent of calcification in a patient correlates closely with their overall atherosclerotic plaque burden but does not correlate with the degree of stenosis or risk of sudden occlusion.

VI-4. **The answer is E.** *(Ch. 35)* VLDLs are too large to enter the artery wall and thus are not responsible for atherosclerosis. Smoking requires the coexistence of cholesterol abnormalities to promote atherogenesis. Studies have shown that serum total cholesterol correlates with the amount of atherosclerosis in all arterial segments in men. Hypertension is also a cholesterol-dependent risk factor. Atherosclerotic plaques progress more rapidly in smokers than nonsmokers.

VI-5. **The answer is C.** *(Ch. 35)* Diabetes is a powerful cholesterol-dependent risk factor. Diabetes is a sex-independent risk factor in that it increases the risk of CAD in women three- to sevenfold and in men two- to threefold. C-reactive protein, serum amyloid A, and fibrinogen are sensitive predictors of coronary events, but are not specific predictors. These blood markers of inflammation are present in all low-grade systemic infections. Elevated homocysteine levels are more closely linked to thrombus-mediated coronary events than with coronary atherosclerosis. The primary mechanism of thrombosis in diabetics is endothelial erosion rather than plaque rupture. The health benefits that are seen in people with regular and moderate alcohol intake are not seen in people with irregular intake.

VI-6. **The answer is A.** *(Ch. 36)* Clinical symptoms develop in plaques of types IV and Va. The majority of these advanced plaques are not visible angiographically and are clinically silent because they do not encroach upon the lumen of a coronary artery. The majority (80 percent) of major coronary thrombi are caused by plaque disruption. Following plaque disruption, a reduction of blood to an area, either by spasm or a large expansion of the plaque by thrombus within the core, increases the likelihood of major thrombosis within the core. Greater numbers of lipid-filled macrophages in the plaque reduce the amount of stress needed to cause plaque disruption. Increases in collagen and glycosoaminoglycans raise the amount of stress required to cause a tear.

VI-7.   **The answer is D.**   *(Ch. 36)*   Thrombus is recovered from the majority of plaques retrieved by atherectomy in patients with unstable angina. Patients with stable angina have thrombus much less often. Women seem to have a larger vasospastic component in acute ischemic events than men. The majority of occlusive coronary thrombi are due to plaque rupture with both an intraplaque and intraluminal component. In radiolabeling studies, only the intraluminal component of the plaque is labeled, showing that some of the formation postdates the infarction. Non ST-segment elevation, compared with transmural infarcts, have a higher frequency of previously established collateral flow and/or restoration of anterograde flow over the plaque.

VI-8.   **The answer is B.**   *(Ch. 36)*   The progression of lesions is often unpredictable. High-grade lesions are not necessarily found in areas where low-grade lesions were present on a previous study. It is not possible to predict the site of future infarctions. Lesions often appear in normal segments of the artery, rather than in those that have an irregular outline. Despite the unpredictability of lesions, high-grade stenoses tend to progress more often to total occlusions. The degree of reduction in the narrowing of established stenosis with lipid lowering trials has been minimal, but the coronary event rates declined precipitously.

VI-9.   **The answer is A.**   *(Ch. 37)*   Myogenic control of vasomotor tone keeps the vessel wall tension constant in response to changes in vascular distending pressure. Perfusion pressure and flow-mediated vasodilatation determine vasomotor tone in prearterioles and large arteries. Vasomotor tone in arterioles is determined by $M\dot{V}O_2$. There is a greater density of nerve endings in prearterioles and arterioles than in epicardial coronary vessels. Abolition of α-adrenergic tone causes an approximate 10 percent increase in resting coronary blood flow. The purinergic receptor, P_2, is most sensitive to ATP and mediates release of endothelial derived relaxing factor (EDRF).

VI-10.   **The answer is D.**   *(Ch. 37)*   A greater basal transstenotic pressure results in a decrease in coronary flow reserve. With this decreased flow reserve, myocardial ischemia will appear at a lower lever of cardiac work. The subendocardium is more vulnerable to ischemia than the subepicardium. The "gold standard" method for assessing the degree of coronary stenosis is the direct measurement of basal transstenotic pressure. Dynamic stenoses are usually eccentric. Some people who have flow-limiting stenoses develop extensive collateral circulation. Others with the same amount of stenoses, however, develop little or no collateral circulation. These differences are likely related to genetic factors.

VI-11.   **The answer is C.**   *(Ch. 37)*   Weak thrombogenic stimuli cause the slow deposition of platelets and formation of platelet-fibrin thrombi, known as white thrombi. An example of a weak thrombogenic stimuli is a local inflammatory activation by infectious or noninfectious stimuli. The first physiologic self-limiting step of vascular injury repair is thrombus formation. Occlusive thrombi can be caused by weak, nonpersistent thrombogenic stimuli, but only when a prothrombotic or deficient fibrinolytic state is present and combined with blood flow stasis. Plaque vulnerability can last anywhere from a few days to a few months.

VI-12.   **The answer is D.**   *(Ch. 37)*   Some of the metabolic consequences of myocardial ischemia are that sodium, calcium, and water accumulate in the cell. There is a loss of intracellular potassium. Protein synthesis is impaired. The accumulation of hydrogen ions causes them to compete with calcium for binding spaces on contractile proteins.

VI-13.   **The answer is B.**   *(Ch. 37)*   There are several components that contribute to myocardial stunning. Among these are a decreased sensitivity of the myofilaments to calcium, calcium overload and free radical generation, slow resynthesis of adenosine nucleotides, microvascular damage with leukocyte activation, myocyte electromechanical uncoupling, and extracellular matrix alterations.

VI-14. The answer is D. *(Ch. 37)* Patients with variant angina generally respond to sublingual nitrates. The anginal episodes are usually of short duration. Patients report pain primarily at rest and often in clusters of two or three in the early morning hours. Calcium channel antagonists and nitrates are treatments for variant angina. Treatment with β-adrenergic blocking agents is totally ineffective.

VI-15. The answer is E. *(Ch. 38)* Secondary prevention (known CAD) with cholesterol lowering in hypercholesterolemic male patients, ages 45 to 54, has been shown to be one of the very few treatments that actually saves, not costs, money. Marked reduction in LDL levels has been shown in one meta-analysis of 13 trials to actually show a tiny (3 percent at 1 year) but significant amount of regression of coronary lesions, although the coronary event rate dropped remarkably. The strategy for treating patients who are at intermediate risk for CAD (i.e., primary prevention) is to lower their cholesterol through diet, weight loss, or medical therapy to <130 mg/dL. The minimum goal for cholesterol levels in patients at low risk for CAD is less the 160 mg/dL. The goal of a level of less than or equal to 100 mg/dL is for patients at high risk of CAD. While the clinical effectiveness of cholesterol lowering therapy has been demonstrated in low and intermediate risk groups (primary prevention), the benefits are small to moderate and are not nearly as cost-effective as treating patients with known CAD. LDL lowering most likely results in lesion stabilization, rather than a change in the size of the lesion.

VI-16. The answer is A. *(Ch. 38)* Pipe smoke and cigar smoke, when not inhaled, carry a low risk for CAD, but increase the risk of oropharyngeal cancer. Pipe smoking and cigar smoking are, however, associated with later resumption of cigarette smoking. The first-line treatment for atherogenic dyslipidemia is weight control and physical activity. These will both often correct the lipoprotein abnormalities. Both the individual and population-wide approaches for dietary intervention are cost-effective. The population-wide approach, however, costs $20 per year of life saved, and the individual approach costs $20,000 per year of live saved. The benefits seen from abstaining from an atherogenic diet are similar and sometimes better than those seen in lipid-lowering drugs, although compliance with an appropriate diet is low. Nothing less than a total cessation of smoking is acceptable for patients with cardiovascular disease.

VI-17. The answer is E. *(Ch. 38)* Insulin sensitivity is associated with endothelial nitric oxide production in healthy persons, thus insulin resistance may promote CAD directly. There are many risk factors for insulin resistance, including obesity, physical inactivity, and inherited factors. Only moderate-intensity physical activity is required to decrease mortality risk. Obesity has not been consistently shown to be an independent risk factor. The consequences of obesity are primarily manifested through its effect on lipid levels, blood pressure, and insulin resistance. Because of recent conflicting data, it is currently not recommended that postmenopausal women with CAD have estrogen replacement therapy to prevent CAD events.

VI-18. The answer is C. *(Ch. 38)* Socioeconomic status is considered an unmodifiable risk factor. Less affluent groups are at higher risk for CAD, probably due to a higher prevalence of risk factors such as smoking, hypertension, obesity, and sedentary lifestyle. There are many other unmodifiable risk factors. All other risk factors listed are modifiable to some extent.

VI-19. The answer is B. *(Ch. 38)* Fibrinogen levels do not correlate with dyslipidemia, thus providing additional risk information beyond lipid and lipoprotein measurement. The risk-to-benefit ratio for aspirin use in women to prevent MI is different from that of men. Evidence is not currently available to support fibrinogen reduction for CAD prevention. β-Adrenergic blocking agents reduce the incidence and complexity of ventricular arrhythmias, while ACE inhibitors probably slow the process of ventricular remodeling and may also bring about endogenous fibrinolysis. It is unclear whether ACE inhibitors are useful in prevention of MI in patients with normal left ventricular function, but are certainly indicated post MI in patients with ejection fractions less than 40 percent. However, a recently published study demonstrated a decrease in the risk of stroke in patients with cerebrovascular disease treated prophylactically with an ACE inhibitor.

VI-20.   The answer is E. *(Ch. 39)*   Origin of both right and left coronary arteries from the same sinus of Valsalva results in an ostium that is slit-like in shape. The acute angle of takeoff causes the normally round or oval ostium to become slit-like.

VI-21.   The answer is D. *(Ch. 39)*   Aneurysm formation in the coronary arteries can result from a number of conditions, including congenital abnormalities, atherosclerosis, trauma, complications of coronary intervention, arteritis, mycotic emboli, mucocutaneous lymph node syndrome, systemic lupus erythematosus, or dissection. The most common location for coronary artery emboli is the left anterior descending artery. Emboli to the left main coronary artery are rare and usually fatal. Secondary coronary artery dissections are more frequent than primary, especially those that are extensions of aortic root dissection. In coronary artery dissection, spiral dissections are among the most serious dissection injuries. There is a diminished potential for vasospasm in arteries that have advanced degrees of luminal narrowing by atherosclerotic plaques and coronary artery muscle depletion.

VI-22.   The answer is D. *(Ch. 39)*   The coronary adventitial layer is usually involved in a direct extension route of entry. The intimal layer is involved in a hematogenous route. Syphilitic arteritis, not tuberculosis, is characterized by chronic inflammation with adventitial fibrosis and patchy destruction of media with lymphoplasmacytic infiltrate. Takayasu's arteritis mainly effects young to middle-aged Asian females. Buerger's disease is a rare complication from placement of a saphenous vein bypass graft. Classic polyarteritis nodosa is manifest as infarction or hemorrhage in various target organs as the result of necrotizing vasculitis. In the infantile form, sparing of vessels other than the coronary arteries is seen.

VI-23.   The answer is B. *(Ch. 39)*   The major epicardial coronary arteries are affected by Hunter's and Hurler's diseases (mucopolysaccharidoses). Other disorders, such as primary oxalosis and Fabry's disease, affect smaller coronary vessels. Accelerated intimal fibrous hyperplasia is believed to be a result of damage from immunologic rejection. Metastatic myocardial lesions from various tumors are found in locations unrelated to coronary arterial supply zones and are usually surrounded by areas of normal myocardium. The intimal lesions seen in radiation-induced CAD consist of fibrous tissue without extracellular lipid deposits. Cocaine users may have coronary artery spasm and thrombosis. A disproportion of myocardial oxygen demand and supply is seen in conditions such as carbon monoxide poisoning, prolonged shock, and aortic valve stenosis.

VI-24.   The answer is A. *(Ch. 40)*   Baye's theorem states that the pretest prevalence of any condition influences the posttest likelihood of having the condition. A pretest prevalence of 50 percent is associated with the greatest accuracy of the posttest results. It is a fortunate coincidence that the pretest prevalence of CAD in middle-aged men who have atypical chest pain is about 50 percent. A resting 12-lead ECG will be normal in approximately 50 percent of patients with chronic stable angina. Simple clinical observations such as pain type, age, and sex are powerful predictors of the probability of CAD. For instance, in a middle-aged man, the presence of classical angina indicates a 95 percent likelihood of CAD. Chest roentgenograms are often normal in patients with stable angina pectoris. Exercise ECG has a relatively high specificity but a fairly low sensitivity for predicting CAD.

VI-25.   The answer is C. *(Ch. 40)*   Exercise stress testing is most valuable when the pretest probability is an intermediate risk of obstructive CAD (see previous answer). There are other reasons to perform exercise stress testing in patients with classical angina, foremost of which is to stratify the patient as to the risk of having a coronary event. Most patients do not need to undergo resting echocardiography for diagnostic evaluation of angina, unless there are physical examination findings suggesting a high-risk condition such as aortic stenosis or hypertrophic obstructive cardiomyopathy. Patients with LBBB should have cardiac stress testing for CAD diagnosis as opposed to having only ECG. Thallium-210 SPECT is more sensitive than planar imaging for diagnosing CAD. Coronary angiography will be most appropriate for a patient with a high-risk exercise stress test outcome.

VI-26. The answer is B. *(Ch. 40)* Myocardial contractility is a major determinant of MV_{O_2}, but is not usually a primary factor for therapeutic intervention. Nitrate therapy acts by decreasing preload, thus decreasing ventricular size and oxygen consumption. The vasodilator reserve is exhausted at coronary perfusion pressures less than 60 mm Hg. Blood flow at this pressure is directly related to perfusion pressure. There is a loss of some of the vasodilation mechanism in even early atherosclerosis. There is an increased response to vasoconstriction in even minimally diseased coronary arteries. Diseased arteries exhibit decreased vasodilation and increased vasoconstriction.

VI-27. The answer is E. *(Ch. 40)* The coronary microvasculature is likely the most important factor in angina pectoris, but lesions in the large epicardial coronaries are almost always responsible for acute coronary syndromes. There is no difference in the response to nonendothelial-dependent vasodilators between patients with capillary narrowing and controls, suggesting that the intrinsic ability of the capillaries to dilate is not affected by CAD. The phenomenon of mixed angina involves constriction in an epicardial stenosis and, sometimes simultaneously, in the microvasculature. The threshold for precipitating an anginal episode (or having an MI) has a circadian variation and is lowest in the morning hours. Anginal pain impulses from the heart travel in unmyelinated or small myelinated fibers through the spinothalamic tract to the thalamus and then to the cortex.

VI-28. The answer is D. *(Ch. 40)* A normal stress echocardiogram is consistent with a very low risk of having an MI. A Duke treadmill score of −11 indicates high risk. Features of a high-risk thallium-201 study are the stress-induced induction of one or more defects of at least moderate size, increased left ventricular size, or increased lung uptake of the radionuclide. An patient with an LVEF of 35 percent and known CAD is at high risk.

VI-29. The answer is C. *(Ch. 40)* β-Adrenergic blocking agents should be avoided in patients with asthma, COPD with bronchospasm, Raynaud's syndrome, severe peripheral vascular disease with rest ischemia, sinus bradycardia, and AV block. β-Adrenergic blocking agents may precipitate or worsen depression, but they are so effective in secondary prevention in the post MI state that their cautious use may be indicated. Many patients may require concomitant antidepressant therapy.

VI-30. The answer is D. *(Ch. 40)* Ticlopidine, a thienopyridine derivative that inhibits platelet aggregation, has not been shown to reduce cardiovascular events. In patients with known CAD, lipid lowering therapy has been shown to be effective in reducing cardiac events for any elevated level of cholesterol. The reduction in events and cost-effectiveness of this therapy, however, is greatest in patients with high cholesterol levels. β-Adrenergic blocking agents have the potential to increase coronary vascular resistance through cyclic AMP formation, although the clinical relevance of this has not been demonstrated. β-Adrenergic blocking agents combined with nitrates are more effective in decreasing the frequency of anginal episodes than treatment with β-adrenergic blocking agents alone, but nitrates have not been shown to decrease the risk of MI or death. Short-acting calcium channel antagonists have been shown to increase the risk of cardiac events. Treatment of hypertension in patients with known CAD should include β-adrenergic blocking agents and/or ACE inhibitors, since these agents have been shown to prolong survival in certain patients with CAD. A long-acting calcium antagonist may be appropriate as well.

VI-31.   **The answer is B.**   *(Ch. 41)*   Plaque erosion is more common in female smokers and diabetics, while hyperlipidemic men are more prone to plaque rupture. Interferon-gamma is produced by T lymphocytes and inhibits collagen production around the plaque. NF-κB is found in an inactive state in the cytoplasm of lymphocytes, monocytes, endothelial cells, and smooth muscle cells. After stimulation, it activates the transcription of interleukins, interferon, tumor necrosis factor-alpha, and adhesion molecules. It is a marker of inflammation and is elevated in patients with unstable angina. It is not elevated in patients with stable angina. Antibodies to cytomegalovirus or *Helicobacter* are not useful in predicting future coronary events; however, total mortality is higher in individuals with antibodies to *Helicobacter*. Two-thirds of lesions that progress to cause acute coronary events are less than 50 percent stenotic and are thus not targets for revascularization.

VI-32.   **The answer is E.**   *(Ch. 41)*   Unstable angina does not usually occur at rest and may not be relieved by nitroglycerin. Episodes of unstable angina are usually longer in duration than stable angina. A description of chest pain as sharp, jabbing, or knifelike is uncommon in unstable angina, although one study showed that 22 percent of people who described their pain in this way were found to have acute ischemia. All patients under age 50 who are suspected of having unstable angina, regardless of social class or ethnicity, should be questioned about cocaine use.

VI-33.   **The answer is C.**   *(Ch. 41)*   Women who present with unstable angina are less likely than men to have significant coronary lesions at coronary angiography. When ST depression is a persistent feature of unstable angina on ECGs recorded with or without chest pain, the finding is less specific for unstable angina. Myocardial stunning distal to the culprit lesion is probably responsible for the persistent T wave depression over the involved area. Only a minority of patients admitted with unstable angina will have elevated troponin levels. Troponin levels remain elevated for 1 week and are thus useful in making a diagnosis when a patient presents late following a coronary event.

VI-34.   **The answer is B.**   *(Ch. 41)*   Nitroglycerin reduces thrombin-induced platelet aggregation, and this effect does not disappear when nitroglycerin tolerance develops. Tolerance to the hemodynamic effects of intravenous nitroglycerin develops in as little as 24 to 48 h. Administration of captopril or *N*-acetylcysteine, both sulfhydryl donors, may be effective in avoiding nitrate tolerance, although unstable angina which fails to respond quickly to medical therapy is usually an indication for coronary angiography. Although β-adrenergic blocking agents are effective in reducing symptoms in patients with unstable angina, there is insufficient evidence to show that they reduce the risk of myocardial infarction in this setting. The calcium channel blockers diltiazem and verapamil are negative chronotropes and isotropes which decrease myocardial oxygen demand. Studies have shown that nifedipine is harmful when used in unstable angina patients who are not receiving β-adrenergic blocking agents.

VI-35.   **The answer is A.**   *(Ch. 41)*   Platelet GP IIb/IIIa inhibition at the time of angioplasty reduces ischemic complications. Symptoms in patients who have not previously taken antianginal drugs are much easier to control than those who have. Aspirin has a relatively large risk reduction rate for the prevention of death or nonfatal MI. There are some negative interactions between aspirin and ACE inhibitors, but studies demonstrating the great benefit of these agents make it reasonable to give them together. Clopidogrel has virtually replaced ticlopidine because of its better safely profile. A recent study has shown that there is a small but significant improvement in acute coronary syndrome outcomes using the combination of aspirin and clopidogrel together over aspirin alone. The cost-effectiveness of this combination has not been explored.

VI-36.   **The answer is D.**   *(Ch. 41)*   Unfractionated heparin has equivalent activity against factor Xa and thrombin, while LMWHs have greater activity against factor Xa. A disadvantage of regular heparin is that it inhibits activation of the protein C anticoagulant pathway more than a LMWH. For reasons that are unclear, thrombolytic therapy has been shown to increase event rates in unstable angina and non-ST-segment elevation myocardial infarctions. Hirudin is not recommended for use in patients with unstable angina, despite early benefits seen as compared to heparin. Hirudin has been shown to be more effective than both heparin and LMWHs in preventing venous thrombosis following total hip replacement. Hirudin has also been approved for use in patients with heparin-induced thrombocytopenia.

VI-37.   The answer is B.   *(Ch. 41)*   The underlying coronary lesion in variant angina, as demonstrated by coronary angiography, varies from subtotal occlusion to very mild stenosis. Surgery almost always eliminates variant angina and has an excellent long-term outcome. It was thought that either parasympathetic nervous system overactivity or reduced sympathetic activity contributed to coronary spasm, but evidence of coronary spasm in a denervated, transplanted heart has made this explanation unlikely. All patients with variant angina should undergo coronary angiography unless this is absolutely contraindicated, since angiography is the only method to distinguish between patients with organic multivessel disease and those with only mild narrowings or angiographically normal arteries. β-Adrenergic blockers should never be used in variant angina patients due to their propensity to increase the frequency and duration of attacks. Calcium channel blockers are very effective in preventing variant angina attacks.

VI-38.   The answer is B.   *(Ch. 42)*   The morning hours (6:00 A.M. to noon) are the time that the largest number of myocardial infarctions occurs. Pulmonary emboli can bring about a myocardial infarction by increasing an excess of catecholamines and adrenergic stimulation. Although a patient may not feel pain, it is highly unusual for a myocardial infarction to go unnoticed, as there are usually some symptoms, such as a dyspnea, nausea, palpitations, malaise, or fatigue. The majority of patients over age 75 who present with a documented MI do not have chest pain as their principal symptom. Sinus tachycardia present 12 to 24 h following a myocardial infarction is predictive of a high mortality rate. An inspiratory rise in jugular venous pressure (Küssmaul's sign) in patients with an acute inferior MI is highly abnormal and quite specific for right ventricular infarction.

VI-39.   The answer is D.   *(Ch. 42)*   The use of total CK without CK-MB is discouraged because of its poor specificity. Cardiac troponin I is a very specific test for an acute MI, since, as opposed to CK-MB, it is not up regulated in injured skeletal muscle. Myoglobin has only 26.3 percent sensitivity 2 h following an acute MI. If CK-MB accounts for less than 5 percent of total CK, skeletal muscle injury should be considered as the reason for the elevation. It has been traditional to use LDH enzymes to assess for myocardial infarction 48 to 72 h after symptoms, but the preferred diagnostic markers are now troponins I or T.

VI-40.   The answer is C.   *(Ch. 42)*   Segmental wall motion abnormalities of the left ventricle occur very rapidly after the onset of an acute MI and are best detected by echocardiography because of the quality of images, the wide availability of the study, and portability of the equipment. Unless pulmonary edema is present due to a severe complication of an MI (cardiogenic shock, papillary muscle dysfunction causing acute mitral regurgitation, or a new ventricular septal defect), there are usually no acute changes on a roentgenogram. This study, however, may be useful in detecting other causes of chest pain such as pneumothorax or aortic dissection. Magnetic resonance imaging and computed tomography are limited by the logistics of having to transport an acutely ill patient to the imaging facility. Radionuclide scintigraphy is limited in its use for patients with suspected MI to unusual cases where history, electrocardiographic changes, and plasma markers are unreliable or unavailable.

VI-41.   The answer is E.   *(Ch. 42)*   Despite the era of enhanced appreciation for atypical presentation, increased potential for litigation, and decreased threshold for admission, the missed diagnosis rate of an acute MI has remained relatively constant around 4 percent. The administration of nitroglycerin may relieve esophageal spasm in patients with gastrointestinal disturbances. It has been routine to give oxygen to patients with an acute MI for several days, although elevated concentrations may cause vasospasm, oxygen is expensive to administer, and there is no data to suggest that it effects outcomes in patients with normal O_2 concentrations. Thus, there is little justification for extending oxygen use in uncomplicated MIs beyond 2 to 3 h. The bulk of evidence does not justify the routine, long-term use of nitrates in uncomplicated acute MI. However, intravenous nitroglycerin early after acute infarction is justified for pain management. All patients who present with acute ST-segment elevation should be considered for rapid reperfusion, since this strategy has been demonstrated to prolong survival and help preserve LV function.

VI-42. **The answer is D.** *(Ch. 42)* Recent studies have shown that primary angioplasty has equivalent or slightly better outcomes than thrombolytic therapy. Primary angioplasty should be performed only by operators skilled at this technique and in facilities which have appropriate equipment and staff. Primary angioplasty has basically the same indications as thrombolytic therapy and may also be useful in patients with contraindications to thrombolytic therapy, such as severe hypertension. Patients who present with an acute coronary syndrome and ST-segment depression do not benefit and may be harmed by thrombolytic therapy, the reasons for which are unclear. There is much controversy surrounding the use of primary PCI in ST-segment depression infarcts.

VI-43. **The answer is E.** *(Ch. 42)* Primary angioplasty has at least equivalent or possibly superior outcomes to thrombolytic therapy, but it must be performed by skilled clinicians supported by experienced personnel in an appropriate laboratory within 2 h of the onset of symptoms. The time delay in transferring a patient to an appropriate facility and the increased cost of this therapy may limit its benefits. Intravenous heparin is preferred in patients with a large or anterior myocardial infarction, atrial fibrillation, a known left ventricular thrombus, or a previous embolism. Rescue angioplasty is not recommended as a routine strategy for failed thrombolysis, since the adverse event rate has been shown to be the same as not undertaking PCI. Atropine should be used in patients with symptomatic bradycardia or significant AV block. Prognosis in acute MI is related primarily to the amount of myocardium lost. Inferior infarctions with relatively little myocardial loss may cause ischemia of the AV node and thus significant AV block. Anterior infarctions cause heart block by damaging both bundle branches, a complication of a large amount of muscle loss, and hence have a much worse diagnosis.

VI-44. **The answer is A.** *(Ch. 42)* Non-ST-segment elevation MI is the current preferred term for what was previously called non-Q-wave MI. This change has been suggested because the American Heart Association/American College of Cardiology practice guidelines for the management of acute chest pain utilize the initial ECG as a decision point for evaluation and treatment. Before the results of cardiac enzymes are available, it may not be possible to determine whether infarction has occurred. In any case, recent studies have shown that enoxiparin is modestly superior to unfractionated heparin for treating patients with unstable angina or non-ST-segment elevation MI. Non-ST-segment elevation infarctions usually involve less myocardial loss, probably because there is less than total compromise of blood flow to a region of myocardium or because early reperfusion occurs. Due to the residual noninfarcted myocardium at risk distal to a disrupted plaque in patients with non-ST-segment elevation MI, there is a high risk for recurrent ischemia, infarction, and death. Secondary prevention is essential after any type of MI. Diltiazem and particularly verapamil are contraindicated in the treatment of acute MI with associated left ventricular failure. β-Adrenergic blocking agents have not been shown to reduce the reinfarction rate in patients recovering from non-ST-segment elevation infarctions.

VI-45. **The answer is D.** *(Ch. 42)* The recurrence of chest pain following any acute MI, particularly if accompanied by ECG changes, is associated with an increased mortality rate and increased incidence of reinfarction. Indomethacin relieves the symptoms of postinfarction pericarditis, but it causes thinning of the developing scar, which may increase the likelihood of ventricular aneurysm or even rupture. Diastolic dysfunction generally precedes systolic dysfunction in heart failure in acute MI. Abnormal right ventricular function following an inferior MI returns to normal in most patients; thus it is attributed to stunning rather than substantial muscle loss. One of the major objectives in the treatment of a patient with right ventricular infarction is to maintain preload, so diuretics should be used with caution.

VI-46. **The answer is B.** *(Ch. 42)* Digoxin is a relatively weak inotropic agent and is not the drug of choice for heart failure in MI. It is more useful to control the ventricular rate in atrial fibrillation. Invasive monitoring is not necessary in uncomplicated acute MI as long as there is careful clinical observation. Dobutamine is a positive inotrope which increases myocardial contractility. Dopamine, on the other hand, is a peripheral vasoconstrictor at moderate to high doses. The most common cause of in-hospital death following MI is cardiogenic shock. Afterload reduction therapy, typically with an ACE inhibitor, should be utilized before diuretics in patients with pulmonary congestion in AMI. Acute MI patients may be critically dependent on adequate preload for the maintenance of cardiac output.

VI-47. **The answer is B.** *(Ch. 42)* Prophylactic anticoagulant therapy should be given to patients following MI who have risk factors for deep venous thrombosis and pulmonary embolism. A pseudoaneurysm, a narrow-based, sac-like structure, is more likely to rupture than a true aneurysm. A ventricular thrombus is much more likely to form in an anterior MI. The location of aneurysms is usually anterior, anteroapical, or apical. It is rare to find them posteriorally. The prognosis for patients with an aneurysm is related to left ventricular function, not the aneurysm, as the risk of rupture is low.

VI-48. **The answer is E.** *(Ch. 42)* Sinus tachycardia following acute MI is common and is an unfavorable prognostic sign. Episodes of paroxysmal supraventricular tachycardia occur commonly, but are usually transient and are unrelated to prognosis. Atrial flutter is relatively uncommon. Right coronary occlusion is responsible for more than 80 percent of inferior infarctions. SA and AV nodal dysfunction is common in patients with an inferior MI. The development of AV conduction abnormalities in this setting does not adversely effect prognosis.

VI-49. **The answer is C.** *(Ch. 44)* In saphenous vein graft disease, the intermediate phase is characterized by intimal hyperplasia, but the late phase involves atherosclerosis similar to that which occurs in the native coronary arteries. Macrophages and T lymphocytes found at the site of a disrupted plaque are in the activated state. A platelet monolayer forms the first layer in a thrombus. Of all plaque types, the lipid-rich plaque displays the most atherogenicity. The extrinsic pathway of the coagulation cascade, initiated by the release of tissue factor, is the predominant mechanism for initiating hemostasis.

VI-50. **The answer is D.** *(Ch. 44)* Tissue factor X must make contact with blood to function. Factors V and VIII require activation by minor proteolysis. A congenital deficiency of the three contact factors (factor XII, prekallikrein, and HMW kininogen) is not associated with bleeding problems. A deficiency of factor VIII and IX, however, results in a severe bleeding condition. Factor VII is activated by tissue factor as well as by phospholipids on platelet membranes, in conjunction with factor Xa. This feature represents a bridge between the intrinsic and extrinsic pathways. For factor Xa to be fully active, it must form a complex with factor Va. Factor XIII contributes to the stability of the fibrin network.

VI-51. **The answer is A.** *(Ch. 44)* The presence of fibrin greatly enhances the plasminogen activating property of t-PA. Vascular endothelial cells synthesize t-PA. The effect of thrombin on fibrinolysis is mediated through the activation of protein C. Various stimuli, such as physical exercise, catecholamines, bradykinin, or desmopressin, produce a rapid increase in t-PA levels in the blood. PAI-1 mRNA has been demonstrated in a wide variety of tissues, suggesting that common cells in these tissues may be the sites of production. PAI-1 is found in plasma, platelets, placenta, and extracellular matrix. PAI-1 binds to its target in a 1:1 stoichiometric reversible complex.

VI-52. **The answer is E.** *(Ch. 44)* Aspirin does not inhibit the adherence of the initial layer of platelets to the subendothelium or atherosclerotic plaque, nor does aspirin oppose the release of granules from the platelet. Aspirin does not appear to have a dose-related response in its efficacy, as doses between 75 and 1300 mg/day have produced similar reductions in cardiovascular events. The antiaggregating effects of thienopyridines are concentration dependent. The rate of recovery is linked to platelet survival, which suggests that effect on platelets is permanent. Clopidogrel is six times more potent than ticlopidine in the inhibition of ADP-induced aggregation of human platelets. Ticlopidine combined with aspirin has been shown to reduce thrombosis and recurrent ischemic attacks in patients undergoing coronary stent implantation.

VI-53. **The answer is B.** *(Ch. 44)* Abciximab binds the GP IIb/IIIa receptor very tightly, thus its effects last much longer than the infusion period. If bleeding occurs, stopping the drug will not reverse the antiplatelet effect immediately. In a recent study in patients with an evolving non-ST-elevation MI, GP IIb/IIIa inhibitors may reduce the size of or even prevent the development of myocardial necrosis. In another study, abciximab used in the setting of an acute MI treated with primary coronary intervention a decrease in the 30-day event rate of death, new MI, or need for revascularization. However, there were no differences in these endpoints at 6 months. Data from several studies shows that GP IIb/IIIa inhibitors should be administered concomitantly with heparin. Tirofiban and eptifibatide both have short half-lives, so antiplatelet activity reverses a few hours after stopping the drug.

VI-54. **The answer is C.** *(Ch. 44)* Sibrafan has a relatively high incidence of minor bleeding at levels that achieve effective, chronic platelet inhibition. Sibrafan also had twice the rate of minor bleeding when given twice, rather than once, per day. There is a moderate amount of evidence that there is a synergistic effect of aspirin and oral GP IIb/IIIa in combination. For one thing, aspirin and GP IIb/IIIa inhibitors inhibit different steps in the formation of a platelet thrombus. Thrombocytopenia generally occurs early in treatment with oral GP IIb/IIIa inhibitors but is well tolerated during long-term follow-up. There has been interpatient variability observed in drug level and degree of platelet inhibition. The strategy of dosing oral GP IIb/IIIa inhibitors by monitoring the degree of platelet inhibition or drug level in patients may need to be employed.

VI-55. **The answer is E.** *(Ch. 44)* It has been shown that in plasma about 20 times more heparin is needed to inactivate fibrin-bound thrombin than to inactivate free thrombin. Therefore, more heparin is needed to prevent the extension of venous thrombosis than to prevent formation of the initial thrombus. The bioavailability of unfractionated heparin after subcutaneous injection is about 30 percent, as opposed to LMWH which has a bioavailability after subcutaneous injection of >90 percent. The risk of bleeding is higher when unfractionated heparin is give by intermittent infusion, rather than continuous infusion or subcutaneously. There is an increase in vascular permeability with unfractionated heparin. Lower initial doses of heparin in the setting of thrombolytic therapy reduce the risk of major bleeding.

VI-56. **The answer is D.** *(Ch. 44)* Factor Xa bound to the platelet membrane in the prothrombinase complex is resistant to inactivation by unfractionated heparin, but is not resistant to inactivation by LMWHs. LMWHs have a longer half-life than unfractionated heparins. LMWHs exhibit less interpatient variability of the anticoagulant response than unfractionated heparins. There is no difference in the rate of recurrence of ischemic events between high and low doses of enoxaparin, but high doses (1.25 mg/kg twice per day) have an unacceptably high rate of major hemorrhage. Danaparoid sodium may be associated with fewer and briefer bleeding episodes than heparin.

VI-57. **The answer is C.** *(Ch. 44)* Warfarin depresses the synthesis of four vitamin K-dependent procoagulants, factors II, VII, IX, and X. It also depresses the synthesis of two natural inhibitor proteins C and S.

VI-58. **The answer is B.** *(Ch. 44)* All thrombolytic drugs, whether they are endogenous to humans or not, are plasminogen activators. A few days following streptokinase administration, the antistreptokinase titer rises significantly and remains elevated for 4 to 6 months. During this time, it may be hazardous to use streptokinase again. Patients who have a high titer of streptokinase antibodies do not respond well to treatment with anistreplase, as the latter also causes an increase in the streptokinase antibody titer. Plasmin that is formed on the fibrin surface is inhibited slowly by α_2-antiplasmin, while free plasmin is inhibited rapidly. The plasmin-staphylokinase complex is rapidly inhibited by α_2-antiplasmin, but not the plasmin (ogen)-streptokinase complex.

VI-59.   The answer is D.   *(Ch. 45)*   Aspirin and ticlopidine were shown to have a lower rate of stent thrombosis than aspirin alone or aspirin combined with warfarin. Later studies, however, showed that ticlopidine was associated with about 20 deaths due to thrombotic thrombocytopenic purpura. Since then, clopidogrel has been widely used instead. The Gianturco-Roubin flex stent made balloon angioplasty much safer, but was still complicated by stent thrombosis in 5 to 10 percent of patients and bleeding was a common complication. The original Palmaz-Schatz stent revolutionized interventional cardiology. The 1-year survival free of death, MI, and reintervention rates are higher in the surgical group as opposed to the stent group, but at an increased cost. Patients treated with IIb/IIIa platelet receptor inhibitors have shown decreased composite endpoints of death or nonfatal MI in the setting of coronary intervention and in acute coronary syndromes. Diabetics who were treated with abciximab while undergoing stent placement had lower rates of repeat target vessel revascularization.

VI-60.   The answer is C.   *(Ch. 45)*   The favorable cost-effectiveness of percutaneous intervention is seen mostly in single-vessel disease. Patients with multivessel disease are more likely to have recurrence and need repeat procedures. Complete revascularization has superior long-term results, with fewer late interventions after angioplasty, but it is achieved in only a minority of patients with multivessel disease. The risk of percutaneous coronary intervention increases in the presence of unstable angina, advanced age, poor left ventricular function, extensive coronary artery disease, comorbid conditions, and female gender. The risk of mortality is higher in stented diabetics than in stented nondiabetics. Patients with unstable angina account for a majority of coronary interventions, but they have an increased risk of abrupt closure.

VI-61.   The answer is A.   *(Ch. 45)*   A lesion with heavy calcification is a type B lesion and has a moderate success rate at 60 to 85 percent and moderate risk. An eccentric lesion is also a type B lesion. A diffuse (>2 cm length) lesion is a type C lesion which has a low success rate and high risk. In-stent restenosis is a new "disease." It is characterized by neointimal proliferation as opposed to a combination of negative remodeling and intimal proliferation that is seen in nonstented lesions.

VI-62.   The answer is D.   *(Ch. 45)*   Complication rates in coronary intervention have declined, despite the increasingly difficult cases being performed. The strongest predictor of a major complication is the appearance of an intimal dissection during the procedure. Dissection has a six-fold increase in the risk of a major complication. The risk of perforation with laser angioplasty is highest in right coronary lesions. One of the newest causes of perforation is the use of the hydrophilic coronary guidewire, which easily penetrates the wall of small distal arteries. Patients at increased risk of microparticular embolization from rotational atherectomy are those who have bulky or long native vessel lesions and nonfocal or thrombotic saphenous vein graft lesions.

VI-63.   The answer is E.   *(Ch. 46)*   Low-risk patients have no survival benefit from primary angioplasty, but they do benefit from less reinfarction, less recurrent ischemia, higher infarct artery patency rates, and better left ventricular function without the risk of intracranial hemorrhage. A greater proportion of patients are eligible for primary coronary intervention than thrombolytic therapy, as 75 to 80 percent of patients are ineligible for thrombolytic therapy. Reperfusion therapy is not useful in most patients presenting 12 h or more after the onset of symptoms, except for patients who have persistent ischemic chest pain. These patients frequently have collateral flow from another coronary artery and have been shown to have substantial recovery of left ventricular function following primary angioplasty. Reperfusion rates in patients with acute MI due to saphenous vein graft occlusion are much lower than those with native vessel occlusion. The cost of primary angioplasty is less than that for thrombolytic therapy, due to shorter, less complicated hospital courses. Thrombolytic therapy is associated with higher drug costs and more need for subsequent cardiac catheterization and possible intervention.

VI-64.   The answer is C. *(Ch. 46)*   Patients with acute MI at highest risk for mortality include patients with cardiogenic shock, elderly patients, patients with anterior wall myocardial infarction, and women. Patients with nonanterior wall infarctions have no mortality benefit from primary angioplasty.

VI-65.   The answer is B. *(Ch. 46)*   TIMI 3 flow is achieved in more than 90 percent of patients who undergo primary angioplasty, regardless of the time to treatment. If reperfusion cannot be established by passing a guidewire through the occlusion, the occlusion should be crossed with the balloon and then withdrawn, without inflating the balloon. More gradual reperfusion may result in fewer reperfusion arrhythmias. With few exceptions, only the infarct artery should be dilated in primary angioplasty. Dilating noninfarct arteries places too much myocardium acutely in jeopardy. Trials with intraaortic balloon counterpulsation in high-risk patients show little benefit when used alone without reperfusion or revascularization. With the advent of coronary stenting, there is now little benefit gained from intraaortic balloon counterpulsation after primary angioplasty in hemodynamically stable patients.

VI-66.   The answer is D. *(Ch. 47)*   The early, subtle changes in atherosclerosis, like fatty streaks, are not visible with current ultrasound devices. Lipid-laden lesions are usually hypoechoic. Fibromuscular lesions produce soft, low-intensity echoes. Visualizing a zone of reduced echogenicity is not diagnostic of a thrombus, because lipid deposition, thrombus, and necrotic degeneration all exhibit this finding. If no calcification is visible on angiogram, there is little chance of detecting a superficial arc of calcium on ultrasound. In vitro studies have shown limitations in reliably detecting thrombi.

VI-67.   The answer is E. *(Ch. 47)*   There is only moderate correlation between angiographic and ultrasonic dimensions on atherosclerotic arteries. The greatest disparities are seen in vessel segments with a noncircular lumen shape. Trailing-edge measurements are unreliable, but leading edge measurements accurately describe the location of a boundary. Studies have shown poor correlation between the apparent circumferential pattern seen by angiography and the actual plaque distribution shown by ultrasound. Ultrasound is frequently better than angiography for quantifying left main coronary artery lesions. There has been no worse prognosis in patients with atherosclerosis that was only detected by ultrasound.

VI-68.   The answer is A. *(Ch. 47)*   Ultrasound detection of superficial calcium predicts poor tissue retrieval in directional atherectomy. It is untested whether production of a larger postprocedure lumen by ultrasound-guided atherectomy results in a lower restenosis rate without an increase in complications. Demonstration of a heavily calcified lesion by either angiography or ultrasound is an indication for rotational ablation. Ultrasound imaging results in additional procedures in approximately 20 to 40 percent of cases following high-pressure coronary stenting. Interventions designed to reduce chronic recoil, such as stenting, may be more important in preventing restenosis than interventions designed to prevent intimal hyperplasia.

VI-69.   The answer is D. *(Ch. 48)*   Grafts occluded within 1 to 2 months following surgery exhibit thrombosis. Grafts examined more than a few months following surgery show hypercellular, proliferative hyperplasia involving the intima. Vein graft atherosclerosis is distributed throughout the length of vein grafts, is circumferential, is not encapsulated, and is extremely friable. Native coronary artery atherosclerosis is a proximal, eccentric, and intermittent lesion that is covered by a fibrous cap. Bilateral internal mammary grafting has not become widespread in use, takes longer, and may increase wound complications. However, there is evidence that bilateral internal mammary grafting does offer incremental benefit because of the superior graft patency rate with these vessels. The gastroepiploic artery has been shown to function well as a graft to the posterior descending branch of the right coronary artery or branches of the circumflex coronary artery. Left internal mammary grafts are superior to radial artery grafts in terms of patency. Radial artery grafts, however, may be superior to vein grafts over the long term if they prove to be resistant to graft atherosclerosis.

VI-70. The answer is B. *(Ch. 48)* Three variables have the greatest predictive value of in-hospital death following bypass surgery: acuteness of operation, age and previous surgery. Lesser indicators of risk include gender, left ventricular ejection fraction, left main coronary artery percent stenosis, and number of coronary systems with more than 70 percent stenosis.

VI-71. The answer is B. *(Ch. 48)* There seems to be a decrease in hospital mortality with the use of internal mammary grafts. Obesity and diabetes are implicated in increasing the risk of sternal complications following bypass surgery. Cold cardioplegia in patients undergoing bypass surgery in the face of acute ischemia seems to provide incremental benefit. The most important predictor for type I neurologic abnormalities is proximal aortic atherosclerosis. Patients with unstable angina and a history of stroke are also at increased risk of type I deficits.

VI-72. The answer is C. *(Ch. 48)* Very young and very elderly patients have a decreased survival rate following bypass surgery. Typical candidates for reoperation underwent primary surgery more 10 years ago, had triple-vessel disease at that time, and need reoperation at least in part due to graft failure. Emergency operation produces a large increase in risk. Late stenoses in vein grafts are more dangerous lesions than native coronary lesions. Patients who had early vein graft stenoses did not have an improved survival rate with surgery, although they did have fewer symptoms at follow-up.

VI-73. The answer is E. *(Ch. 49)* The transient myocardial depression is attributed to the inflammatory state induced by cardiopulmonary bypass (CPB). Depressed myocardial function is unrelated to the CPB time, number of coronary artery grafts, preoperative medications, or postoperative core temperatures. Hypothermia causes peripheral vasoconstriction, and may contribute to the hypertension frequently observed following cardiac surgery. There is generally no localized bleeding site found on exploration when severe postoperative bleeding occurs. If vasodilatation with increased venous capacitance is responsible for hypotension following bypass surgery, colloid administration will provide a longer-lasting augmentation of intravascular volume.

VI-74. The answer is A. *(Ch. 49)* Sinus tachycardia is the most common rhythm disturbance following bypass surgery and should be managed by treatment of the underlying cause. Frequent causes include pain, anxiety, low cardiac output, anemia, fever, or beta-blocker withdrawal. Ventricular ectopy is the second most common rhythm disturbance. Although increases in systemic vasculature resistance can impede ventricular ejection and lower cardiac output, the most common cause of low cardiac output postoperatively is due to decreased left ventricular preload. Nitroglycerin should be given to patient with high filling pressures and active myocardial ischemia. Hydralazine, a direct arterial vasodilator, is usually more appropriate several days following surgery in hemodynamically stable patients with hypertension. Ventricular fibrillation or sustained ventricular tachycardia following surgery can be seen in the absence of evidence of acute myocardial ischemia or infarction or electrolyte imbalance.

VI-75. The answer is D. *(Ch. 49)* Pulmonary problems are the most significant cause of morbidity following cardiac surgery. Lung water is usually normal following routine CPB. If increased capillary permeability does exist, it is generally related to elevated cardiac filling pressures. A common mistake is to not give patients opioids during bypass surgery or postoperatively, due to fear of respiratory depression. Atelectasis is the most common pulmonary complication following bypass surgery. The inhaled form of potent bronchodilators given to patients with bronchospasm following bypass surgery have minimal effects on the cardiovascular system.

VI-76. **The answer is D.** *(Ch. 49)* Transient elevations in liver function tests may occur after cardiac surgery, but the appearance of jaundice has a poor prognosis. Hypomagnesemia is a relatively common occurrence following cardiac surgery using CPB. The most common cause of fever following surgery is atelectasis, since 70 percent of patients have this complication following surgery. The risk of postbypass renal failure is related to the patient's underlying renal function. Development of encephalopathy or delirium following bypass surgery is generally transient.

VI-77. **The answer is A.** *(Ch. 50)* Although young patients usually have an increase in stroke volume during exercise, elderly patients have an increased heart rate without an increased stroke volume. An improvement in resting ejection fraction frequently occurs in both exercising and control patients, probably because of the recovery of hypofunctioning myocardium following revascularization and not exercise per se. Activity related symptoms, like angina, dyspnea, and claudication are usually reduced following exercise training. Patients were previously advised to exercise to a heart rate of 70 to 85 percent of the heart rate safely achieved during exercise testing, but recent data suggest that a more appropriate rate is 50 to 70 percent. The latter produces comparable improvements in functional capacity and endurance with less risk of cardiovascular complications. Beta-blocker therapy decreases the heart rate and blood pressure response to exercise, but does not attenuate the improvement in physical work capacity gained during exercise training.

VI-78. **The answer is C.** *(Ch. 50)* Continuous ECG monitoring has not been shown to provide added safety to low-risk patients during supervised exercise. No complications or adverse outcomes have been shown in elderly patients in cardiac rehabilitation, but the rates of referral, however, are lower in elderly than in young patients. Elderly patients who have been referred to cardiac rehabilitation have shown high adherence to exercise training and significant reduction in risk factors. The 6-month mortality rate in patients with coronary heart disease who live alone is double that of patients who live with others, perhaps due to depression. Left ventricular ejection fraction is a poor predictor of exercise capacity and potential for improvement of symptoms. Some patients with substantial left ventricular dysfunction have a normal exercise capacity. The rate at which patients return to work following a coronary artery bypass graft is less favorable than anticipated, despite a decrease in symptoms, improvement in functional capacity, and reported enhancement of life quality.

PART VII
SYSTEMIC ARTERIAL HYPERTENSION

VII. SYSTEMIC ARTERIAL HYPERTENSION

QUESTIONS

DIRECTIONS: Each question listed below contains five suggested responses. Select the **one best** response to each question.

VII-1. Which of the following statements regarding the pathophysiology of hypertension is true?

(A) the sympathetic nervous system is responsible for long-term blood volume and blood pressure control

(B) a defect in sodium excretion in hypertensive patients is most likely genetically determined

(C) vasopressin is involved in the genesis of hypertension

(D) endothelin plays an important role in the etiology of essential hypertension

(E) atherosclerosis plays a major role in the development of hypertension

(pages 1556–1558)

VII-2. Which of the following statements regarding the pathophysiology of hypertension is true?

(A) increases in intracellular sodium cause an elevated systolic blood pressure

(B) there is a correlation between high-risk groups associated with salt-dependent essential hypertension and tubulointerstitial disease

(C) in salt-sensitive individuals, the sympathetic nervous system is inhibited with salt loading

(D) there need not be a genetic predisposition to develop insulin resistance

(E) several "hypertensive genes" have been located

(pages 1558–1560)

VII-3. Which of the following statements best describes blood pressure measurements?

(A) an inaccurately low blood pressure may be measured if the cuff is too small

(B) blood pressure measurements can underestimate true intraarterial pressure in elderly patients with extensive peripheral atherosclerosis

(C) blood pressure differences of 20 to 30 mm Hg are often found when blood pressure is measured in both arms, even in the absence of advanced atherosclerosis

(D) the normal blood pressure response to standing is a slight decrease in systolic and a slight increase in diastolic pressure with little change in mean arterial pressure

(E) orthostatic hypertension has been associated with abnormally low norepinephrine levels

(pages 1561–1562)

VII-4. Which of the following statements regarding the diagnosis of hypertension is true?

(A) a nurse measuring blood pressure in a physician's office would not cause "white coat" hypertension

(B) blood pressure measurements in the leg are not necessary in hypertensive patients

(C) there has been no correlation between lower home blood pressure measurements, as compared to those in the physician's office, and reduced cardiovascular events

(D) there is no difference in risk of cardiovascular events in those who display nocturnal dipping of blood pressure and those who do not

(E) blood pressure measurements in a physician's office more accurately predict left ventricular hypertrophy or cardiac damage resulting from high blood pressure than ambulatory blood pressure measurements

(pages 1562–1564)

VII-5. Which of the following statements regarding the evaluation of the hypertensive patient is true?

(A) a diagnosis of hypertension should be made on the first recording of an elevated blood pressure

(B) left ventricular hypertrophy (LVH) among hypertensive patients is the most powerful predictor of death, myocardial infarction (MI), and stroke

(C) papilledema in most patients results from a hypertensive emergency

(D) an ECG is not necessary in most persons with hypertension

(E) elderly patients with elevated blood pressure from "stiff" arteries, do not benefit from blood pressure lowering treatment

(pages 1565–1569)

VII-6. Which of the following statements regarding evaluation for identifiable causes of hypertension is true?

(A) primary aldosteronism is the most common identifiable cause of hypertension

(B) fibromuscular dysplasia causes the majority of renovascular hypertension

(C) when renal activity is initially normal and becomes abnormal after captopril in isotopic renography, the likelihood of a cure or improvement after revascularization is low

(D) patients with a history of hypertension that has been easy to control and then has become refractory are most likely to have atherosclerotic renal artery stenosis

(E) the presence of an anatomic renal artery stenosis is an indication that that is the cause of the elevated blood pressure

(pages 1569–1571)

VII-7. Which of the following statements best characterizes patients with hypertension secondary to fibrous dysplasia?

(A) the onset of symptoms occurs typically in the fifth decade

(B) a positive family history of hypertension is more likely than in essential hypertension

(C) women are more often afflicted than men

(D) obesity is common

(E) severe retinopathy (grade III or IV) is evident on fundoscopic examination

(pages 1569–1573)

VII-8. Which of the following statements regarding evaluation for identifiable causes of hypertension is true?

(A) an elevated blood pressure may be the first sign for a variety of unusual conditions, such as

17-α-hydroxylase deficiency, Ask-Upmark kidney, or Cushing's disease

(B) pallor is a typical finding in patients with an epinephrine-producing pheochromocytoma

(C) the measurement of plasma catecholamines is the most useful test for detecting pheochromocytoma

(D) the most common cause of primary aldosteronism is hyperplasia of the zona glomerulosa layer of the adrenal cortex

(E) patients rarely become normotensive following surgical excision of an aldosterone-producing adenoma

(pages 1571–1573)

VII-9. Which of the following hypertensive patients would be the most likely to lower his or her blood pressure?

(A) a patient taking antihypertensives alone

(B) a patient lowering Na^+ intake and reducing his or her weight

(C) a patient reducing his or her stress level and taking antihypertensives

(D) a patient taking antihypertensives and reducing his or her weight

(E) a patient reducing alcohol intake to two drinks a day

(pages 1573–1575)

VII-10. Which of the following statements regarding the pharmacologic treatment of hypertension is true?

(A) the goal for blood pressure reduction in patients is a systolic blood pressure of 130 mm Hg and diastolic blood pressure of 85 mm Hg

(B) more aggressive therapy to achieve a greater reduction in blood pressure is not cost-effective

(C) it has not been proven that changes in serum lipids caused by certain antihypertensives are harmful in patients with dyslipidemias

(D) centrally acting alpha agonists are appropriate for initial treatment of hypertension

(E) moderate- and high-dose thiazides improve insulin sensitivity

(pages 1577–1583)

VII-11. The preferred drug given as monotherapy in managing the hypertension associated with preeclampsia is

(A) hydralazine

(B) methyldopa

(C) minoxidil

(D) prazosin

(E) phentolamine

(pages 1577–1583)

VII-12. Which of the following statements regarding pharmacologic treatment of hypertension is true?

(A) patients with hypertension and low ejection fractions (systolic heart failure) have both improved blood pressure control and long-term prognosis with diltiazem or verapamil

(B) positive inotropic agents are most effective in treating aortic insufficiency in hypertensives

(C) short-acting dihydropyridine calcium channel antagonists are effective agents in reducing microalbuminuria in hypertensives

(D) following a stroke, blood pressure should always be reduced quickly to prevent a hypertensive emergency

(E) β-adrenergic blocking agents and calcium channel antagonists are effective antihypertensive treatment in patients with coronary artery disease

(pages 1584–1586)

VII-13. Which of the following statements regarding the special considerations involved in the pharmacologic treatment of hypertension is true?

(A) the incidence of clinical side effects rises with increasing doses in all classes of antihypertensives

(B) suddenly lowering blood pressure in a patient with a hypertensive crisis may be detrimental

(C) peripheral alpha blockers and calcium channel antagonists are more effective in blacks than in whites

(D) higher doses of antihypertensives are generally necessary in older patients

(E) hypertension during pregnancy does not predict future health problems for the woman

(pages 1587–1589)

VII. SYSTEMIC ARTERIAL HYPERTENSION

ANSWERS

VII-1. The answer is E. *(Ch. 51)* The kidney is responsible for the long-term regulation of blood volume and blood pressure. The sympathetic nervous system and the renin-angiotensin-aldosterone system are responsible for short-term changes in blood pressure. It has been shown that salt restriction is not important in normotensive patients and hypertensive patients under age 40. This supports the fact that defects in sodium excretion are more likely acquired than genetically determined. It has been shown that vasopressin is not involved in the genesis of hypertension, but it does play a role in the maintenance of established hypertension. The role of endothelin in essential hypertension is minimal. It plays a greater role in cyclosporine-induced hypertension and decreased renal function. Atherosclerosis plays a major role in the development of hypertension. It does so through interference with nitric oxide release or synthesis, which is vital to the maintenance of normal blood pressure.

VII-2. The answer is B. *(Ch. 51)* Increased intracellular sodium is highly correlated with an elevated diastolic blood pressure. A correlation exists between tubulointerstitial disease and high-risk groups associated with salt-dependent essential hypertension, particularly the elderly, African Americans, and obese patients. The normal response to a salt load is inhibition of the sympathetic nervous system. In salt-sensitive individuals, however, the sympathetic nervous system is not inhibited but may even be activated by a salt load. There appears to be a genetic predisposition to insulin resistance. Despite intense ongoing efforts, there has been no success to date in locating "hypertensive genes."

VII-3. The answer is D. *(Ch. 51)* False elevations of blood pressure occur frequently if regular-sized blood pressure cuffs are used in adult patients whose midarm circumference exceeds 33 cm. Auscultatory measurements can also overestimate intraarterial pressure in some elderly patients, presumably because of "pipe stem" arteries stiffened by extensive peripheral atherosclerosis. Blood pressure should be measured initially in both arms, and all subsequent determinations should be performed in the arm with the highest pressure. Differences greater than 10 mm Hg are unusual in the absence of advanced arteriosclerosis. The normal blood pressure response to standing is a slight decrease in systolic and slight increase in diastolic pressure with little change in mean arterial pressure. The usual criteria for orthostatic hypotension is a standing reduction in systolic pressure of 20 mm Hg or more, or a mean arterial pressure of 10 percent or more. Orthostatic hypertension (i.e., an increase in diastolic pressure exceeding 8 to 10 mm Hg upon standing) is associated with elevated norepinephrine levels and evidence of increased neurogenic tone.

VII-4. The answer is A. *(Ch. 51)* "White coat" hypertension results from an approaching physician who is not previously known to the patient. A nurse taking a patient's blood pressure usually does not provoke "white coat" hypertension. Blood pressure measurements should routinely be performed in the leg of young hypertensive patients. There has been a correlation between lower cardiovascular events and patients with much lower home blood pressure measurements, as compared with those in the physician's office. There is a higher risk of a cardiovascular event in patients who do not display nocturnal dipping of blood pressure. Ambulatory blood pressure measurements are a better predictor of left ventricular hypertrophy and cardiac function than blood pressure measurements obtained in a physician's office.

VII-5. **The answer is B.** *(Ch. 51)*   There is considerable normal variation in blood pressure, so a diagnosis of hypertension should not be made without at least two or three separate measurements on different occasions. LVH in hypertensive patients is the most powerful predictor of death, MI, stroke, heart failure, and other cardiovascular end points. Papilledema, when seen in the absence of exceedingly high blood pressure and no other evidence of target organ damage, most likely has another cause. An ECG is recommended as part of the initial evaluation of patients with hypertension. It is a useful and cost-effective way to diagnose and/or exclude LVH. There is strong evidence that elderly patients with hypertension and "stiff" arteries benefit from lowering their blood pressure.

VII-6. **The answer is D.** *(Ch. 51)*   The most common identifiable cause of hypertension is chronic renal failure. The majority of cases of renovascular hypertension are due to renal artery atherosclerosis. Only a small percentage are due to either fibromuscular dysplasia or unusual causes. When activity of the kidneys is initially normal and becomes abnormal after captopril in isotopic renography, the likelihood of a cure or improvement after revascularization is high. Renal artery atherosclerotic stenosis is the most common cause of loss of blood pressure control. The presence of an anatomic renal artery stenosis does not correlate well as the cause of an elevated blood pressure.

VII-7. **The answer is C.** *(Ch. 51)*   Several features help to differentiate the hypertension of fibrous dysplasia from other types of hypertension. Patients with fibrous dysplasia are likely to present with hypertension before 35 years of age, to be women, and to be white. In a recent study, 80 percent of patients with fibrous dysplasia were women and 90 percent were white. Patients with fibrous dysplasia are likely to be thin and have abdominal bruits. They are not likely to have severe retinopathy, cardiomegaly, or a creatinine of greater than 1.5 mg/dL.

VII-8. **The answer is A.** *(Ch. 51)*   An elevated blood pressure may be the first sign in a variety of unusual clinical conditions, including 17-α-hydroxylase deficiency, Ask-Upmark kidney, Cushing's syndrome, Cushing's disease, and renal tuberculosis. An epinephrine-producing pheochromocytoma produces flushing. Pallor is seen in a norepinephrine-producing pheochromocytoma. The measurement of plasma catecholamines is only a useful test for pheochromocytoma when the urinary assays are borderline. The most common cause of primary aldosteronism is an aldosterone-producing adenoma. Patients often become normotensive following surgical excision of an aldosterone-producing adenoma. Within 5 years postoperatively, however, only about half remain normotensive.

VII-9. **The answer is D.** *(Ch. 51)*   The two lifestyle modifications most likely to lower blood pressure are weight reduction and reduction of Na^+ intake. Reducing alcohol intake has been shown to provide some reduction of blood pressure. Studies with stress reduction have not yet shown a consistent decrease in blood pressure. The greatest lowering of blood pressure occurs in patients who take antihypertensives, lose weight, and reduce Na^+ intake.

VII-10. **The answer is C.** *(Ch. 51)*   The goal of blood pressure reduction in nondiabetic patients is a systolic blood pressure of 140 mm Hg and a diastolic blood pressure of 90 mm Hg. In diabetic patients, the systolic blood pressure goal is <130 mm Hg and the diastolic goal is <85 mm Hg. It is cost-effective to lower blood pressure to normal, despite increased use of medications. It has not been proven that changes in serum lipids caused by certain antihypertensives are harmful in patients with dyslipidemias. However, it seems prudent to choose lipid-neutral agents or agents that may improve the lipid profile. There are four classes of drugs that have been shown to reduce cardiovascular events when used as initial therapy for hypertension: thiazide diuretics, β-adrenergic blocking agents, long-acting dihydropyridine calcium channel antagonists, and angiotensin-converting enzyme (ACE) inhibitors. Centrally acting alpha agonists should not be used as initial therapy or should be taken in combination with diuretics. Moderate- and high-dose thiazides worsen insulin sensitivity and can precipitate glucose intolerance. Some ACE inhibitors have been shown to reduce urinary protein excretion and improve insulin sensitivity.

VII-11. **The answer is B.** *(Ch. 51)* Hydralazine and minoxidil are direct vasodilators with a poorly understood mechanism of action. They cause reflex tachycardia and fluid retention. Methyldopa is a centrally acting α_2-adrenoreceptor agonist and, when given as monotherapy, is the preferred drug in managing the hypertension associated with preeclampsia. Prazosin is a selective α_1-adrenergic blocker, and phentolamine is a nonselective α_1-adrenergic blocker.

VII-12. **The answer is E.** *(Ch. 51)* Patients who have systolic heart failure or a low ejection fraction have both improved blood pressure control and prognosis with ACE inhibitors, β-adrenergic blocking agents, and spironolactone. Treatment of hypertension with diastolic dysfunction and heart failure has not been well studied, but treatment with drugs that reduce heart rate, increase diastolic filling time, and allow the myocardium more time to relax seems reasonable. Recommended drugs are β-adrenergic blocking agents and diltiazem or verapamil. Vasodilators are more effective therapy for aortic insufficiency in hypertensives than positive inotropic agents. Short-acting dihydropyridine calcium channel antagonists increase microalbuminuria and proteinuria. ACE inhibitors have been shown to reduce microalbuminuria. There has been a great deal of concern regarding lowering blood pressure too much or too quickly following a stroke. "Watershed" areas of the brain may be poorly perfused if blood pressure is lowered rapidly. Treatment probably should not be instituted unless mean arterial pressure is >130 mm Hg in the setting of concomitant hemorrhagic transformation or another hypertensive emergency. β-Adrenergic blocking agents, ACE inhibitors, and calcium channel antagonists are effective antihypertensive treatments in patients with coronary artery disease.

VII-13. **The answer is B.** *(Ch. 51)* The incidence of clinical side effects increases with increasing doses of all classes of antihypertensives, with the exception of ACE inhibitors and angiotensin receptor blockers. If blood pressure is reduced below the autoregulatory capacity during a hypertensive crisis, inadequate tissue perfusion may occur. Peripheral alpha blockers, alpha/beta adrenergic blocking agents and calcium channel antagonists are equally effective in all types of hypertensive patients in all ethnic groups. Elderly patients generally need lower doses of antihypertensives. Hypertension during pregnancy carries a prognostic significance for future health problems as the woman ages.

PART VIII
PULMONARY HYPERTENSION
AND PULMONARY DISEASE

VIII. PULMONARY HYPERTENSION AND PULMONARY DISEASE

QUESTIONS

DIRECTIONS: Each question listed below contains five suggested responses. Select the **one best** response to each question.

VIII-1. Which of the following statements regarding pulmonary hypertension is true?

(A) pulmonary congestion and edema are the hallmarks of pulmonary arterial hypertension
(B) the degree of pulmonary hypertension is usually less severe in patients with chronic lung disease than in those with connective tissue diseases
(C) the "gold standard" method for diagnosing pulmonary hypertension is echocardiography
(D) autonomic innervation of the vascular tree plays the largest role in modulating vasomotor tone
(E) the ECG is most reliable in diagnosing obstructive airway diseases and parenchymal lung disease

(pages 1607–1610)

VIII-2. Which of the following statements regarding secondary pulmonary hypertension due to cardiac disease is true?

(A) the pulmonary hypertension that results from left ventricular failure brings about right ventricular failure
(B) in the presence of left-to-right shunting, pulmonary vasoconstriction contributes a large portion of the resistance to blood flow
(C) occlusion of small muscular arteries and arterioles by organized thrombi is the most common presentation of thromboembolic disease
(D) increases in pulmonary vascular tone brought on by hypoxia offer the largest amount of resistance to blood flow in patients with congenital heart disease
(E) patients with proximal pulmonary thromboembolism will show two or more segmental perfusion defects on ventilation-perfusion lung scanning

(pages 1611–1613)

VIII-3. Which of the following statements regarding secondary pulmonary hypertension due to respiratory diseases and disorders is true?

(A) cough is frequently present in patients with interstitial fibrosis

(B) systemically administered vasodilators are beneficial in treating pulmonary hypertension associated with interstitial fibrosis
(C) right ventricular enlargement is the primary diagnostic sign on a roentgenogram of pulmonary hypertension in patients with chronic obstructive pulmonary disease
(D) the histopathologic lesions seen with connective tissue diseases resemble those of primary pulmonary hypertension
(E) vasodilator agents are equivocal in their treatment of both primary and secondary hypertension

(pages 1614–1615)

VIII-4. Which of the following clinical signs would most likely lead to a diagnosis of primary pulmonary hypertension?

(A) examination of the jugular venous pulse shows a decreased *a* wave
(B) there is a widely split second heart sound
(C) an ejection sound is heard over the second right intercostal space
(D) there is an audible midsystolic murmur along the sternal border
(E) a fourth heart sound can be heard over the apex

(page 1618)

VIII-5. Which of the following statements regarding primary pulmonary hypertension (PPH) is true?

(A) PPH mainly affects the intermediate pulmonary arteries
(B) sudden death accounts for a significant portion of all PPH-related deaths
(C) PPH is often recognized early by abnormal chest radiograph or ECG showing right ventricular hypertrophy
(D) obtaining a family history is not beneficial in the diagnosis of PPH
(E) α-adrenergic antagonists are useful in the treatment of PPH

(pages 1617–1619)

VIII-6. Which of the following statements regarding the diagnosis of deep venous thrombosis (DVT) and pulmonary embolism (PE) is true?

(A) a diagnosis of PE would be incorrect in a patient who presents with dyspnea and is found to have leukocytosis

(B) there is often no elevation of the alveolar-arterial difference in patients with acute PE who are otherwise normal

(C) pulmonary arteriography is the "gold standard" method for diagnosing PE

(D) a chest radiograph can generally diagnose or exclude PE

(E) pulmonary arteriography is useful for diagnosing subsegmental emboli

(pages 1628–1631)

VIII-7. Which of the following statements regarding therapy of pulmonary embolism is true?

(A) heparin-associated thrombocytopenia usually occurs within 24 h of onset of heparin therapy

(B) a 62-year-old man being treated for a pulmonary embolus has a recurrent pulmonary embolus 2 weeks after the initial event; his prothrombin time on warfarin is 14 s with a control of 11.9 s; appropriate therapy is venous interruption

(C) embolic obstruction of a pulmonary artery resolves by 10 to 20 percent during the first 24 h after acute pulmonary embolism

(D) thrombolytic therapy reduces the mortality of patients with pulmonary embolism when compared with heparin therapy alone

(E) the preferred therapy of fat embolism is heparin infusion

(pages 1633–1635)

VIII-8. Which of the following statements regarding chronic obstructive pulmonary disease (COPD) is true?

(A) oxygen desaturation frequently increases during sleep

(B) patients who have dyspnea on exertion generally develop cor pulmonale earlier than those who do not

(C) one hypothesis of the difference between "blue bloaters" and "pink puffers" is that the former have more pure emphysema

(D) asthma is a form of COPD that commonly leads to chronic cor pulmonale

(E) the exercise limitation of patients with COPD is usually due to a decrease in cardiac reserve

(pages 1645–1646)

VIII-9. Which of the following statements regarding chronic cor pulmonale and pulmonary vascular disease is true?

(A) patients with pulmonary vascular disease also often have the Pickwickian syndrome

(B) chronic cor pulmonale is a feature of Goodpasture's syndrome

(C) sickle cell disease will not bring about chronic cor pulmonale

(D) idiopathic pulmonary hemosiderosis is often associated with chronic cor pulmonale

(E) chronic cor pulmonale has been associated with HIV infection

(pages 1646–1647)

VIII-10. Which of the following statements regarding the pathophysiology of chronic cor pulmonale is true?

(A) as little as a 10 percent reduction in effective cross-sectional area of the pulmonary vascular bed will result in detectable changes in the pulmonary artery systolic pressure at rest

(B) alveolar hypoxia is the most important cause of pulmonary vasoconstriction

(C) hypercarbia decreases plasma renin activity

(D) patients with chronic cor pulmonale usually demonstrate an abnormal pulmonary artery wedge pressure

(E) hypoxic vasoconstriction is enhanced by alkalosis

(pages 1648–1650)

VIII-11. Which of the following statements regarding the clinical manifestations and treatment of cor pulmonale is true?

(A) the most sensitive physical sign of pulmonary hypertension is the presence of a right-sided systolic ejection sound and right ventricular S_3 gallop

(B) the absence of changes on an ECG can rule out cor pulmonale

(C) right bundle branch block occurs in the majority of patients with cor pulmonale

(D) diuretics are appropriate treatments for right ventricular failure

(E) vasodilators are widely used to reduce right ventricular afterload

(pages 1650–1653)

VIII. PULMONARY HYPERTENSION AND PULMONARY DISEASE

ANSWERS

VIII-1. **The answer is B.** *(Ch. 52)* Pulmonary congestion and edema are the hallmarks of pulmonary *venous* hypertension. Patients with chronic lung disease generally have less severe pulmonary hypertension than those with connective tissue diseases, chronic thromboembolic disease, or primary pulmonary hypertension. The "gold standard" for the diagnosis of pulmonary hypertension is right heart catheterization. However, if the quality of an echocardiogram is sufficient and tricuspid regurgitation is present, echocardiography provides an accurate noninvasive alternative. The largest role in modulation of vasomotor tone is contributed by local stimuli; autonomic innervation plays much less of a role. The ECG is most reliable in diagnosing respiratory disorders that do not involve the parenchyma of the lungs.

VIII-2. **The answer is E.** *(Ch. 52)* Left ventricular failure is the most common cause of right ventricular failure. The pulmonary hypertension that results from left ventricular failure, however, is insufficient to account for the extent of the right ventricular failure. Instead, right ventricular failure is generally attributed to failure of the myocardium in the shared ventricular septum. When right-to-left shunting occurs, pulmonary vasoconstriction contributes to the resistance to blood flow. Occlusion of the intermediate pulmonary arteries by emboli is the most common thromboembolic disease. The predominant factor contributing to increases in pulmonary resistance in patients with congenital heart disease is changes in the walls of small muscular arteries and arterioles. An increase in pulmonary vascular resistance elicited by hypoxia accounts for much less of the resistance. It is important to recognize patients with proximal pulmonary thromboembolism, as this can be relieved by surgical intervention (or, possibly, thrombolytic therapy). As a rule, patients with proximal pulmonary thromboembolism have two or more segmental perfusion defects on ventilation-perfusion lung scanning.

VIII-3. **The answer is D.** *(Ch. 52)* Patients with interstitial fibrosis have dyspnea and tachypnea, but rarely have a prominent cough. Systemic vasodilators are not beneficial and may worsen intrapulmonary gas exchange in patients with pulmonary hypertension associated with interstitial fibrosis. It is often difficult to discern right ventricular enlargement in patients with chronic obstructive pulmonary disease, due to hyperinflation and cardiac rotation. The "gold standard" for diagnosis of right ventricular enlargement is echocardiography. The histopathologic lesions seen in connective tissue diseases resemble those seen in primary pulmonary hypertension. The efficacy of vasodilator agents in patients with secondary pulmonary hypertension is much less impressive and predictable than in primary pulmonary hypertension.

VIII-4. **The answer is D.** *(Ch. 52)* A patient with primary pulmonary hypertension would have a jugular venous pulse with a prominent *v* wave because of the presence of severe tricuspid regurgitation. The second heart sound is narrowly split because of delayed right ventricular emptying and late pulmonic valve closure. A pulmonic ejection sound could be heard over the pulmonic area in the second left intercostals space. It is important to note that the pulmonic ejection sound is the *only* right-sided heart sound that is softer during inspiration. A right-sided fourth heart sound can often be heard at the lower left sternal border. A midsystolic murmur can be audible along the sternal border as well as sometimes in the pulmonic area.

VIII-5.   The answer is B.   *(Ch. 52)*   Primary pulmonary hypertension (PPH) mainly affects small pulmonary arteries and arterioles. In its early stages, the disease is often difficult to recognize. In its late stages, PPH is usually diagnosed by abnormal radiography, ECG, or, more specifically, echocardiography. Sudden death accounts for 10 to 15 percent of all PPH-related deaths. A family history can be quite beneficial in the diagnosis of PPH because there is a genetic component to the disease. Most vasodilator agents have not been proven to be beneficial in the treatment of PPH. Calcium channel antagonists, arachidonic acid metabolites, and nitric oxide have shown some promise for treatment.

VIII-6.   The answer is C.   *(Ch. 53)*   Although a patient who presents with dyspnea and is found to have leukocytosis most likely has pneumonia, acute pulmonary embolism (PE) can occur in the setting of other cardiopulmonary disorders. The presence of pneumonia does not exclude the possibility of concomitant PE. In acute PE, the alveolar-arterial difference is usually elevated, even in patients without preexisting cardiopulmonary disease. A chest radiograph can generally not be used definitively to diagnose or exclude PE. Pulmonary arteriography is the "gold standard" method for the diagnosis of PE, although the noninvasive ventilation/perfusion nuclear scan may be very useful. Pulmonary angiography has excellent agreement between observers for the diagnosis of main, lobar, and segmental emboli, but has low agreement on subsegmental emboli.

VIII-7.   The answer is C.   *(Ch. 53)*   Intravenous heparin can cause an immunologically mediated thrombocytopenia in 5 to 22 percent of patients. Onset of this usually occurs 6 to 12 days after initiation of therapy. Heparin-associated thrombocytopenia may be associated with life-threatening arterial thrombosis. The patient presented in choice B should have more aggressive anticoagulation before considering vena caval interruption. The indications for venous interruption are (1) recurrent emboli on adequate anticoagulation, (2) contraindication of anticoagulants, (3) persistent disease state predisposing to emboli, (4) septic embolization from below the heart, and (5) certain patients with massive emboli in whom a further embolus would be fatal. Resolution of pulmonary embolus occurs by fibrinolysis and mechanical changes in the location of clots within the vascular bed. Embolic obstruction resolves by about 10 to 20 percent in the first 24 h, and can be completely resolved as early as 14 days after the acute event. Thrombolytic therapy is potentially most useful in a small group of patients with documented massive pulmonary embolism with severe hemodynamic compromise. Except for this situation, thrombolytic therapy has not reduced the mortality in pulmonary embolism when compared with heparin therapy alone. Fat embolization occurs usually after fractures of long bones and consists of the development of acute respiratory distress syndrome with altered levels of consciousness, delirium, seizures, coma, and development of petechiae. The most important therapy is maintenance of oxygenation. Heparin is not beneficial and may even be detrimental in that increased lipase activity might increase the toxic fatty acids in the lungs.

VIII-8.   The answer is A.   *(Ch. 54)*   Oxygen desaturation frequently increases during exercise and sleep. Patients whose primary symptom is dyspnea on exertion have less hypoventilation and less hypoxemia at rest and develop cor pulmonale later than others. One hypothesis of the difference between "blue bloaters" and "pink puffers" is that the latter suffer more from pure emphysema, while the former have more inflammatory bronchitis. Asthma is a form of COPD that rarely leads to chronic cor pulmonale. The exercise limitation seen in COPD results from a decrease in ventilatory capacity, rather than from a decrease in cardiac reserve.

VIII-9.   The answer is E.   *(Ch. 54)*   Patients who have the Pickwickian syndrome (hypoventilation, cyanosis, polycythemia, and somnolence) are usually extremely obese. These patients suffer from hypoventilation syndromes associated with cor pulmonale. Cor pulmonale is not a feature of Goodpasture's disease or idiopathic pulmonary hemosiderosis. Sickle cell disease, resulting from either SS or SC hemoglobinopathy, can cause cor pulmonale, usually after multiple episodes of pulmonary infarction. Cor pulmonale has definitely been associated with HIV infection.

VIII-10.   The answer is B.   *(Ch. 54)*   There must be a 25 to 50 percent reduction in effective cross-sectional area of the pulmonary vascular bed to cause a detectable change in pulmonary artery systolic pressure at rest. Alveolar hypoxia is the most important cause of pulmonary vasoconstriction. Hypercarbia stimulates plasma renin activity. Patients who are edematous and hypercarbic have increased plasma levels of aldosterone and antidiuretic hormone. Patients with chronic cor pulmonale generally demonstrate a normal resting cardiac output, normal pulmonary artery wedge pressure, and normal resting left ventricular ejection fraction. Hypoxic vasoconstriction is enhanced by acidosis and decreased by alkalosis.

VIII-11.   The answer is D.   *(Ch. 54)*   The most sensitive physical sign for pulmonary hypertension is an accentuated pulmonary component of S_2, which may also be palpable in the pulmonic area. With very high pulmonary artery systolic pressure, the diastolic and systolic murmurs of pulmonary valvular and tricuspid valvular regurgitation may be heard in combination with a systolic ejection sound and a right ventricular S_3 gallop. The latter is very specific but not sensitive for pulmonary hypertension. The ECG can be normal in advanced cor pulmonale. Right bundle branch block occurs in about 15 percent of patients with cor pulmonale. Diuretics are appropriate treatments for right ventricular failure. Vasodilators are not widely used to reduce right ventricular afterload, as there have been observed reductions in pulmonary hypertension and worsening of gas exchange.

PART IX
VALVULAR HEART DISEASE

IX. VALVULAR HEART DISEASE

QUESTIONS

DIRECTIONS: Each question listed below contains five suggested responses.
Select the **one best** response to each question.

IX-1. Which of the following statements regarding the clinical manifestations of acute rheumatic fever is true?

(A) carditis is the most common manifestation of rheumatic fever
(B) patients with valvulitis may exhibit a Carey Coombs murmur, a mid-diastolic murmur preceded by an opening snap and an S_3 gallop
(C) MRI may reveal abnormalities in the putamen
(D) group A streptococci can be cultured from the synovial fluid of patients with rheumatic fever
(E) it is common for patients to have myocarditis in the absence of valvulitis with rheumatic fever

(pages 1659–1661)

IX-2. Which of the following statements regarding the laboratory findings of rheumatic fever is true?

(A) throat cultures of patients with rheumatic fever are usually positive for group A streptococci
(B) patients will often have a moderate normochromic, normocytic anemia
(C) patients often have sinus tachycardia that resolves during sleep
(D) the etiology of heart failure in patients with rheumatic fever is from myocarditis
(E) myocardial biopsy generally provides the diagnosis of rheumatic fever

(page 1661–1662)

IX-3. Which of the following statements regarding valvular aortic stenosis is true?

(A) atrial fibrillation may precipitate heart failure
(B) in patients aged 70 years and older with aortic stenosis, the most common finding is bicuspid aortic valve
(C) cardiac muscle cells usually degenerate
(D) elevated left ventricular end-diastolic pressure is a marker for left ventricular systolic failure
(E) coronary blood flow per 100 g of left ventricular mass remains normal

(pages 1667–1670)

IX-4. Which of the following statements regarding clinical findings of aortic stenosis (AS) is true?

(A) patients with AS do not usually have classic angina pectoris unless they have concomitant coronary artery disease
(B) two-dimensional echocardiography does not reliably estimate the severity of the AS
(C) patients with mild AS will have a single or paradoxical second heart sound
(D) thickened aortic cusps seen with echocardiography are diagnostic for valvular aortic stenosis
(E) left ventricular ejection fraction provides a good estimate of myocardial function after aortic valve replacement

(pages 1670–1673)

IX-5. Which of the following statements regarding the surgical treatment for aortic stenosis is true?

(A) aortic valve replacement does not significantly alter the subsequent risk of sudden death
(B) in the evaluation of patients for aortic valve replacement, all men and women over the age of 35 years should undergo coronary arteriography
(C) when mechanical or ultrasonic debridement of the aortic valve is successfully performed, the results generally last well over 15 years
(D) if complete coronary revascularization is performed, the operative risk is not significantly different than that of aortic valve replacement alone
(E) the probability of freedom from valve reoperation at 10 years in patients with cryopreserved homografts is about 90 percent

(pages 1675–1678)

IX-6. In patients undergoing valve replacement for aortic regurgitation, a high-risk group can be identified by which of the following?

(A) an Austin Flint murmur is present

(B) the pulse pressure exceeds 50 percent of the peak systolic pressure

(C) a third heart sound (S_3) is present

(D) left ventricular end-systolic dimension is greater than 55 mm

(E) there is premature closure of the mitral valve before onset of the QRS complex

(pages 1679–1682)

IX-7. Which of the following statements regarding acute aortic regurgitation (AR) is true?

(A) tachycardia is not present in all symptomatic acute severe AR patients

(B) peripheral diastolic pressure is usually elevated

(C) vasodilators are useful in the management of patients with acute AR

(D) the aorta will not be dilated on a roentgenogram

(E) the usefulness of transthoracic echo/Doppler ultrasound is limited in this condition

(pages 1679–1681)

IX-8. Which of the following statements regarding chronic aortic regurgitation is true?

(A) total coronary blood flow is increased in severe AR

(B) cardiac muscle cells do not degenerate

(C) clinical heart failure is generally a result of left ventricular diastolic dysfunction

(D) the jugular venous pressure is usually abnormal

(E) inhalation of amyl nitrate causes an increase in the Austin Flint murmur

(pages 1683–1686)

IX-9. Which of the following statements regarding the management of patients with chronic aortic regurgitation is true?

(A) only patients with moderate to severe AR need to be treated with prophylactic antibiotics

(B) patients with asymptomatic, moderate AR and normal left ventricular function do not need to be treated with a vasodilator

(C) asymptomatic patients with mild AR should be followed up every 1 to 2 years

(D) patients with severe symptoms will have abnormal ventricular function

(E) vasodilators are of short-term benefit in patients in functional classes III and IV heart failure

(pages 1689–1690)

IX-10. Which of the following statements regarding mitral stenosis (MS) is true?

(A) the pressure gradient between the left atrium (LA) and the left ventricle (LV) decreases with increased heart rate

(B) examination in the left lateral decubitus position is essential to diagnosing MS

(C) the hemoglobin-O_2 dissociation curve is shifted to the left

(D) shortly after the event of acute rheumatic fever, the patient shows symptomatic MS

(E) infective endocarditis is a common complication of pure MS

(pages 1698–1701)

IX-11. Which of the following statements regarding mitral stenosis is true?

(A) the opening snap occurs early in diastole in mild stenosis

(B) the severity of the stenosis is inversely proportional to the length of the diastolic murmur

(C) mitral commissurotomy should be offered to patients with functional class II symptoms

(D) it is difficult to make a diagnosis from a chest film

(E) digitalis is an effective treatment, even for patients with normal sinus rhythm and left ventricular function

(pages 1701–1706)

IX-12. Which of the following echocardiographic appearances would be seen in a patient with mitral regurgitation (MR) with rheumatic etiology?

(A) thickened chordae/leaflets

(B) reduced motion of leaflets

(C) prolapsing/flail leaflet

(D) normal leaflets

(E) ruptured chordae

(page 1709)

IX-13. Which of the following statements regarding mitral regurgitation is true?

(A) when the regurgitant orifice is small, most of the regurgitation occurs in late systole

(B) in chronic MR, the atrial *v* wave tends to limit the regurgitant volume

(C) severe MR is most commonly seen in females

(D) about half of patients with surgically corrected MR have atrial fibrillation

(E) in posterior leaflet prolapse, the murmur may radiate to the axilla

(pages 1711–1714)

IX-14. Which of the following statements regarding the treatment of mitral regurgitation is true?

(A) α-adrenergic blockers are the drug of choice for patients with mitral valve prolapse and palpitations
(B) vasodilator therapy is recommended for chronic treatment of MR
(C) valve repair is more feasible in patients with rheumatic valvulitis than in those with degenerative valve disease
(D) even in patients with a low left ventricular ejection fraction (LVEF) (<50 percent), surgical treatment is better than medical treatment
(E) the risk of surgery is much greater for patients in their sixth decade and above as compared to younger patients

(pages 1720–1722)

IX-15. Which of the following statements regarding mitral valve prolapse (MVP) is true?

(A) MVP is inherited as a recessive trait
(B) serum and 24-h urine epinephrine are decreased in patients with MVP
(C) there is no association between patients with MVP and patients with tricuspid valve prolapse
(D) panic attacks occurring in patients with MVP are just as likely to be by chance than as a part of the MVP syndrome
(E) the diagnosis of MVP is most commonly made in patients presenting with chest pain

(pages 1730–1732)

IX-16. Which of the following statements regarding mitral valve prolapse is true?

(A) when a patient with MVP is in the squatting position, the midsystolic click and the murmur move closer to S_1
(B) patients with or without symptoms, who have negative cardiac auscultation findings and mild MVP found on echocardiography, should be diagnosed as having MVP
(C) infective endocarditis is a serious complication
(D) the incidence of stroke is higher among patients with leaflet thickening and redundancy as compared to those without leaflet thickening
(E) in patients with a definite diagnosis of MVP, antibiotic prophylaxis is recommended in only those with class III symptoms when undergoing procedures associated with bacteremia

(pages 1732–1738)

IX-17. The most common valvular lesion resulting from external blunt chest trauma (as in an automobile accident) is which of the following?

(A) tricuspid stenosis
(B) tricuspid regurgitation
(C) aortic stenosis
(D) aortic regurgitation
(E) mitral regurgitation

(pages 1741–1742)

IX-18. Which of the following statements regarding tricuspid regurgitation is true?

(A) any regurgitant flow from the right ventricle (RV) to the right atrium (RA) is pathologic tricuspid regurgitation (TR)
(B) the most common etiology of isolated TR is myocardial infarction
(C) paroxysmal nocturnal dyspnea is usually present in patients with TR and left ventricular failure
(D) in patients with TR due to pulmonary hypertension, there are large *a* waves in the jugular veins
(E) a characteristic finding of TR due to pulmonary hypertension is a holosystolic murmur at the left sternal border that increases during inspiration

(pages 1741–1748)

IX-19. Which of the following statements regarding tricuspid valve disease is true?

(A) atrial fibrillation is not often present in patients with TR
(B) accurate documentation of TR is not readily obtained with angiography
(C) TR is rarely associated with a left parasternal lift
(D) when severe TR is present, with only a modest elevation of pulmonary artery pressure, valve replacement is not necessary
(E) mild TR significantly increases the risk of surgery involving the mitral valve or both the aortic and mitral valves

(pages 1749–1754)

IX-20. Which one of the following statements regarding tricuspid valve disease is true?

(A) atrial myxomas are more common in the RA than in the LA
(B) the most frequent symptoms in tricuspid stenosis are syncope and chest pain
(C) elevation of the mean right atrial pressure above 10 mm Hg produces peripheral edema
(D) tricuspid stenosis is the dominant valve lesion seen in Ebstein's anomaly
(E) tricuspid stenosis aggravates the symptoms of mitral stenosis

(pages 1751–1754)

IX-21.   Malignant carcinoid tumor with metastases most frequently involves which of the following valves?

(A)   aortic and mitral valves
(B)   aortic and tricuspid valves
(C)   aortic and pulmonic valves
(D)   tricuspid and pulmonic valves
(E)   tricuspid and mitral valves

(pages 1742–1743)

IX-22.   Which of the following statements regarding pulmonic valve disease is true?

(A)   congenital lesions are the most common cause of pulmonic regurgitation (PR)
(B)   the radiographic finding of pulmonary artery prominence is not diagnostic for pulmonic regurgitation
(C)   pulmonic stenosis is the most frequently acquired lesion of the pulmonic valve
(D)   the murmur of acquired PR is a low-pitched, decrescendo murmur along the left sternal border, which peaks shortly after P_2
(E)   patients with congenital valve stenosis are best treated surgically, rather than medically

(pages 1743–1752)

IX-23.   Which of the following statements regarding prosthetic heart valves is true?

(A)   acetaldehyde is used to sterilize, destroy antigenicity, and stabilize the collagen of valve tissue for porcine heterografts
(B)   nonstructural dysfunction of heart valves does not need to be reported according to the American Academy of Thoracic Surgery/Society of Thoracic Surgeons (AATS/STS) guidelines
(C)   there is an intrinsic problem with using bovine pericardial tissue to form a valve
(D)   bleeding events, according to the AATS/STS guidelines, are those that occur in all patients, regardless of anticoagulant or antiplatelet use
(E)   valvular thrombosis, according to the AATS/STS guidelines, does not need to be reported

(pages 1761–1763)

IX-24.   Which of the following statements regarding the management of patients with prosthetic heart valves is true?

(A)   the most important cause of postoperative ventricular dysfunction is previous myocardial damage
(B)   the most common cause for dysfunction of mechanical prosthetic valves is thrombotic obstruction
(C)   coronary bypass surgery should not be performed at the time of valve replacement, due to the greater risk of operative mortality
(D)   bioprosthetic aortic valve failure is more common and occurs more rapidly in older rather than younger patients
(E)   echocardiography/Doppler ultrasound is not necessary unless the patient shows signs of valve dysfunction

(pages 1768–1771)

IX-25.   Which of the following statements concerning tissue degeneration with valvular regurgitation in patients with artificial heart valves is true?

(A)   this complication occurs most frequently in the first 2 years after implantation due to structural problems
(B)   aortic valves are more frequently affected than mitral valves
(C)   surgical correction of perivalvular leaks can usually be accomplished by additional suturing rather than replacing the entire valve
(D)   the elderly are more often affected than young patients
(E)   all prosthetic valve leaks should be surgically corrected, even if not hemodynamically significant

(pages 1760–1762)

IX. VALVULAR HEART DISEASE

ANSWERS

IX-1. **The answer is C.** *(Ch. 55)*   Arthritis is the most common manifestation of rheumatic fever, occurring in 75 percent of attacks, while carditis occurs in 40 to 50 percent. Increased flow across the mitral valve, in the presence of valvulitis, may produce a Carey Coombs murmur, which is mid-diastolic and follows an S_3 gallop. Mitral stenosis, which develops later, has an opening snap, presystolic accentuation, and a loud first sound. Patients who have Sydenham's chorea may show abnormalities in the caudate nucleus, putamen, and substantia nigra. There are no bacteria isolated from the synovial fluid of patients with rheumatic fever. Patients generally do not have myocarditis in the absence of valvulitis with rheumatic fever.

IX-2. **The answer is B.** *(Ch. 55)*   Throat cultures of patients are usually negative for group A streptococci by the time rheumatic fever appears. Patients often have a mild to moderate normocytic, normochromic anemia. Persistent sinus tachycardia that does not resolve during sleep is common in the presence of myocarditis. Mitral regurgitation is the usual cause of heart failure, rather than myocarditis. Endomyocardial biopsies are diagnostic in only a few cases.

IX-3. **The answer is A.** *(Ch. 56)*   Atrial fibrillation or flutter increase mean atrial pressure and reduce cardiac output. Typically, the sudden onset of these arrhythmias are also accompanied with rapid ventricular response, all of which are powerful precipitators of heart failure. There is a bimodal distribution of AS: in ages 45 to 65, bicuspid aortic valve is the most common finding, while patients over the age of 70 typically have degenerated trileaflet valves. Cardiac muscle cells do not usually degenerate in AS. Many patients maintain normal or hyperdynamic left ventricular function for extended periods of time with severe AS. Diastolic left ventricular dysfunction, manifested by impaired myocardial relaxation and altered chamber compliance, is universal in patients with advanced AS, and is caused by ultrastructural changes including the development of unusually large nuclei, loss of myofibrils, mitochondrial accumulation, large cytoplasmic areas without contractile material, and fibroblast and collagen fibril proliferation in the interstitial space. There is an overall increase in coronary blood flow due to the severe left ventricular hypertrophy, but there is a reduction in blood flow per 100 g of left ventricular mass. Blood flow is reduced due to reduced coronary perfusion pressure (increased left ventricular end-diastolic pressure lowers the diastolic aortic-left ventricular pressure gradient) which may result in inadequate flow to the subendocardium.

IX-4. **The answer is B.** *(Ch. 56)*   Although there is a substantially increased prevalence of coronary artery disease in patients with AS (for reasons which are unclear), classic angina pectoris may be present in the absence of coronary artery disease because of the imbalance between myocardial oxygen supply and demand. Echo Doppler studies are necessary to determine the severity of AS. Patients with mild aortic stenosis have a normal second heart sound. As AS progresses, A_2 is progressively delayed and may lag behind P_2, producing paradoxical splitting. In critical AS, A_2 may disappear altogether. Some patients, particularly the elderly, may have thickened aortic valve leaflets and not have any detectible aortic valve gradient. The left ventricular ejection fraction with severe AS does not correlate well with the amount of improvement in left ventricular function which usually occurs rapidly after aortic valve replacement.

IX-5.   The answer is E.   *(Ch. 56)*   About 50 percent of patients with severe aortic stenosis will die within 5 years of the time of diagnosis. This risk is significantly lowered if successful aortic valve replacement is performed. In the evaluation of patients for aortic valve replacement, all men over age 35 and all *postmenopausal* women should undergo coronary angiography because of the very high rate of coronary artery disease in patients with AS. The results of either mechanical or ultrasonic debridement of the aortic valve have been very disappointing with a rapid recurrence of AS. Complete coronary revascularization should be performed together with aortic valve replacement whenever indicated; however, the risk is significantly increased over that of aortic valve replacement alone. In patients with cryopreserved homografts, the probability of freedom from valve reoperation at 10 years is 90 percent.

IX-6.   The answer is D.   *(Ch. 56)*   Echocardiographic studies before and after aortic valve replacement indicate that a left ventricular end-systolic dimension greater than 55 mm identifies a high-risk surgical group. A third heart sound (S_3), an apical diastolic rumble (the Austin Flint murmur), and premature closure of the mitral valve on echo all indicate severe aortic regurgitation but are not predictive of postoperative outcome. A wide pulse pressure suggests chronic aortic regurgitation in which left ventricular diastolic pressure is not severely elevated.

IX-7.   The answer is C.   *(Ch. 56)*   Tachycardia is present in nearly all symptomatic patients with acute severe AR. Systolic pressure usually remains normal, unless there is severe heart failure. Diastolic pressure is usually normal or slightly decreased. Vasodilators are a useful and important treatment in the management of patients with acute AR. It must be emphasized, however, that acute severe AR has a very high mortality rate unless treated surgically. Depending on what caused the acute AR, the aorta may or may not be dilated. If the acute AR results from dissection or aortic annular/root disease, the aorta will be dilated on a roentgenogram. It may also be dilated in older patients and those who have systemic hypertension. Transthoracic echo/Doppler ultrasound is a valuable noninvasive procedure and should be used in all cases.

IX-8.   The answer is A.   *(Ch. 56)*   Total coronary blood flow is increased in severe AR, but coronary reserve is significantly reduced. This probably occurs because of a reduced diastolic aortic-left ventricular pressure gradient and compression of intramyocardial coronary arteries. An important difference between AS and AR is that cardiac muscle cells degenerate in AR, while they do not in AS. Clinical heart failure in chronic AR is usually a result of abnormal left ventricular systolic pump function. The jugular venous pressure usually remains normal, except in heart failure and in the rare instances when a greatly dilated aorta obstructs the superior vena cava. Inhalation of amyl nitrate causes vasodilation, increased forward flow, less regurgitant volume, and a reduction or disappearance of the Austin Flint murmur. This is a physical examination technique to distinguish between the Austin Flint murmur and the murmur of mitral stenosis, although echocardiography is more definitive.

IX-9.   The answer is E.   *(Ch. 56)*   All patients with AR should be treated with antibiotic prophylaxis to prevent infective endocarditis. Patients with asymptomatic, moderate AR with normal left ventricular function should be treated with a vasodilator such as an angiotensin-converting enzyme inhibitor. Asymptomatic patients with mild AR should have a follow-up every 2 to 5 years. Patients with moderate AR should have a follow-up every 1 to 2 years. Some patients with severe symptoms will have normal left ventricular function, making decisions regarding surgery difficult. In general, surgery for chronic AR should be considered in patients with increasing symptoms, increasing left ventricular size, and decreasing left ventricular systolic function. Vasodilators are of considerable short-term benefit in patients in functional classes III and IV heart failure.

IX-10.   The answer is B.   *(Ch. 57)*   The pressure gradient between the LA and the LV is increased with faster heart rates because of shortening of the diastole filling time of the LV. Many of the features of MS will be missed if the patient is not examined in the left lateral decubitus position. The body accommodates for the decreased cardiac output by extracting more oxygen from the arterial blood, a right-shift of the hemoglobin-O_2 dissociation curve. There is usually a long (10 to 20 years) asymptomatic period between the acute rheumatic fever and symptomatic MS. Infective endocarditis is rarely a complication of pure MS.

IX-11. **The answer is C.** *(Ch. 57)* The duration of the interval between the second heart sound and the opening snap is inversely related to the severity of MS. Greater left atrial pressure causes the mitral valve leaflets to "dome" sooner, allowing less distance for the leaflets to move in early diastole; therefore the opening snap occurs earlier. In general, the longer the diastolic murmur lasts, the more severe the MS. There is a classic and practically diagnostic triad on a chest roentgenogram: large proximal pulmonary arteries and pulmonary congestion, a large left atrium, but *normal* left ventricular size. Mitral commissurotomy is an acceptable treatment for patients with functional class II symptoms, although mitral balloon valvuloplasty may be superior in many of these cases. Transesophageal echocardiography is necessary to determine whether patients are candidates for balloon valvuloplasty, mitral valve repair, or mitral valve replacement. It has been shown that mitral valve repair, rather than valve replacement, has better outcomes if performed by skilled surgeons. The only role of digitalis in MS is to control ventricular rate in patients with atrial fibrillation.

IX-12. **The answer is A.** *(Ch. 57)* A patient with mitral regurgitation of rheumatic etiology would have thickened chordae/leaflets on echocardiogram. MS reduces leaflet mobility. Degenerative changes are most frequently responsible for ruptured chordae and flail of a mitral valve leaflet.

IX-13. **The answer is D.** *(Ch. 57)* When the regurgitant orifice is small, the orifice declines with the ventricular volume, thus limiting regurgitation to early systole. The atrial *v* wave decreases the ventriculoatrial gradient and thus limits the regurgitant volume. When MR becomes chronic, however, the atrial *v* wave is less prominent and does not limit the regurgitant volume. With the decrease in rheumatic heart disease, severe MR is now most commonly seen in males, because of a higher prevalence of coronary artery disease, hypertensive heart disease, and spontaneous rupture of a chordae. About 50 percent of patients with surgically corrected MR have atrial fibrillation. In posterior leaflet prolapse, the murmur can sometimes be heard in the neck, back, and even skull. In rheumatic or anterior leaflet prolapse, the murmur is at maximum intensity in the axilla.

IX-14. **The answer is E.** *(Ch. 57)* β-Adrenergic blocking agents are the drug of choice for the treatment of patients with mitral valve prolapse and palpitations or chest pain. Vasodilator therapy is not recommended for chronic treatment of MR. Valve repair is more feasible in patients with degenerative valve disease than in those with rheumatic valvulitis or endocarditis. A reduced EF (<50 percent) is associated with a high late mortality rate; however, surgery provides a better outcome than medical treatment. Mitral valve repair, as opposed to replacement, has been shown to improve outcomes substantially. The risk of surgery has become almost the same between patients in their sixth decade and older as compared to younger patients.

IX-15. **The answer is D.** *(Ch. 58)* MVP appears to be inherited as an autosomal dominant trait with variable penetrance. The severity of the abnormalities of the mitral valve and its supporting structures vary greatly. Patients with substantial thickening and ballooning of the mitral valve leaflets on echo are at the highest risk for complications, including endocarditis and acute MR due to rupture of a chordae. Rupture of a degenerated chordae is the most common cause of acute MR in middle-aged men. Serum and 24-h urine epinephrine and norepinephrine may be increased in patients with MVP. Tricuspid valve prolapse occurs in about 40 percent of MVP patients. The diagnosis of MVP is most often made in asymptomatic patients by auscultation or echocardiography that is being performed for other purposes. The most common presenting complaint that patients with MVP have is palpitations. Panic attacks and MVP both occur relatively frequently. It is likely that panic attacks occurring in a patient with MVP are by chance, rather than being a part of the MVP syndrome.

IX-16. **The answer is C.** *(Ch. 58)* When a patient with MVP is in the squatting position, they have a decreased end-diastolic left ventricular volume. Thus, the midsystolic click and the murmur move closer to S_2. Patients with or without symptoms, who have negative cardiac auscultation findings and mild MVP found on echocardiography, should not be diagnosed as having MVP. Infective endocarditis is a serious complication of MVP. The incidence of stroke is similar in groups with or without leaflet thickening and redundancy. When the diagnosis of MVP is definite, antibiotic prophylaxis is recommended in all patients undergoing procedures associated with bacteremia.

IX-17. **The answer is B.** *(Ch. 59)* The most common valvular lesion following external blunt trauma as in an automobile accident is traumatic tricuspid regurgitation, the main cause of which is rupture of the papillary muscle or chordae. Laceration of leaflet tissue is less common. Rupture of tricuspid papillary muscles has also been described following external cardiopulmonary resuscitation. There is extensive variability in how well traumatic tricuspid regurgitation is tolerated. Prolonged survival (up to 39 years) has been reported. In general, rupture of a tricuspid papillary muscle is not as well tolerated as rupture of chordae. Acute aortic regurgitation, usually a much more serious condition, can also occur from blunt trauma.

IX-18. **The answer is E.** *(Ch. 59)* Some amount of regurgitant flow from the RV to the RA occurs in 24 to 96 percent of normal individuals by Doppler ultrasound. The most common etiology of isolated TR is infective endocarditis in drug addicts. Other less common causes include myocardial infarction, trauma, carcinoid syndrome, leaflet prolapse, and congenital anomalies. Paroxysmal nocturnal dyspnea is often absent in patients with TR and left ventricular failure, as TR may diminish the pulmonary symptoms of left-sided heart failure. Patients with TR typically have large *v* waves in the jugular veins. A holosystolic murmur at the left sternal border that increases during inspiration is characteristic of TR.

IX-19. **The answer is B.** *(Ch. 59)* Atrial fibrillation is frequently present in patients with TR because of increased right atrial pressure. Accurate angiographic evidence of TR is difficult to obtain, due to the catheter transiting the tricuspid valve, the odd shape of the RV, and right ventricular irritability during contrast injection. TR is essentially an echocardiographic diagnosis. A left parasternal lift is caused by right ventricular pressure or volume overload (as seen in TR), left atrial enlargement, or an ascending thoracic aortic aneurysm. When severe TR is present with only a modest elevation of pulmonary artery pressure, the tricuspid valve leaflets are probably deformed and valve replacement is necessary. Mild TR does not significantly increase the risk of surgery involving the mitral valve or the aortic and mitral valves. Moderate to severe TR, however, does increase the surgical risk.

IX-20. **The answer is C.** *(Ch. 59)* The LA is the site for the majority of myxomas; 15 to 20 percent occur in the RA. The causes of tricuspid valve disease include right ventricular pressure or volume overload, rheumatic tricuspid stenosis, carcinoid syndrome, endocardial fibroelastosis, endomyocardial fibrosis, and systemic lupus erythematosus. Mechanical obstruction of the valve can occur with a right atrial myxoma, tumor metastasis, or right atrial thrombi. The most frequent symptoms of tricuspid stenosis are dyspnea and fatigue. When mitral stenosis coexists, the development of significant tricuspid stenosis can diminish the symptoms of dyspnea, orthopnea, and paroxysmal nocturnal dyspnea by preventing the increase in pulmonary congestion and pulmonary hypertension. Mild elevations of the right atrial pressure to values of 10 mm Hg may lead to marked venous hypertension with concomitant changes, such as jugular venous distention, ascites, and peripheral edema. Ebstein's malformation is a condition that involves an abnormal attachment of the septal tricuspid valve leaflet that leads to significant tricuspid regurgitation in most cases.

IX-21. **The answer is D.** *(Ch. 59)* Malignant carcinoid tumor (usually originating in the ileum) with extensive metastases affects the tricuspid and pulmonary valves about 10 percent of the time. The involvement of the tricuspid valve usually results in regurgitation, although tricuspid stenosis may occur. The carcinoid syndrome with cardiac involvement of the pulmonic valve can create slight pulmonic stenosis and associated regurgitation. Symptoms of the carcinoid syndrome include facial flushing, increased intestinal activity, diarrhea, and bronchospasm.

IX-22. **The answer is B.** *(Ch. 59)* Pulmonic regurgitation (PR) is more common than pulmonic stenosis (PS) and is usually due to acquired pulmonic valve disease. The murmur of acquired PR is a high-pitched diastolic blow along the left sternal border. The murmur of congenital PR is a low-pitched, decrescendo murmur heard along the left sternal border, which peaks shortly after P_2. The radiographic finding of pulmonary artery prominence can be seen in patients with both PR and PS. Once again, these lesions are best demonstrated by echocardiography. Patients with congenital pulmonic valve stenosis are usually best treated by catheter balloon valvotomy.

IX-23. **The answer is D.** *(Ch. 60)* Glutaraldehyde is used to sterilize valve tissue, render it bioacceptable by destroying the antigenicity, and stabilize the collagen cross-links. Early problems with valves formulated from bovine pericardial tissue were due to inadequate valve design, not to difficulties with the tissue. The Carpentier-Edwards Perimount pericardial bioprosthesis largely overcame the previous design problems and was approved by the U.S. Food and Drug Administration (FDA) for the aortic position in 1991. According to the AATS/STS guidelines, all complications of prosthetic valves are reported. Bleeding events are reported as those that occur in any patients, regardless of whether they are on anticoagulants or antiplatelet drugs. Valvular thrombosis should be reported.

IX-24. **The answer is B.** *(Ch. 60)* An important cause of postoperative ventricular dysfunction is perioperative myocardial damage. There have been significant improvements in myocardial protection during valve surgery, including techniques that reduce myocardial oxygen consumption and maintain adequate myocardial perfusion. The most common cause for the dysfunction of mechanical prosthetic valves is thrombotic obstruction. Although coronary bypass surgery performed at the time of valve surgery does increase the risk of perioperative mortality, the long-term mortality benefits of bypass surgery outweigh the additional surgical risk. Bioprosthetic valve failure is more common and occurs more rapidly in younger patients, in any patients with chronic renal failure, and in the mitral position. Echocardiography/Doppler is essential at the first postoperative visit because it gives a baseline for comparison at a later date, when valvular dysfunction may occur.

IX-25. **The answer is C.** *(Ch. 60)* Tissue degeneration with valvular regurgitation is the most frequent hemodynamic form of artificial valve disease. This complication is rare in the first 3 years after implantation, but it occurs at the rate of 2 to 3 percent per year after 3 years of implantation. After 10 years, the rate is about 5 percent per year. Degeneration occurs more commonly in younger patients and in patients with valves in the mitral position. Small perivalvular leaks do not usually require surgical correction. When repair is necessary, additional suturing is usually sufficient.

PART X
CONGENITAL HEART DISEASE

X. CONGENITAL HEART DISEASE

QUESTIONS

DIRECTIONS: Each question listed below contains five suggested responses. Select the **one best** response to each question.

X-1. Which of the following statements regarding the genetics of single-gene disorders is true?

(A) *allele heterogeneity* refers to the same disease being due to single or multiple mutations in two or more genes

(B) an elongated mutant is a result of two genes interacting and part of the nucleotide sequence of one becoming incorporated into the other

(C) to have expressivity, a genetic trait must be penetrant

(D) in a disease with autosomal dominant inheritance, normal children of infected individuals will have affected offspring approximately half of the time

(E) women are affected more often than men in diseases with X-linked inheritance

(pages 1786–1788)

X-2. Which of the following statements regarding chromosomal mapping and the identification of a disease-related gene is true?

(A) homozygous chromosomal markers are informative for genetic linkage

(B) recombination refers to the random assortment of alleles into gametes during meiosis

(C) RFLPs are used more often that STRPs as chromosomal markers

(D) recombination occurs more frequently in males

(E) any two loci that are coinherited more than 50 percent of the time are said to be genetically linked

(pages 1789–1791)

X-3. Which of the following statements regarding familial hypertrophic cardiomyopathy (FHCM) is true?

(A) it is characterized by X-linked inheritance

(B) it has been proposed that FHCM is a disease of the sarcomere

(C) the α-tropomyosin gene is most commonly affected

(D) the incidence of sudden death is higher in older patients

(E) the amount of hypertrophy correlates with the incidence of sudden death

(pages 1793–1794)

X-4. Which of the following statements agrees with a diagnosis of Friedreich's ataxia?

(A) cardiac involvement is rare

(B) the most common cardiac abnormality is pulmonic stenosis

(C) there is a characteristic combination of macroglossia, exopthalmos, and visceromegaly

(D) it is inherited as an autosomal recessive disorder

(E) dilated cardiomyopathy often occurs

(pages 1796–1798)

X-5. Which of the following statements regarding dilated cardiomyopathy (DCM) is true?

(A) Barth syndrome is characterized by DCM and the triad of endocardial fibroelastosis, neutropenia, and skeletal myopathy

(B) the first symptom of idiopathic dilated cardiomyopathy is usually angina

(C) dystrophin is the mutated protein responsible for Barth syndrome

(D) the actin and desmin genes are responsible for X-linked dilated cardiomyopathy

(E) the inheritance of Barth syndrome is autosomal recessive

(pages 1798–1800)

X-6. A patient shows progressive atrial dysfunction that eventually results in permanent paralysis of the atria. Histopathologic studies show myofibril necrosis and interstitial accumulation of fat. The disease shows patterns of autosomal dominant inheritance. What is the most likely diagnosis?

(A) Duchenne's muscular dystrophy

(B) myotubular (centronuclear) myopathy

(C) fascioscapulohumeral muscular dystrophy

(D) Becker's muscular dystrophy

(E) myotonic dystrophy

(pages 1802–1808)

X-7. Which of the following diagnoses is most likely in a patient with cardiomyopathy and ragged-red fibers seen in muscle biopsy specimens?

(A) primary carnitine deficiency
(B) medium-chain acyl-CoA dehydrogenase deficiency
(C) homocystinuria
(D) a complex I mitochondrial cardiomyopathy
(E) Fabry's disease

(pages 1809–1812)

X-8. Which of the following connective tissue disorders shows signs of right-sided heart failure in infancy?

(A) type I Ehlers-Danlos syndrome
(B) type IV Ehlers-Danlos syndrome
(C) pseudoxanthoma elasticum
(D) Marfan's syndrome
(E) cutis laxa

(pages 1813–1815)

X-9. Which of the following autosomal dominant rhythm and conduction disorders may be responsible for a group of children with sudden infant death syndrome (SIDS)?

(A) Romano-Ward long-QT syndrome
(B) Jervell and Lange-Nielsen long-QT syndrome
(C) Brugada syndrome
(D) familial atrial fibrillation
(E) Wolff-Parkinson-White syndrome

(pages 1816–1818)

X-10. An infant in its first 48 h of life has hypocalcemia and truncus arteriosus. What is the most likely diagnosis?

(A) Shprintzen velocardiofacial syndrome
(B) Turner syndrome with monosomy X
(C) DiGeorge syndrome
(D) Down syndrome
(E) Turner syndrome with mosaicism of the X chromosome

(pages 1823–1825)

X-11. Which of the following statements concerning the transition of the fetal circulation to the neonatal circulation is true?

(A) umbilical arterial blood has a higher saturation than the umbilical venous blood
(B) umbilical blood, like maternal venous blood, is usually 50 to 60 percent saturated
(C) despite the extracardiac and intracardiac shunts, left ventricular and right ventricular output must remain equal
(D) the ductus arteriosus normally diverts more than 80 percent of the right ventricular output

(E) less than 5 percent of the cardiac output crosses the foramen ovale, since it is only a potential space not an actual conduit

(pages 1838–1840)

X-12. Which of the following statements regarding the complications of congenital heart disease is true?

(A) in children with congenital heart disease, the onset of heart failure usually occurs after the first year
(B) iron deficiency in hypoxic children may lead to strokes
(C) infants who have congestive heart failure during the first 12 to 18 h of life usually have critical obstruction to systemic arterial flow
(D) hypoxia due to cyanotic defects usually responds well to oxygen administration
(E) children with severe cardiac malformations often have weights that are above the mean percentile for their height

(pages 1841–1843)

X-13. Which of the following statements regarding a ventricular septal defect (VSD) is true?

(A) the majority of VSDs are conal septal defects
(B) VSDs may be associated with coarctation of the aorta
(C) in most infants, VSDs can lead to right ventricular failure
(D) a systolic murmur along the left sternal border that is limited to early or midsystole suggests a defect in the membranous septum
(E) a patient who has improved rate of weight gain, less dyspnea, and a diminution of the precordial hyperactivity has unequivocal signs of a reduction in defect size

(pages 1846–1847)

X-14. Which of the following statements regarding a ventricular septal defect is true?

(A) most VSDs that remain large at age 6 months will still undergo spontaneous closure
(B) females are more likely to develop aortic regurgitation as a result of prolapse of the right, posterior, or both aortic leaflets into the defect
(C) surgical closure of a VSD with aortic regurgitation does not lower the risk of infective endocarditis
(D) patients with a VSD who have survived to 5 to 10 years of age are no longer candidates for surgical closure of the defect
(E) multiple trabeculated septal defects can be successfully be closed or have only trivial leaks by transcatheter closure

(pages 1848–1850)

X-15. Which of the following statements regarding an atrial septal defect (ASD) is true?

(A) one or more of the right pulmonary veins often drains into the right atrium in a coronary sinus defect

(B) heart failure is common in children with atrial septal defects

(C) ASDs should be surgically closed in adults, even if pulmonary resistance approaches 15 Wood units

(D) the left superior vena cava empties directly into the left atrium in a partial atrioventricular canal defect

(E) most children with an ASD exhibit retarded growth and development

(pages 1850–1854)

X-16. A patient presents with cyanosis and clubbing of the toes with sparing of the fingers. A rough murmur is heard at the left upper sternal border. What is the most likely diagnosis?

(A) atrial septal defect

(B) sinus of Valsalva fistula

(C) common atrioventricular canal defect

(D) patent ductus arteriosus

(E) ventricular septal defect

(page 1859)

X-17. Which of the following statements regarding coarctation of the aorta is true?

(A) the narrowing lies proximal to the origin of the left common carotid artery in most of the cases

(B) a 4-year-old child with coarctation would not show notching of the inferior margin of the ribs on chest x-ray

(C) a child under the age of 6 months would best be treated with balloon dilatation

(D) most infants with coarctation also have at least one complicating cardiac abnormality

(E) low-pitched murmurs can be heard over the chest wall in young patients

(pages 1862–1864)

X-18. Which of the following statements regarding pulmonary stenosis with intact ventricular septum is true?

(A) supravalvular stenosis does not usually progress with time

(B) valvular pulmonary stenosis is characterized most often by a dysplastic valve

(C) most infants present with severe shortness of breath and cyanosis

(D) the systolic ejection sound heard at the left upper sternal border increases with inspiration

(E) operation is nearly always indicated for isolated pulmonary valvular stenosis

(pages 1872–1875)

X-19. Which of the following statements regarding the tetralogy of Fallot is true?

(A) a malformed pulmonary valve is commonly the only site of obstruction to pulmonary flow

(B) coronary artery abnormalities are uncommon

(C) a persistent left superior vena cava is the most commonly associated condition with tetralogy of Fallot

(D) a patent foramen ovale is usually closed during surgical repair of patients with tetralogy of Fallot

(E) heart failure is uncommon

(pages 1875–1878)

X-20. Which of the following statements regarding total anomalous pulmonary venous connection is true?

(A) pulmonary venous obstruction is present in nearly all cases of supradiaphragmatic drainage

(B) the physical examination in infants with accompanying pulmonary venous obstruction is substantially abnormal

(C) there is always a patent foramen ovale

(D) the heart is enlarged in obstructed types

(E) there is significant pulmonary edema with the unobstructed types

(pages 1880–1882)

X-21. Which of the following statements regarding dextro transposition of the great arteries is true?

(A) the majority of patients have a large ventricular septal defect

(B) catheter atrial septostomy at is a beneficial procedure for these infants

(C) significant pulmonary stenosis is common in neonates

(D) left ventricular pressure is equal to systemic arterial pressure

(E) a patent ductus is rarely seen in very young infants

(pages 1885–1886)

X-22. Which of the following statements regarding single ventricle is true?

(A) the common type of single ventricle has the morphology of a left ventricle

(B) the majority of patients with single ventricle have a transposition of the great arteries

(C) when there is one large atrioventricular valve, the most common finding is the trabecular features of a right ventricle

(D) this condition can be easily diagnosed from the electrocardiogram

(E) the surgical repair of this condition usually involves dividing the common chamber into the right and left ventricles

(pages 1894–1896)

X-23. Which of the following statements regarding the medical considerations of adult patients with congenital heart disease is true?

(A) most patients with a high hematocrit exhibit a greatly increased risk of stroke

(B) rhythm disturbances that are benign in structurally normal hearts are usually also benign in patients with congenital heart disease

(C) the rate control of arrhythmias is more important than restoring sinus rhythm in congenital heart disease

(D) early surgical repair of tetralogy of Fallot may reduce the incidence of postoperative ventricular arrhythmias

(E) pregnant women with right-to-left shunts tolerate pregnancy better than those with left-to-right shunts

(pages 1909–1911)

X-24. Which of the following statements regarding adults with an ASD is true?

(A) the life expectancy is normal

(B) patients older than 40 do not benefit from surgical repair

(C) transcatheter repair is most widely used for ASD repairs

(D) patients who have had ASD repair in their first two decades of life should exercise caution when taking part in physical activities

(E) changes associated with coronary artery disease may bring about the development of symptoms

(pages 1918–1919)

X-25. Which of the following statements regarding various congenital heart diseases is true?

(A) isolated VSD is more common in adolescents and adults than in infants and children

(B) the noncardiac features of atrioventricular septal defect have the most influence on management in adolescence and adult life

(C) survival in unoperated patients with tetralogy of Fallot is fairly normal until age 40

(D) adults with tetralogy of Fallot are not suitable surgical candidates

(E) the decreasing benefit with age of surgical repair for pulmonary stenosis is dependent on the use of ventriculotomy and outflow patches

(pages 1919–1922)

X-26. Which of the following statements regarding various congenital heart diseases is true?

(A) patients with coarctation of the aorta and well-developed collaterals almost never need surgical repair

(B) once patients with coarctation of the aorta are corrected, they have normal blood pressure

(C) patients who have the Rastelli procedure for correction of transposition of the great arteries rarely need further heart surgery later in life

(D) newborns who present with Ebstein's anomaly have a much poorer prognosis than those who do not present until adulthood

(E) after atrial redirection, loss of sinus rhythm correlates with an increased risk of sudden death

(pages 1925–1930)

X. CONGENITAL HEART DISEASE

ANSWERS

X-1. The answer is C. *(Ch. 62)* *Allele heterogeneity* refers to the fact that the same disease may be due to multiple mutations in the same gene. *Locus heterogeneity* refers to the same disease being due to single or multiple mutations in two or more genes. An elongated mutant results when a stop codon is eliminated by a point mutation. Expressivity refers to the variable nature of the clinical features of a disease. Penetrance refers to the fact that any manifestation of a disease indicates that the person has full penetrance. The disease, therefore, must be penetrant to have expressivity. In an autosomal dominant disease, normal children of affected individuals will have normal offspring. Due to the dominant nature of the disease, anyone who has no manifestation of it does not carry the gene. Men are affected more often than women in diseases that have X-linked inheritance.

X-2. The answer is E. *(Ch. 62)* Additional markers in a region may need to be analyzed in an individual who is homozygous for a genetic marker, as homozygous markers are not informative for genetic linkage. Recombination refers to crossing over between homologous chromosome pairs. Recombination occurs more frequently in females. STRPs are used as chromosomal markers more often that RFLPs. This is because STRPs have rapid and convenient detection by PCR, which also requires only a nanogram of DNA. Any two loci that are coinherited more than 50 percent of the time are said to be genetically linked.

X-3. The answer is B. *(Ch. 62)* FCHM is an autosomal dominant disorder. It has been proposed that it is a disease of the sarcomere and should be known as *sarcomeropathy*. The β-MHC gene is the most common gene affected in FHCM and over 50 mutations have been described. The incidence of sudden death is higher in younger patients with FHCM. The amount of hypertrophy does not correlate with the incidence of sudden death.

X-4. The answer is D. *(Ch. 62)* Cardiac involvement occurs in 50 to 90 percent of patients with Friedreich's ataxia (FA). The most common cardiac abnormality is hypertrophic cardiomyopathy. Dilated cardiomyopathy occurs rarely. FA is inherited as an autosomal recessive disorder. It is characterized by progressive limb ataxia, loss of deep tendon reflexes, sensory abnormalities, and musculoskeletal deformities.

X-5. The answer is A. *(Ch. 62)* Barth syndrome, also known as X-linked cardioskeletal myopathy, is an X-linked recessive disease. It is characterized by DCM and the triad of endocardial fibroelastosis, neutropenia, and skeletal myopathy. The first symptoms of idiopathic dilated cardiomyopathy are usually sudden death and heart failure. The protein tafazzin is mutated in this disorder. Mutations in the actin and desmin genes are responsible for this disorder. There are mutations in the dystrophin gene in X-linked dilated cardiomyopathy.

X-6. The answer is C. *(Ch. 62)* Each of these diseases is a muscular dystrophy with cardiac involvement. This patient has fascioscapulohumeral dystrophy characterized by atrial paralysis and progressive weakness of the facial, shoulder, and upper arm muscles. The pathology is similar to that of Duchenne's muscular dystrophy.

X-7. The answer is D. *(Ch. 62)* Each of these diseases is a defect of metabolism that causes cardiomyopathy. This patient has a complex I mitochondrial cardiomyopathy. Cardiomyopathy occurs in about 40 percent of cases. Mitochondrial cardiomyopathies almost invariably have ragged-red fibers in muscle biopsy specimens. They show mitochondrial inheritance, with only maternal involvement in a family history.

X-8.   The answer is E. *(Ch. 62)*   Cutis laxa is the connective tissue disorder that shows signs of right-sided heart failure in infancy, generally due to pulmonary disease. These patients have lax, nonresilient skin. Mitral valve prolapse has also been noted frequently.

X-9.   The answer is A. *(Ch. 62)*   There is evidence that Romano-Ward long-QT syndrome may be responsible for a group of children with SIDS. Retrospective ECG analysis from infants, taken on their third or fourth days of life, showed that one-half of these infants had QTc prolongation on initial screening ECG. Although no molecular analysis exists, ion channel mutations may play a role in some children with SIDS.

X-10.   The answer is C. *(Ch. 62)*   This patient has DiGeorge syndrome. Eighty percent of affected infants present with congenital heart defects within the first 48 h of life. These defects include conotruncal defects and branchial arch mesenchymal tissue defects. Truncus arteriosus is the most common of the conotruncal defects. Patients also often present with hypocalcemia because the parathyroid glands may be absent or reduced in size or number.

X-11.   The answer is D. *(Ch. 63)*   The placental circulation provides the fetus with all the necessary nutritional requirements, including oxygen. Since the fetal lungs are not expanded, a high flow bypassing them is of no detrimental consequence. Three vascular channels are of extreme importance in the fetal circulation. (1) The foramen ovale allows blood to pass from the right atrium to the left atrium, bypassing the fetal lungs. (2) The ductus arteriosus connects the pulmonary artery to the aorta distal to the left subclavian, bypassing uninflated lung tissue. (3) The ductus venosus shunts blood from the placenta through the umbilical cord to bypass the liver. The return of blood to the heart from the inferior vena cava accounts for 65 to 70 percent of the combined ventricular output. About 25 percent of the total ventricular output crosses the foramen ovale to the left atrium, joining 5 to 10 percent of the combined ventricular output returning from the fetal lungs. Thus, the right ventricle pumps two-thirds of the combined ventricular output, whereas the left ventricle pumps only one-third. About 85 to 90 percent of the blood ejected by the right ventricle is directed through the patent ductus arteriosus. Umbilical venous blood has a P_{O_2} of 26 to 28 mm Hg and an oxygen saturation of 80 percent; umbilical arterial blood has a P_{O_2} of 26 to 28 mm Hg and an oxygen saturation of 55 to 60 percent. The calculated fetal pulmonary vascular resistance is quite high but falls progressively until term. After birth, pulmonary vascular resistance drops due to decreased kinking (with lung expansion) and decreased vasoconstriction (due to increased P_{O_2}). Adult resistance levels are reached by 6 to 8 weeks of age.

X-12.   The answer is B. *(Ch. 63)*   The onset of congestive heart failure in children with congenital heart disease is usually within the first 6 months of life. It occurs rarely after 1 year of age, unless accompanied by serious problems like infective endocarditis, pneumonia, and anemia. The majority of infants who have heart failure in the first 12 to 18 h of life have malformations that involve pressure or volume overload, independent of pulmonary flow. Examples are severe valvular regurgitation or a systemic arteriovenous fistula. Iron deficiency leads to stiff red cells, and, in hypoxic children who are polycythemic, the stiff red cells cause sludging to occur, even with a fairly normal hematocrit. Hypoxia that is due to cyanotic defects does not respond to oxygen administration. Hypoxia due to heart failure or to lung disease with intrapulmonary shunting does respond to oxygen administration. Children with severe cardiac malformations have retardation of growth and development, with heights and weights below the third percentile.

X-13.   The answer is B. *(Ch. 63)*   The majority of VSDs (80 percent) are paramembranous defects. Conal septal or subarterial doubly committed defects account for 5 to 7 percent. There may be associated coarctation of the aorta. As pulmonary resistance begins to decrease after birth, an increasing amount of blood returns to the left atrium and left ventricle.

This left ventricular volume overload eventually leads to left ventricular failure, with elevated left ventricular end-diastolic pressure, increased left ventricular pressure, and pulmonary congestion. A systolic murmur along the lower left sternal border that is limited to early or midsystole suggests a defect in the muscular septum rather than the membranous septum. The signs of clinical improvement, such as less dyspnea, improved weight gain, and a diminution of the precordial hyperactivity, can indicate that either the defect is getting smaller, there is development of subvalvular pulmonary stenosis with little or no change in the defect size, or there is development of pulmonary vascular obstructive disease with continued severe pulmonary hypertension.

X-14. **The answer is E.** *(Ch. 63)* VSDs that are still large at age 6 months will undergo spontaneous closure in only 50 percent of cases. Males are more likely than females to develop aortic regurgitation as a result of the prolapse of the right, posterior, or both aortic valve leaflets into the defect. Aortic regurgitation more than doubles the risk of infective endocarditis in patients with VSDs, but surgical closure reduces the risk to less than half that of unoperated patients. Patients with VSDs between the ages of 5 and 10 years may still be candidates for surgical closure if a significant volume overload is present. Transcatheter closures have had some success at closing or leaving only trivial residual leaks in multiple trabeculated septal defects.

X-15. **The answer is C.** *(Ch. 63)* One or more of the right pulmonary veins may drain into the right atrium commonly in a defect at the fossa ovalis. The left superior vena cava may enter directly into the left atrium in a coronary sinus defect. ASDs should be surgically closed in adults, even if pulmonary resistance approaches 15 Wood units, because there is excessive morbidity and mortality associated with a persistent interatrial communication. Heart failure is uncommon in children with ASDs. Heart failure becomes more common in the fourth and fifth decades and is usually associated with the onset of arrhythmias. Many children with ASDs have normal growth and development.

X-16. **The answer is D.** *(Ch. 63)* The patient has a patent ductus arteriosus. The differential cyanosis exists from the shunting of hypoxemic blood from the pulmonary artery into the descending aorta. The murmur is described as a "machinery" murmur and peaks at or near the second heart sound.

X-17. **The answer is B.** *(Ch. 63)* The narrowing is usually at the ligamentum arteriosum. Rarely, it lies proximal to the origin of the left common carotid artery or involves a segment of the abdominal aorta. About half of affected infants have uncomplicated coarctation and the other half have at least one complicating cardiac abnormality. Low-pitched, continuous murmurs of collateral circulation can be heard over the chest wall, but can rarely be heard before adolescence. Similarly, a child under the age of 7 or 8 years would not show notching of the inferior margin of the ribs on chest x-ray. The rate of restenosis is up to 75 percent after balloon dilatation of children under 6 months of age, so surgical repair is the favored approach.

X-18. **The answer is A.** *(Ch. 63)* Valvular pulmonary stenosis is characterized most often by a dome-shaped stenosis of the pulmonary valve. Less often, it is characterized by dysplasia of the valve. Most infants and young children are asymptomatic. The only right-sided sound that becomes louder on expiration is the pulmonic ejection sound heard. Balloon valvuloplasty is nearly always successful in eliminating the obstruction.

X-19. **The answer is E.** *(Ch. 63)* The pulmonary valve is often malformed, but it is uncommonly the only site of obstruction to pulmonary flow. Coronary artery abnormalities are not uncommon. The left anterior descending coronary artery may arise from the right coronary sinus or even the right coronary itself. This abnormality should be corrected at the time of surgery. Due to the typical presence of a large ventricular septal defect, the right ventricle is "protected" from excessive pressure and work and heart failure is uncommon. The condition most commonly associated with tetralogy of Fallot is a persistent right aortic arch. Persistent left superior vena cava is seen in about 11 percent of cases. A patent foramen ovale is often left open during surgical repair to allow decompression during the perioperative period.

X-20. **The answer is C.** *(Ch. 63)*   Pulmonary venous obstruction is present in nearly all cases of infradiaphragmatic connection, but is rare in with supradiaphragmatic or supracardiac drainage. The physical examination of total anomalous pulmonary venous connection with pulmonary venous obstruction is usually unimpressive. Cardiomegaly is more likely without concomitant pulmonary venous obstruction, while pulmonary edema is more typical when obstruction is present. A patent foramen ovale must be present in all cases of total anomalous pulmonary venous connection.

X-21. **The answer is B.** *(Ch. 63)*   The ventricular septum remains intact in half of patients with dextro transposition of the great arteries. If there is a ventricular septal defect, it is small in 10 percent of patients and the remainder have a large defect. Atrial septostomy by catheterization can benefit all newborns, due to the increased mixing of the pulmonary and systemic venous circulation and the decompression of the left atrium. Significant pulmonary stenosis is not seen in many neonates with an intact ventricular septum, but develops in time in patients with a right ventricle connected to be the systemic ventricle. Because the right ventricle is functioning as the systemic ventricle, its pressure is equivalent to systemic arterial pressure. A patent ductus arteriosus and a narrow patent foramen are commonly seen in very young infants.

X-22. **The answer is A.** *(Ch. 63)*   The common type of single ventricle has the morphology of a left ventricle. The majority of patients with a single ventricle have a type I deformation, with normally related great vessels. Only about one-third of patients have a type II deformation with transposition. The most common finding when there is one large atrioventricular valve is a trabecular pattern of the left ventricle. The findings on ECG are those of either right or left ventricular hypertrophy, and therefore are not diagnostic. The study of choice is echocardiography. This condition used to be repaired by dividing the common chamber into right and left ventricles. Repair of this anomaly previously involved separating the two chambers, but this practice has been mostly abandoned due to unacceptably high mortality. The current approach allows the functional chamber to act as the ventricle for systemic circulation and the right side of the heart is bypassed.

X-23. **The answer is D.** *(Ch. 64)*   Chronic cyanosis can lead to erythrocytosis and hyperviscosity, but many patients with a stable high hematocrit have a low risk of stroke and do not require venesection. Rhythm disturbances that are benign in a structurally normal heart can be life-threatening for a patient with congenital heart disease. Restoring sinus rhythm is the most important treatment option. Early surgical repair for tetralogy of Fallot may reduce the incidence of postoperative ventricular arrhythmias. Pregnant women with left-to-right shunts tolerate pregnancy much better than those with right-to-left shunts or valvular stenosis.

X-24. **The answer is E.** *(Ch. 64)*   After the age of 40, mortality rates in patients with an ASD increase about 6 percent per year. Patients who have ASD repair after the age of 40 have a significantly poorer late survival, but they still benefit from surgical repair. The only real contraindication to repair is excessive pulmonary vascular disease. Surgical repair is the most widely used, although the transcatheter approach may someday supplant surgery as the method of choice. Patients who have had ASD repair during their first two decades of life can lead a normal life and need not be restricted from physical activity in the absence of hemodynamic or electrophysiologic sequelae. Changes associated with coronary artery disease or superimposed hypertension may increase the shunt and cause symptoms to appear.

X-25. **The answer is B.** *(Ch. 64)*   Isolated VSD is more common in infants and children than in adolescents and adults because most patients with a significant defect have it repaired during their childhood, spontaneous closure or reduction in size occurs, or patients who had large, unoperated defects die early in life. Noncardiac features, particularly mental retardation, have a major influence on the management of atrioventricular septal defect in adolescence and adulthood. Survival in unoperated patients with tetralogy of Fallot is poor. Only 25 percent of patients reach the age of 10 years, and only 3 percent reach age 40. Most adults with tetralogy of Fallot are suitable candidates for repair. The decreasing benefit with age for the surgical repair of pulmonary stenosis is independent of the use of ventriculotomy or outflow patches, but is attributed to long-standing pressure overload on the right ventricle.

X-26. The answer is D.   *(Ch. 64)*   Patients with coarctation of the aorta who have well-developed collaterals still may need surgical repair because of excessive upper extremity hypertension. Patients who have corrected coarctation of the aorta often have late hypertension, despite the early fall in blood pressure after the surgery. The Rastelli procedure involves closing the ventricular septal defect and inserting a valved conduit from the right ventricle to the pulmonary artery. Although the long-term results are good, surgery to replace the extracardiac conduit in adolescence and adult life is inevitable. A loss of sinus rhythm after atrial redirection does not appear to correlate with an increased risk of sudden death, but a more worrisome sign is the development of atrial tachyarrythmias. Newborns who present with Ebstein's anomaly often have a poorer outcome than those who do not present until they are adults.

PART XI
CARDIOMYOPATHY AND SPECIFIC HEART MUSCLE DISEASES

XI. CARDIOMYOPATHY AND SPECIFIC HEART MUSCLE DISEASES

QUESTIONS

DIRECTIONS: Each question listed below contains five suggested responses. Select the **one best** response to each question.

XI-1. According to the endomyocardial biopsy histology classification, which of the following is classified as an infiltrative cardiomyopathy?

(A) cytomegalovirus
(B) giant cell myocarditis
(C) right ventricular lipomatosis
(D) Fabry's disease
(E) lymphocytic myocarditis

(page 1944)

XI-2. Which of the following statements regarding myocardial dysfunction in dilated cardiomyopathies is true?

(A) other organs, such as the kidney or brain, exhibit modulated function in a similar manner to the heart
(B) signals responsible for abnormal cellular and chamber remodeling are examples of abnormalities of modulated function
(C) the inhibition component of modulated function remains normal in a failing heart
(D) inhibition of the autonomic nervous system and renin-angiotensin system does not prevent deterioration in or improve myocardial function
(E) β-adrenergic receptors can support intrinsic myocardial activity in the absence of an agonist

(pages 1950–1951)

XI-3. Which of the following statements regarding hypertensive cardiomyopathy is true?

(A) hypertensive cardiomyopathy could be put into the WHO/ISFC classification as a "dilated," "restrictive," or "unclassified" disorder
(B) the prognosis is worse than for other types of dilated cardiomyopathy
(C) intracardiac thrombi and mural endocardial plaques are present at necropsy in a majority of these patients

(D) interstitial parenchymal and perivascular focal infiltrates of small lymphocytes are diagnostic of hypertensive cardiomyopathy on histologic examination
(E) there is little variation among the phenotypic expression

(pages 1954–1956)

XI-4. Which of the following statements best describes the β-adrenergic pathway in idiopathic dilated cardiomyopathy (IDC)?

(A) there is decreased activation of the adrenergic nervous system in chronic heart failure
(B) β_1 receptors are up-regulated
(C) the inotropic response to Ca^{2+} administration is unchanged
(D) the response to exogenous β agonists is unchanged
(E) the β_2-agonist responsiveness is unchanged

(pages 1955–1957)

XI-5. Which of the following statements is characteristic of the cardiomyopathy caused by the anthracycline chemotherapeutic agents?

(A) about half of the subjects who develop anthracycline cardiomyopathy will recover completely
(B) subjects who present early have a better prognosis
(C) there is a characteristic extracellular deposition of proteins
(D) there is a relative absence of hypertrophy and dilatation and a higher heart rate than that usually seen in ambulatory heart failure
(E) anthracycline cardiomyopathy usually has a much better cardiac output than idiopathic dilated cardiomyopathy

(pages 1957–1960)

XI-6. Regarding alcohol-induced cardiomyopathy, which of the following is true?

(A) in the early, presymptomatic stages of alcoholic cardiomyopathy, global systolic dysfunction is the predominant physiologic abnormality

(B) chest pain is rare and angina indicates the presence of atherosclerotic coronary artery disease

(C) patients who drink mixed drinks are more likely to develop alcoholic cardiomyopathy than patients who consume beer and wine

(D) patients with alcohol-induced cirrhosis and peripheral neuropathy rarely develop alcohol-related cardiomyopathy

(E) by the time symptoms of alcohol-induced cardiomyopathy ensue, the left ventricular walls are usually hypertrophied

(page 1960)

XI-7. Which of the following statements regarding the gross morphologic features of hypertrophic cardiomyopathy (HCM) is true?

(A) the hypertrophy is usually distributed around the ventricle in a symmetric pattern

(B) necropsy examination of the heart will typically show dilated atria

(C) hypertrophy is usually seen in both the septum and the posterior segment of the free wall

(D) most cases of idiopathic hypertrophy presenting within the first 2 years of life are due to sarcomere protein mutations

(E) the magnitude of left ventricular hypertrophy in symptomatic adults increases further with time

(pages 1968–1970)

XI-8. Which of the following statements regarding the etiology and genetics of hypertrophic cardiomyopathy is true?

(A) routine echocardiographic screening is not productive in individuals less than 12 years of age with a family history of HCM

(B) HCM is inherited as an autosomal recessive trait

(C) a mutation in the β-myosin heavy chain is responsible for all cases of familial HCM

(D) individuals with a proven genetic abnormality, regardless of their phenotypic manifestations, should be advised not to take part in competitive athletics

(E) genotyped pedigrees of different families affected with HCM show the same genetic mutation

(pages 1974–1975)

XI-9. Which of the following statements regarding the pathophysiology of hypertrophic cardiomyopathy is true?

(A) increasing myocardial contractility reduces or abolishes subaortic obstruction

(B) systolic dysfunction is the most important pathophysiologic mechanism responsible for symptoms

(C) obstruction to right ventricular outflow is common in infants and young children

(D) myocardial ischemia in patients with HCM is most likely a result of atherosclerotic coronary artery disease

(E) the early filling phase of diastole is shortened

(page 1976)

XI-10. Which of the following statements concerning the murmur of left ventricular outflow obstruction in hypertrophic cardiomyopathy is true?

(A) the murmur is due to diastolic anterior motion of the mitral valve and mid-diastolic contact with the ventricular septum

(B) the murmur is louder with by beta-blocking drugs

(C) the murmur is increased by squatting due to an increase in arterial pressure

(D) the murmur is louder during the strain phase of the Valsalva maneuver

(E) the murmur decreases with exercise

(page 1979)

XI-11. Which of the following statements regarding the treatment of hypertrophic cardiomyopathy is true?

(A) prophylactic drug treatment to prevent sudden death has been highly effective

(B) alcohol septal ablation may increase the risk for life-threatening ventricular tachyarrhythmias and sudden death

(C) the vegetations of bacterial endocarditis are most likely to affect the aortic valve

(D) a reduction in the basal subaortic gradient with the myotomy-myectomy operation does not seem to be permanent

(pages 1979–1982)

XI-12. Which of the following statements regarding restrictive cardiomyopathy is true?

(A) a diastolic arterial pulse may be detected

(B) restrictive cardiomyopathy is always a primary disease of heart muscle

(C) Doppler shows a decreased E/A ratio for mitral valve flow

(D) hepatic venous flow reversals occur in expiration

(E) there is a higher right ventricular than left ventricular filling pressure

(pages 1989–1992)

XI-13. Which of the following statements regarding restrictive myocardial diseases is true?

(A) deposition of the intermediate filament desmin has been linked to pseudoxanthoma elasticum

(B) coronary artery disease commonly accompanies hemochromatosis

(C) pulmonary hypertension is the leading cause of death in patients with scleroderma

(D) cardiac involvement is most common in secondary amyloidosis

(E) myocyte hypertrophy and fibrosis on endomyocardial biopsy characterize Fabry's disease

(pages 1993–1997)

XI-14. Which of the following is a restrictive cardiomyopathy that affects the endocardium?

(A) sarcoidosis

(B) Gaucher's disease

(C) pseudoxanthoma elasticum

(D) carcinoid syndrome

(E) hemochromatosis

(page 1999)

XI-15. The effects of alcohol on the heart are correctly characterized by which of the following?

(A) ventricular arrhythmias are more common than atrial arrhythmias

(B) mechanisms of cardiac arrhythmias in alcoholics include high levels of circulating catecholamines, electrolyte abnormalities, and abnormal delays in normal conduction

(C) alcohol does not have a direct toxic effect on cardiac myocytes, but indirectly causes cardiac pathology by neurohormonal influences on the heart

(D) in female alcoholics, alcohol-induced cardiomyopathy is more common in premenopausal women

(E) in experimental animals, alcohol impairs protein synthesis in myocytes

(pages 2019–2020)

XI-16. Which of the following statements regarding the pathogenesis of infective myocarditis is true?

(A) cardiac dysfunction decreases after eradication of the infectious agent

(B) the effects of T cell-mediated injury are permanent

(C) high levels of IgM with cardiac specificity have been detected in patients with myocarditis

(D) attempts at culturing viruses from human myocardial tissue have been highly successful

(E) several viruses can trigger apoptosis

(pages 2003–2004)

XI-17. Which of the following statements regarding infective myocarditis is true?

(A) the degree of left ventricular dysfunction at initial presentation is most predictive of recovery

(B) there is no familial tendency for the development of myocarditis

(C) noninvasive techniques are the diagnostic standard

(D) immune modulatory therapy results in significant improvement in left ventricular ejection fraction

(E) laboratory findings are generally diagnostic

(pages 2005–2008)

XI-18. Which of the following statements regarding non-viral myocarditis is true?

(A) *Borrelia burgdorferi* is responsible for Chagas' disease

(B) the initial presenting symptom in patients with Lyme carditis is left ventricular dysfunction

(C) only a minority of patients will develop the chronic form of Chagas' disease

(D) the inflammatory infiltrate in Chagas' disease consists mainly of CD4+ T cells

(E) the Aschoff body is present during only the acute phase of rheumatic carditis

(pages 2008–2010)

XI-19. Which of the following statements regarding infiltrative cardiomyopathy due to amyloid is true?

(A) amyloid protein deposition due to chronic inflammatory processes occurs primarily in the heart

(B) systolic left ventricular dysfunction is not usually seen until late in the disease process

(C) left-sided symptoms of congestive heart failure occur more frequently

(D) digoxin is a recommended treatment

(E) heart transplantation has shown promising results

(pages 2013–2014)

XI-20. Which of the following statements regarding infiltrative cardiomyopathy due to sarcoidosis is true?

(A) the initial lesion consists of natural killer cells and B lymphocytes
(B) transplantation is a successful treatment
(C) the effects of the disease on the body are always widespread
(D) pericardial involvement is much more frequent than myocardial involvement
(E) endomyocardial biopsy has a high sensitivity and specificity

(pages 2015–2016)

XI-21. Which of the following statements regarding the systemic arterial hypertension found in patients with primary hyperparathyroidism is true?

(A) hypertension is a distinctive entity associated with the disease state
(B) hypertension responds dramatically to surgical removal of the parathyroid gland
(C) hypertension should be treated with thiazides as the diuretic of choice
(D) primary hyperparathyroidism is usually associated with concomitant Hashimoto's thyroiditis
(E) hypertension should be treated with loop diuretics as the diuretic of choice

XI-22. Compared to an ethnic-, age-, and sex-matched population, a predominant cardiovascular manifestation in patients with acromegaly is which of the following?

(A) high plasma renin activity
(B) accelerated coronary atherosclerosis
(C) dilated cardiomyopathy
(D) systemic arterial hypertension
(E) mitral valve prolapse

(page 2019)

XI-23. The cardiomyopathy seen with doxorubicin is best characterized by which of the following?

(A) significant increases in QRS voltage often indicate the onset of heart failure
(B) a total dose of over 550 mg/m^2 is associated with a high incidence of heart failure
(C) preexisting heart disease does not appear to increase the incidence
(D) prior radiation therapy does not increase the incidence
(E) most patients improve clinically with discontinuation of doxorubicin

(pages 2021–2022)

XI-24. Which of the following statements regarding acquired immune deficiency syndrome (AIDS) and cardiomyopathy is true?

(A) symptomatic cardiomyopathy is commonly associated with human immunodeficiency virus type 1 (HIV-1) infection
(B) echocardiographic evidence of left ventricular dysfunction is seen less commonly than symptoms are reported
(C) heart failure is responsible for a significant number of AIDS-related deaths
(D) there is a greater mean intensity of tumor necrosis factor α (TNF-α) in HIV patients compared with idiopathic cardiomyopathy patients
(E) most cardiac damage is as a result of the HIV virus invading the myocyte using the CD4+ receptor

(pages 2036–2038)

XI-25. Which of the following statements regarding AIDS and the cardiovascular system is true?

(A) cardiopulmonary bypass may accelerate the progression of HIV disease
(B) in most patients with AIDS and cardiomyopathy, drugs, both therapeutic and recreational, are the most common cause
(C) in the workup of patients with AIDS, screening echocardiograms and electrocardiograms should be performed
(D) interventional procedures should not be performed in patients with medically uncontrollable symptoms, due to the risk to the patient and health care provider
(E) protease inhibitors have no effect on the cardiovascular system

(pages 2037–2039)

XI-26. Which of the following statements regarding the effect of chemotherapeutic drugs on the heart is true?

(A) the occurrence of early ECG abnormalities in patients taking anthracyclines is a good predictor of cardiomyopathy
(B) mitoxantrone has features similar to doxorubicin, but is more cardiotoxic
(C) the most common cardiovascular effect of paclitaxel is transient asymptomatic bradycardia
(D) herceptin exerts an imperceptible effect on the heart
(E) a decreased resting left ventricular ejection fraction is a sensitive method for detecting early cardiotoxicity with anthracyclines

(pages 2045–2047)

XI-27. Which of the following statements regarding psychotropic agents and the cardiovascular system is true?

(A) selective serotonin reuptake inhibitors (SSRIs) have greater toxicity than tricyclic antidepressants (TCAs)

(B) orthostatic hypertension in older patients taking TCAs will improve with a dosage reduction

(C) TCAs are a good antidepressant for patients following myocardial infarction

(D) orthostatic hypertension is a common side effect seen in patients taking SSRIs

(E) the major concern in patients taking monoamine oxidase inhibitors (MAOIs) is interaction with other drugs

(pages 2047–2048)

XI-28. The cardiovascular effects of electrical injuries, including lightning, are best characterized by which of the following statements?

(A) the path of the electrical current (entry to exit sites) is not important in determining the cardiac effects

(B) evidence of myocardial damage is very unusual

(C) both significant left ventricular dysfunction and a return to normal ventricular function can be seen following successful recovery of the patient

(D) despite catecholamine release following the injury, hypertension and tachycardia are not seen

(E) direct current even of low voltage is of greater hazard than an alternating current because of the "let go" phenomenon

(page 2052)

XI. CARDIOMYOPATHY AND SPECIFIC HEART MUSCLE DISEASES

ANSWERS

XI-1. **The answer is C.** *(Ch. 65)* According to the endomyocardial biopsy histology classification of cardiomyopathies, there are four disorders classified as infiltrative cardiomyopathies: glycogen storage disease, hemochromatosis, right ventricular lipomatosis, and amyloidosis. Giant cell myocarditis and lymphocytic myocarditis are both inflammatory/immune cardiomyopathies. Cytomegalovirus is an infectious cardiomyopathy. Fabry's disease is classified as a miscellaneous nonspecific cardiomyopathy.

XI-2. **The answer is E.** *(Ch. 66)* Modulated function is defined as stimulation or inhibition of myocardial contraction or relaxation by endogenous bioactive compounds. Other organs do not exhibit modulated function. The signals responsible for abnormal cellular and chamber remodeling are abnormalities of intrinsic function, not modulated function. The inhibition component of modulated function is abnormal in a failing heart because of a reduction in parasympathetic drive. Inhibition of the autonomic nervous system and the renin-angiotensin system can prevent deterioration or possibly improve myocardial function, as well as reducing mortality. β-Adrenergic receptors have intrinsic activity. Some receptors can remain in an activated state, without the presence of an agonist.

XI-3. **The answer is A.** *(Ch. 66)* Hypertensive cardiomyopathy within the WHO/ISFC classification can be in either the "dilated," "restrictive," or "unclassified" categories. In subjects with a controlled afterload, the prognosis is probably better than for other types of dilated cardiomyopathy. Intracardiac thrombi and mural endocardial plaques present at necropsy are seen in about half of patients with idiopathic dilated cardiomyopathy (IDC). Interstitial parenchymal and perivascular focal infiltrates of small lymphocytes are also seen on histologic exam of patients with IDC. There is a great deal of variation in phenotypic expression in patients with hypertensive cardiomyopathy.

XI-4. **The answer is C.** *(Ch. 66)* There is substantial activation of the adrenergic nervous system in chronic heart failure. There is a 30 percent reduction in β_2-agonist responsiveness. β_1 receptors are down-regulated. Although there is a reduction in the responsiveness to exogenous β agonist, the inotropic response to Ca^{2+} administration is unchanged.

XI-5. **The answer is D.** *(Ch. 66)* Patients with anthracycline cardiomyopathy have a relative absence of hypertrophy and dilatation and a higher heart rate than those usually seen with ambulatory heart failure. About half of the subjects who develop postpartum cardiomyopathy will recover completely; anthracycline cardiomyopathy is usually irreversible. Patients with anthracycline cardiomyopathy who present late (several months to several years) have a better prognosis. There is a characteristic extracellular deposition of protein in amyloid cardiomyopathy. Anthracycline cardiomyopathy and idiopathic dilated cardiomyopathies have reduced cardiac output. Alcoholic cardiomyopathy is similar to IDC but usually presents with a relatively high cardiac output.

XI-6. **The answer is D.** *(Ch. 66)* Chronic alcohol abuse can cause significant myocardial dysfunction prior to the onset of clinical symptoms. In the early, preclinical phases of the disease, myocardial hypertrophy and diastolic dysfunction predominate. Only late in the disease process, when symptoms finally appear, does the ventricle dilate and the ventricular walls thin and systolic function decline. Symptoms of left-sided heart failure are often the presenting symptoms, but it is not uncommon for the first symptoms to be chest pain (occasionally anginal in nature). The etiology of the chest pain is not clear since most patients do not have occlusive coronary disease by angiography. The pattern of alcohol intake (i.e., binge versus regular, constant imbibing) and the type of alcohol consumed (i.e., beer versus wine versus mixed drinks) do not predict who will develop the dilated cardiomyopathy of alcoholism. However, it has been observed that patients who develop neuropathy and cirrhosis rarely acquire alcoholic cardiomyopathy.

XI-7.   **The answer is B.**   *(Ch. 67)*   The distribution of the hypertrophy is almost always asymmetric, with certain segments of the left ventricular wall thickened to a dissimilar degree. Necropsy examination of the heart typically reveals atrial dilation but virtually every other form of heart failure also demonstrates this feature. Hypertrophy generally affects both the septum and the lateral portion of the free wall. Rarely is the posterior portion of the free wall affected. Most cases of idiopathic left ventricular hypertrophy that present in the first 2 years of life are not due to sarcomere protein mutations, but are associated with other conditions, such as Noonan syndrome. In symptomatic adult patients with HCM, the magnitude of the left ventricular hypertrophy may decrease over time.

XI-8.   **The answer is A.**   *(Ch. 67)*   Routine echocardiographic screening is unproductive in individuals less than 12 years of age, as phenotypic expression of the mutant is rarely present at that age. Family screening can usually be deferred until individuals reach adolescence, unless they are involved in intense athletic programs or are members of families with HCM-related sudden deaths. HCM is inherited as an autosomal dominant trait. There can be mutations in any one of the nine genes that encode contractile proteins of the cardiac sarcomere. Most genotyped pedigrees show mutations that are apparently unique to that particular family. There is not currently enough evidence to recommend individuals with a proven gene defect, but no physical manifestations, to abstain from competitive athletics.

XI-9.   **The answer is C.**   *(Ch. 67)*   Interventions that increase myocardial contractility or decrease arterial pressure or ventricular volume will increase or provoke the subaortic obstruction. Infants and young children will commonly have obstruction to right ventricular outflow. Diastolic dysfunction is most likely to be responsible for symptoms. The early filling phase of diastole is significantly prolonged and has a decreased rate and volume of rapid filling. There is some evidence that myocardial ischemia occurs in HCM as part of the underlying cardiomyopathic process, but the ischemia is unrelated to coronary artery disease.

XI-10.   **The answer is D.**   *(Ch. 67)*   In hypertrophic cardiomyopathy, left ventricular outflow obstruction and its consequent murmur is a dynamic process caused by *systolic* anterior motion of the mitral valve and *midsystolic* contact with the ventricular septum. Interventions or circumstances that decrease myocardial contractility (beta-blocking) drugs or increase ventricular volume or arterial pressure (vasoconstrictor agents or squatting) reduce or abolish the murmur. Interventions or circumstances that increase contractility (exercise or isoproterenol) or that decrease arterial pressure or ventricular volume (Valsalva maneuver or administration of an agent producing hypotension) increase the loudness of the murmur.

XI-11.   **The answer is B.**   *(Ch. 67)*   There is little evidence that drug treatment prevents sudden death. The implantable cardiac defibrillator has been shown to effective in preventing sudden death, but the indications for this device in asymptomatic patients are not clear. The vegetations of bacterial endocarditis most commonly involve the anterior mitral leaflet or septal endocardium at the site of mitral valve contact. Many patients tolerate chronic atrial fibrillation well, as long as ventricular rate is well controlled. Alcohol septal ablation may increase the future long-term risk of life-threatening ventricular tachyarrhythmias and sudden death. The reduction in the basal subaortic gradient with the myotomy-myectomy operation appears to be permanent, but does not reduce mortality.

XI-12.   The answer is A.   *(Ch. 68)*   In severe cases of restrictive cardiomyopathy, a diastolic arterial pulse may be detected, due to a reduced stroke volume and tachycardia. Restrictive cardiomyopathy may occur in the setting of systemic or iatrogenic disease, thus it is not always a primary disease of heart muscle. Doppler evaluation of mitral valve inflow shows an increased E/A ratio, a short deceleration time, and a short isovolumic relaxation time without respiratory variation. Hepatic venous flow reversal in expiration is seen in constrictive pericarditis, not restrictive cardiomyopathy. The left ventricular filling pressure is usually higher than the right ventricular filling pressure, as opposed to constrictive pericarditis where the filling pressures are equal.

XI-13.   The answer is C.   *(Ch. 68)*   Deposition of the intermediate filament desmin, myocyte hypertrophy, and fibrosis are present on endomyocardial biopsy in idiopathic restrictive cardiomyopathy. Coronary artery disease is very common in patients with pseudoxanthoma elasticum. Pulmonary hypertension is the leading cause of death for patients with scleroderma. Cardiac involvement is most likely in primary amyloidosis.

XI-14.   The answer is D.   *(Ch. 68)*   In carcinoid syndrome, restrictive physiology is produced by infiltration of the endocardium. Pseudoxanthoma elasticum is a noninfiltrative cardiomyopathy affecting the myocardium. Sarcoidosis and Gaucher's disease are both infiltrative cardiomyopathies that affect the myocardium. Hemochromatosis is an iron storage disease that affects the myocardium.

XI-15.   The answer is B.   *(Ch. 69)*   Arrhythmias are common in patients who abuse alcohol and are often the precipitators of the first episode of overt heart failure. Atrial arrhythmias predominate, although ventricular premature contractions and sudden cardiac death have been reported. The mechanisms of cardiac dysrhythmias in the alcoholic are not known with certainty, but elevated levels of catecholamines, delays in native conduction, and electrolyte abnormalities (hypokalemia and hypomagnesemia) have been implicated. There is a direct toxic effect of alcohol on myocytes, but in animals, alcohol does not impair protein synthesis of cardiac myocytes. Female alcoholics are more likely to develop cardiomyopathy after menopause.

XI-16.   The answer is E.   *(Ch. 69)*   Cardiac dysfunction has been shown to increase after eradication of the infectious agent, thus leading to the speculation that immune processes, rather than infectious agents, are responsible for the damage. T cell-mediated injury caused by perforin cytotoxicity is permanent, but the injury mediated by cytokines is reversible. High levels of IgG with cardiac specificity have been detected in patients with myocarditis. Attempts at culturing viruses from human myocardial tissue have been unsuccessful. Several viruses have been reported to trigger apoptosis.

XI-17.   The answer is A.   *(Ch. 69)*   The degree of left ventricular dysfunction at initial presentation is most predictive of recovery. There seems to be a familial tendency for the development of myocarditis. Endomyocardial biopsy is the diagnostic standard, despite the promise of noninvasive techniques. Immune modulatory therapy is not routinely recommended for infective endocarditis because no randomized study has yet demonstrated the efficacy of this treatment. Therapy is still that of standard heart failure. Laboratory finding are not generally diagnostic of myocarditis. About 60 percent of patients will have an elevated erythrocyte sedimentation rate and 25 percent will have an elevated white blood cell count.

XI-18.   The answer is C.   *(Ch. 69)*   *Trypanosoma cruzi* is responsible for Chagas' disease. The inflammatory infiltrate in these patients consists mainly of CD8+ T cells with a low number of CD4+, suggesting that there is some degree of immunologic depression in the host. Only 20 to 30 percent of patients will develop a chronic form of Chagas' disease. The initial presenting symptom for Lyme carditis is complete heart block. The Aschoff body, which is pathognomic for rheumatic carditis, can persist for years after an acute attack.

XI-19. **The answer is B.** *(Ch. 69)*   Amyloid deposition due to chronic inflammatory processes is usually limited to the intima and media of arterioles and not the heart. Abnormalities of left ventricular diastolic function always precede systolic dysfunction, which is generally not seen until late in the disease process. Symptoms of right heart failure are more are typical. Digoxin is not recommended because of increased myocardial concentrations due to binding of the drug to amyloid fibrils. Heart transplants have been disappointing, due to the recurrence of amyloid in the transplanted heart.

XI-20. **The answer is B.** *(Ch. 69)*   The initial lesion consists of activated helper-inducer T lymphocytes and abundant cytokine-secreting macrophages. The disease can be either widespread or limited to a singe organ. Myocardial involvement is much more frequent than pericardial involvement. Heart transplantation has been a successful treatment, as the recurrence of sarcoid is low. Due to the scattered nature of the granulomas, endomyocardial biopsy lacks sensitivity but is very specific.

XI-21. **The answer is E.** *(Ch. 69)*   The incidence of systemic arterial hypertension appears to be higher in hypercalcemic patients compared to the normal population, but there is uncertainty whether there is a true association between hypertension and hyperparathyroidism. Surgical removal of the hyperactive parathyroid gland does not have a distinctive beneficial effect on hypertension but may improve the management of hypertension with medical therapy. When diuretics are necessary for the treatment of hypertension associated with hyperparathyroidism, thiazides should be avoided since they may further increase serum calcium levels. There is no relationship to Hashimoto's thyroiditis. Loop diuretics are the agents of choice since they are calciuric diuretics.

XI-22. **The answer is D.** *(Ch. 69)*   Autopsy studies in acromegalic patients have been unable to show a characteristic form of cardiac pathology. Although cardiac enlargement is evident, this is usually reflected in hypertension rather than a dilated cardiomyopathy. Hypertension occurs in acromegaly three times more frequently than in the general population. It tends to be mild, responsive to conventional therapy, and regression may occur after successful treatment of growth hormone excess. The etiology of the hypertension in acromegaly is thought to be secondary to growth hormone-mediated sodium retention associated with low plasma renin. However, the possibility of a pheochromocytoma or hyperaldosteronism should also be kept in mind since acromegaly could be a variant of a multiple endocrine neoplasia syndrome. Ironically, in spite of the high incidence of glucose intolerance and hypertension, the occurrence of coronary artery disease or peripheral vascular disease is not higher than that of a comparable matched population.

XI-23. **The answer is B.** *(Ch. 69)*   Doxorubicin is a very commonly used chemotherapeutic agent. There is a tendency to have decreased QRS voltage after doxorubicin therapy, but QRS voltage changes are unreliable in determining the severity of the cardiomyopathy. Cardiomyopathy is a very serious effect of doxorubicin. There is a 14 percent incidence of clinical heart failure with doses of 430 mg/m^2, and 30 percent with doses over 550 mg/m^2. Factors that may increase the chance of cardiomyopathy, even with lower doses, include prior radiation therapy, preexisting heart disease, hypertension, and associated use of other chemotherapeutic agents. A higher incidence is also noted in young children and older adults. The clinical presentation of doxorubicin cardiomyopathy is similar to that of idiopathic dilated cardiomyopathy. The clinical course is variable, but only a few patients improve with medical therapy. The value of radionuclide determination of left ventricular ejection fraction at rest and with exercise has been reported. Serial determinations of ejection fraction may allow for higher doses without additional risk of heart failure.

XI-24. **The answer is D.** *(Ch. 70)*   Symptomatic cardiomyopathy in HIV-1 infection is uncommon, but echocardiographic evidence of left ventricular dysfunction may be present. The incidence of heart failure has been extremely small. Cardiac causes of death are in fact quite rare. There is little evidence supporting the fact that the HIV virus can invade myocardial cells.

Myocytes do not have the CD4+ receptor, thus the virus must enter via a different receptor or through a different mechanism. There is evidence that the cardiomyopathy is due to auto-immune mechanisms. There is a greater mean intensity of TNF-α and inducible nitric oxide synthase in HIV patients compared to idiopathic cardiomyopathy patients.

XI-25. The answer is A. *(Ch. 70)* There is some evidence that cardiopulmonary bypass may accelerate the progression of HIV disease, and this should be taken into consideration before surgery. In most patients with AIDS and cardiomyopathy, drugs, whether recreational or therapeutic, do not seem to be the cause. There does not seem to be a therapeutic advantage to detecting subclinical cardiovascular involvement, so there is little justification for performing screening electrocardiograms or echocardiograms in AIDS patients. Interventional procedures that can ameliorate symptoms should be performed. Protease inhibitors, in their ability to cause metabolic abnormalities, have caused an increasing incidence of extensive coronary artery disease.

XI-26. The answer is C. *(Ch. 71)* The occurrence of early ECG abnormalities in patients taking anthracyclines does not predict cardiomyopathy and should not indicate a need for the discontinuation of therapy. Mitoxantrone has features similar to doxorubicin, but is less cardiotoxic. The most common cardiovascular side effect of paclitaxel is transient asymptomatic bradycardia. Herceptin has caused cardiac dysfunction in patients and its use requires close cardiac monitoring. Resting left ventricular ejection fraction is not a sensitive test for detecting early cardiotoxicity from anthracyclines.

XI-27. The answer is E. *(Ch. 71)* Tricyclic antidepressants inhibit the uptake of both norepinephrine and serotonin, resulting in greater toxicity compared to SSRIs. Orthostatic hypertension is a common side effect of TCAs, especially in older patients, and does not usually improve with dosage reduction. TCAs are relatively contraindicated in patients following a myocardial infarction, because of evidence of a proarrhythmic effect in patients with serious structural heart disease. Orthostatic hypertension and bradycardia are rarely seen in patients taking SSRIs. The major concern in patients taking monoamine oxidase inhibitors is their potential interaction with other drugs.

XI-28. The answer is C. *(Ch. 71)* The path of electrical current through the body (entry to exit sites) is very important in determining the cardiac and central nervous system effects of electricity. A current path from arm to arm or arm to leg is more likely to cause direct cardiac effects. Extensive body surface burns are also a predictor of myocardial damage. Electrocardiographic changes, such as sinus tachycardia and nonspecific ST-segment and T-wave changes, cardiac arrhythmias, and myocardial damage are common findings. The catecholamine release often produces hypertension and tachycardia and can be successfully managed with intravenous beta-blocking drugs. Many patients develop significant left ventricular dysfunction but some may return to near normal. Alternating current, regardless of the voltage, is more hazardous than a direct current because tetanic muscle contractions prevent the "let go" phenomenon.

PART XII
PERICARDIAL DISEASES
AND ENDOCARDITIS

XII. PERICARDIAL DISEASES AND ENDOCARDITIS

QUESTIONS

DIRECTIONS: Each question listed below contains five suggested responses. Select the **one best** response to each question.

XII-1. Which of the following regarding the anatomy and histology of the pericardium is true?

(A) the superior and inferior pericardiosternal and diaphragmatic ligaments anchor the heart during positional changes but do not neutralize the effects of respiration on the position of the heart

(B) the pericardial space normally contains up to 150 mL of pericardial fluid

(C) the pericardium is composed primarily of elastin fibers and stretches considerably more in the long axis than the short axis

(D) the phrenic nerves run superficial to the parietal layer along the surface of the pericardium

(E) the left atrium is largely extrapericardial

(page 2061)

XII-2. Which of the following is true about the function of the pericardium?

(A) the pericardium shifts gravitational, inertial, and hydrostatic pressures to the left side of the heart

(B) the pericardium influences right and left ventricular filling equally

(C) the pericardium modulates myocyte structure, function, and gene expression

(D) the small concentrations of various substances in pericardial fluid are useful in determining the severity of heart failure

(E) the pericardium prevents maximum drug delivery and gene therapy to the coronary arteries

(page 2062)

XII-3. Which of the following is a typical presentation in acute pericarditis?

(A) anginal chest pain and an ECG showing ST-segment elevation with downward concavity

(B) pleuritic chest pain, a friction rub, and an ECG showing ST-segment depression

(C) pleuritic chest pain, an echo showing a small pericardial effusion, and an ECG showing T-wave inversions

(D) anginal chest pain and diffuse T-wave inversions on an ECG

(E) pleuritic chest pain and a biphasic or triphasic friction rub

(pages 2064–2065)

XII-4. Which of the following is the best therapy for acute pericarditis?

(A) oral nonsteroidal anti-inflammatory agents and colchicine

(B) oral nonsteroidal anti-inflammatory agents and indomethacin

(C) oral nonsteroidal anti-inflammatory agents and corticosteroids

(D) corticosteroids, colchicine, and indomethacin

(E) corticosteroids

(page 2066)

XII-5. In which of the following patients with pericardial effusions would analysis of pericardial fluid be LEAST beneficial?

(A) a 45-year-old woman with possible tuberculosis

(B) a 60-year-old male with adenocarcinoma of the lung

(C) a 28-year-old female with breast cancer

(D) a 73-year-old white male with severe chronic heart failure

(E) a 51-year-old male with recurrent pericardial effusion of unknown cause

(page 2067)

XII-6. Which of the following regarding the physical examination of cardiac tamponade is true?

(A) there is elevation of pericardial pressures, pulsus paradoxus, and arterial hypertension
(B) Küssmaul's sign is typically present
(C) there is a rapid *x* descent in the jugular venous pulse, arterial hypotension, and pulsus paradoxus
(D) there are rapid *x* and *y* descents in the jugular venous pulse
(E) there are normal jugular venous pressures and pulsus alternans

(page 2069)

XII-7. Which of the following is diagnostic for cardiac tamponade on echocardiography?

(A) right atrial collapse exceeding one-third of the cardiac cycle
(B) a decrease of tricuspid flow velocity during inspiration
(C) absent respiratory variations in the mitral flow velocity
(D) extreme enlargement of the right and left atria
(E) apparent calcification of the pericardium

(pages 2069–2070)

XII-8. Which of the following regarding constrictive pericarditis is true?

(A) echocardiography shows flattening of the LV posterior wall and abnormal septal motion
(B) constrictive pericarditis is often misdiagnosed as hepatic failure
(C) the most common cause in the United States is tuberculosis
(D) there is a large cardiac silhouette on a chest roentgenogram
(E) there is no adequate test for detecting pericardial thickening

(pages 2073–2074)

XII-9. Which of the following statements regarding pericardial heart disease is true?

(A) pericardial disease is present in up to 50 percent of HIV-positive patients but is not indicative of poor prognosis
(B) pericarditis is associated with HIV infection, Lyme disease, tuberculosis, uremia, and immunosuppression
(C) bacterial infections are the most common cause of pericarditis in hospitalized patients
(D) thrombolytic therapy increases the incidence of postinfarction pericarditis
(E) congenital malformation of the pericardium usually require surgical repair within the first year of life

(pages 2077–2080)

XII-10. Which of the following statements regarding the history and epidemiology of endocarditis is true?

(A) cases of endocarditis were only described in literature after the discovery of penicillin
(B) antibiotics have successfully cured infective endocarditis and dramatically reduced the incidence
(C) recent major changes in the clinical features and epidemiology of infective endocarditis are mainly from the widespread use of antimicrobial agents
(D) It is cost-effective to treat patients with a relatively high risk of endocarditis prophylactically with antibiotics
(E) Children under age 2 and intravenous drug users who develop infective endocarditis are likely to have preexisting heart disease

(page 2088)

XII-11. Which of the following statements regarding infective endocarditis in children is true?

(A) it affects more females than males
(B) most cases are found in children with rheumatic heart disease
(C) surgical repair of patent ductus arteriosus and ventricular septal defect increases the risk of getting infective endocarditis
(D) The three most common causative agents, in order, are viridans streptococci, *Staphylococcus aureus,* and enterococci
(E) Endocardial infections with enterococci have a worse prognosis than other types

(pages 2081, 2089–2090)

XII-12. Which of the following statements concerning infective endocarditis and intravenous drug users is true?

(A) intravenous drug users are 50 times more likely to die suddenly with infective endocarditis than nonusers
(B) *Pseudomonas* species account for more than 50 percent of the endocardial infections in intravenous drug users
(C) the mitral and aortic valves are the most common locations for vegetations to form
(D) mortality rates are lower for intravenous drug users with endocarditis than for nonusers
(E) the spectrum of infectious agents is similar in intravenous drug users and nonusers

(page 2090)

XII-13. Which of the following statements regarding infective endocarditis in postcardiac surgery patients is true?

(A) gram-negative bacilli and fungi infect native valves more frequently than prosthetic valves

(B) the peak of onset of prosthetic valve endocarditis is 3 to 4 months postsurgery

(C) patients with prosthetic valves remain at a higher risk for infective endocarditis for the rest of their lives

(D) the total number of cases of postsurgical endocarditis has increased recently with rates now as high as 2 percent

(E) the most common organism involved in early-onset prosthetic valve endocarditis is group B streptococci

(page 2091)

XII-14. Which of the following statements regarding endocarditis is true?

(A) hemodialysis and pacemaker patients are at high risk for infective endocarditis

(B) hospital-acquired infective endocarditis is rare and is mostly connected to cardiac surgery

(C) up to two-thirds of patients with nosocomial endocarditis have preexisting cardiac abnormalities

(D) cardiac catheterization procedures account for about 10 percent of nosocomial endocarditis cases

(E) patients with nosocomial endocarditis have a better prognosis than other patients with endocarditis because the infection is detected in its early stages

(page 2092)

XII-15. Which of the following statements regarding organisms for infective endocarditis is true?

(A) staphylococcus organisms cause more cases of endocarditis than any other organism

(B) *Streptococcus viridans* is the most common cause of infective endocarditis and usually infects more than one valve in older patients

(C) up to 30 percent of patients with *Staphylococcus aureus* bacteremia have an associated endocarditis

(D) *Haemophilus* endocarditis usually causes large vegetations with arterial emboli but represents a small fraction of endocarditis infections

(E) fungal infections are more common in nonintravenous drug users

(pages 2093–2094)

XII-16. Which of the following statements regarding the distribution of valvular involvement in infective endocarditis is true?

(A) the right heart valves are involved more than the left heart valves

(B) the frequency of involvement is directly proportional to the mean blood pressure across the valve

(C) intravenous drug users are more likely to have left heart valve involvement than nonusers

(D) vegetations tend to be occur just upstream from anatomic abnormalities in the heart

(E) the aortic valve has a higher frequency of infection than the mitral valve

(page 2097)

XII-17. Which of the following is true regarding the complications of infective endocarditis?

(A) only about 50 percent of patients with infective endocarditis present with a heart murmur

(B) in the past, 25 percent of patients with infective endocarditis had heart failure as a complication

(C) up to 50 percent of patients with infective endocarditis have major arterial emboli

(D) conduction abnormalities occur in over 75 percent of cases

(E) few patients experience involvement of the nervous system during the course of infective endocarditis

(page 2101)

XII-18. According to the Duke criteria, which of the following patients is most likely to have infective endocarditis?

(A) the patient in whom the manifestations of endocarditis have resolved fully by the 4th day of antibiotic therapy

(B) the patient who has Roth's spots, fever, and a predisposition to infective endocarditis

(C) the patient who has an oscillating intracardiac mass and a predisposition to infective endocarditis

(D) the patient who has an oscillating intracardiac mass and two positive blood cultures

(E) the patient who fulfills three minor Duke criteria

(page 2104)

XII-19. Which of the following statements regarding currently recommended therapy of infective endocarditis is true?

(A) patients with penicillin-sensitive streptococci should be given penicillin and vancomycin for 6 weeks

(B) patients with penicillin-resistant streptococci should be given ampicillin and vancomycin for 4 weeks

(C) patients with methicillin-sensitive staphylococci on prosthetic valves should be given vancomycin plus gentamicin for 4 to 6 weeks

(D) patients with methicillin-resistant staphylococci on prosthetic valves should be given vancomycin, gentamicin, and rifampin

(E) patients with methicillin-resistant staphylococci on prosthetic valves should be given ceftriaxone, ampicillin, and gentamicin

(pages 2108–2109)

XII-20. Which of the following situations is most likely to require prompt surgical intervention?

(A) the development of moderate heart failure in a patient being treated for acute endocarditis

(B) an intravenous drug user diagnosed with acute staphylococcal endocarditis

(C) a laboratory report indicating a serum bactericidal titer of 1:32 during the 1 week of antibiotic treatment for a patient with streptococcal endocarditis

(D) a patient with a relapsed case of streptococcal endocarditis 2 weeks after completing a 4-week antibiotic regimen

(E) the 1 week of acute bacterial endocarditis to prevent emboli from developing

(pages 2111–2113)

XII-21. Which of the following statements regarding prophylactic use of antibiotics to prevent endocarditis is true?

(A) antibiotics should be given long-term at low doses for prevention of endocarditis

(B) prophylactic antibiotics should be given prior to root canal procedures in patients without valvular heart disease

(C) prophylactic antibiotics should be given prior to dental extraction procedures in patients with mild to moderate valvular heart disease

(D) antibiotic prophylaxis is similar in patients with prosthetic valves to those with mild to moderate native valve abnormalities

(E) erythromycin should be used for patients allergic to penicillin before undergoing procedures with high risk of causing high-grade bacteremia

(page 2115)

XII. PERICARDIAL DISEASES AND ENDOCARDITIS

ANSWERS

XII-1. **The answer is E.** *(Ch. 72)* The superior and inferior pericardiosternal and diaphragmatic ligaments limit displacement of the pericardium and neutralize the effects of respiration and changes of body position. The pericardial space normally contains up to 50 mL of pericardial fluid. The pericardium is composed mostly of compact collagen layers with some interspersed elastin fibers. The pericardium is capable of stretching more in the short axis than the long axis. The phrenic nerves are embedded in the parietal pericardium. The left atrium is anterior to the oblique sinus and is therefore largely extrapericardial.

XII-2. **The answer is C.** *(Ch. 72)* The pericardium helps to equalize the various external forces operating on the heart, not shift them to the left heart, although the pericardium influences filling of the thin-walled right ventricle and atrium more than the thicker-walled left ventricle and atrium. The pericardial fluid contains substances that modulate myocyte structure, function, and gene expression. While the pericardial fluid contains substances that influence the growth and remodeling of the myocardium, there is no clinical utility in their measurement. In spite of the multiple contributions of the pericardium, it is not essential to the normal functioning of the heart.

XII-3. **The answer is E.** *(Ch. 72)* Acute pericarditis is characterized by pleuritic chest pain, a biphasic or triphasic friction rub, possibly a small pericardial effusion on echocardiography, and an ECG which shows diffuse ST-segment elevation with a downward concavity and possibly PR-segment depression. The ST-segment elevation of pericarditis must be differentiated from other causes of ST elevation, the most important of which is acute myocardial injury. The latter is usually localized to the area of injury and has upward concavity. The chest pain is anginal, and an echo will show left ventricular segmental wall motion abnormalities. Cardiac enzymes are usually elevated within an hour of the onset of chest pain. It is essential to make this differential diagnosis, as thrombolytic therapy may be indicated in an acute ST-segment elevation myocardial infarction (MI), while thrombolytic therapy in acute pericarditis may cause life-threatening hemorrhagic tamponade.

XII-4. **The answer is A.** *(Ch. 72)* Acute pericarditis usually responds to oral nonsteroidal anti-inflammatory agents. Colchicine is effective for acute episodes and may prevent recurrences. Indomethacin reduces coronary blood flow and should probably be avoided. Corticosteroids should not be first-line therapy for acute pericarditis unless there is another reason to use them, such as uremia or a connective tissue disease. Corticosteroids may be necessary in recurrent pericarditis.

XII-5. **The answer is D.** *(Ch. 72)* It is appropriate to analyze pericardial fluid in certain clinical situations, including possible infectious or neoplastic disease. Otherwise, the diagnostic yield of pericardial fluid when the etiology is unknown is only 20 percent. Pericardial fluid in some conditions, such as renal failure with chronic hemodialysis or chronic heart failure, does not need analysis.

XII-6. **The answer is C.** *(Ch. 72)* The physical examination of cardiac tamponade demonstrates elevated jugular venous pressure with a single rapid x descent, arterial hypotension, pulsus paradoxus, and possibly pulsus alternans. An elevated jugular venous pressure with rapid *x* and *y* descents, Küssmaul's sign, and an early diastolic sound (the pericardial "knock") are indicative of constrictive pericarditis.

XII-7. **The answer is A.** *(Ch. 72)* The echocardiographic findings of cardiac tamponade include a pericardial effusion, diastolic collapse of the right atrium and possibly the right ventricle, and more than a 25 percent respiratory variation of the transtricuspid flow velocity. Right atrial and ventricular collapse occurs during diastole when the pressure in the chambers is lower than the elevated pressure in the pericardium. Lesser variation of the transmitral flow is usually also present. Flow across both atrioventricular valves is greater during inspiration. Extreme enlargement of the right and left atria is typical of restrictive cardiomyopathy. Calcification of the pericardium may be detected in some patients with constrictive pericarditis due to tuberculosis. These two diseases are mentioned here because they and cardiac tamponade usually share the common feature of equalization of diastolic pressures in the cardiac chambers.

XII-8. **The answer is B.** *(Ch. 72)* Flattening of the left ventricular posterior wall and abnormal septal motion are suggestive of restrictive cardiomyopathy. Constrictive pericarditis is frequently misdiagnosed as chronic hepatic failure because of hepatomegaly, elevated liver enzymes, mildly elevated bilirubin, possibly ascites, and certainly peripheral edema. The most common cause in developed counties is idiopathic, presumably postviral infection. Tuberculosis is still the most common cause in developing countries. A chest roentgenogram usually shows normal cardiac size. Calcification of the pericardium strongly suggests tuberculosis. A CT scan usually reveals the thickened pericardium.

XII-9. **The answer is B.** *(Ch. 72)* The most common pericardial disease is metastatic cancer. The most common infectious cause of pericardial disease is viral. The spectrum of pericardial infections has been changing since the appearance of AIDS, with unusual bacterial and other microbes as causative agents. Pericardial disease is present in up to 21 percent of AIDS patients and a pericardial effusion may signal end-stage HIV disease. Thrombolytic therapy reduces the incidence of post-MI pericarditis by half because of smaller areas of myocardial necrosis. Although congenital malformations of the pericardium are rare and often asymptomatic, a medium-sized defect can allow cardiac herniation.

XII-10. **The answer is D.** *(Ch. 73)* Cases of infective endocarditis were described as early as the 1600s and the microbial origin was demonstrated in 1869. Antibiotics are effective cures for endocarditis but have not decreased the overall incidence of the disease. Recent changes in the clinical features and epidemiology are due primarily to changes in the populations at risk. Many cases of endocarditis are found in patients with no underlying heart disease, especially children under age 2 and intravenous drug users. Some studies have shown that it is cost-effective to administer antibiotics prophylactically to those patients at high risk for endocarditis.

XII-11. **The answer is D.** *(Ch. 73)* Infective endocarditis in children is relatively uncommon and affects more males (65 percent) than females. Most cases (77 percent) occur in children with chronic heart diseases other than rheumatic heart disease. Repair of patent ductus arteriosus and ventricular septal defect decreases the risk of infective endocarditis. The three most common infective agents are viridans streptococci (38 percent), *Staphylococcus aureus* (32 percent), and enterococci (7 percent). There are more complications and a worse prognosis with *Staph. aureus* infections than any other type.

XII-12. **The answer is D.** *(Ch. 73)* Intravenous drug users are at least 300 times more likely to die suddenly from infective endocarditis than nonusers. Most cases of infective endocarditis originate from the user's skin and over 60 percent are *Staph. aureus*. The majority of vegetations are formed in the right side of the heart and the tricuspid valve is involved in up to 70 percent of the cases. Mortality from infective endocarditis is lower among intravenous drug users (4 percent) than in other populations, probably because of the more benign nature of tricuspid involvement as opposed to mitral and aortic endocarditis. The spectrum of infectious agents in intravenous drug users is very different from nonusers, and includes skin contaminants, *Pseudomonas,* and fungal agents.

XII-13.   The answer is C.   *(Ch. 73)*   Intracardiac operations have created a new population at risk for infective endocarditis. There are two forms of prosthetic valve endocarditis: early (less than 6 months postoperatively) and late. The peak time for onset of early endocarditis is 3 to 9 weeks postoperation and is usually caused by *Staphylococcus epidermidis.* Gram-negative bacilli and fungal infections also occur in this time interval. These agents affect prosthetic valves much more often than native valves. Late prosthetic endocarditis usually involves infection with organisms typical of native valve endocarditis. The prognosis for early prosthetic endocarditis is considerably worse than late endocarditis. Although the total number of postsurgery endocarditis cases has increased, the incidence per patient has decreased and is about 0.5 percent. Patients with valve replacements will remain at higher risk for endocarditis for their lifetime.

XII-14.   The answer is A.   *(Ch. 73)*   The incidence of nosocomial endocarditis was as high as 28 percent of cases in one study. Up to 75 percent of cases are related to vascular access sites. The majority of cases had no predisposing cardiac disease. Cardiac catheterization has an extremely low risk of infective endocarditis, whereas patients with solid organ transplants, flow-directed pulmonary artery catheters, arteriovenous shunts, and permanent pacemakers are at high risk. Patients with nosocomial infective endocarditis have a much worse prognosis than other forms of valve infection, with up to 50 percent mortality.

XII-15.   The answer is D.   *(Ch. 73)*   Streptococcus causes more cases of endocarditis than any other group of organisms. Although *Streptococcus viridans* accounts for the majority of the cases, *Streptococcus bovis* more commonly infects older patients and multiple valves. *Staphylococcus aureus* is the most common cause of acute endocarditis, but only 6 to 15 percent of patients with *Staph. aureus* bacteremia have endocarditis. *Haemophilus* endocarditis usually causes large vegetations with arterial emboli but represent a small fraction of endocarditis infections. Fungal infections, most frequently with *Candida* and *Asperigillus,* are more common in intravenous drug users.

XII-16.   The answer is B.   *(Ch. 73)*   The frequency of involvement on each valve is directly proportional to the mean blood pressure across that valve. Therefore, the left-sided valves are more frequently involved than the right heart valves. The mitral valve is the most often involved valve, except for intravenous drug users in whom the tricuspid valve is most often involved. Vegetations are usually found downstream from cardiac lesions, such as the lateral right ventricular wall in patients with a ventricular septal defect.

XII-17.   The answer is C.   *(Ch. 73)*   Over 95 percent of patients with infective endocarditis have a heart murmur sometime during the course of the infection, but up to 15 percent do not have a murmur when they are first seen. Heart failure is the most important complication of infective endocarditis, previously occurring in up to 55 percent of cases. The incidence of heart failure has been declining, however, probably due to earlier detection and antibiotic therapy, as well as earlier surgical intervention. Emboli are a significant complication for 12 to 40 percent of subacute cases and 40 to 60 percent of acute cases. Conduction abnormalities are an uncommon complication (4 to 16 percent) of endocarditis, but are indicative of extension of the infection into the conduction system, usually with abscess formation, and thus of a poor prognosis. There is a substantial risk (29 to 50 percent) of neurologic complications, including infarct, hemorrhage, aneurysm formation and rupture, and meningoencephalitis.

XII-18.   The answer is D.   *(Ch. 73)*   It can be difficult to tell with certainty that a patient has infective endocarditis because many of the symptoms appear with a wide variety of other diseases. The Duke criteria have received the most attention, but it should be recognized that the criteria were designed to favor specificity, not sensitivity. A diagnosis of infective endo-carditis requires two major criteria, one major and three minor criteria, or five minor crite-ria. An oscillating intracardiac mass and two positive blood cultures are both major criteria. Refer to Tables 73-7 and 73-8 on page 2104 in *Hurst's The Heart,* 10th edition.

XII-19. **The answer is D.** *(Ch. 73)* The treatment regimen, dose, and route for various organ-isms responsible for infective endocarditis are listed in Table 73-9 on pages 2108–2109 in *Hurst's The Heart,* 10th edition.

XII-20. **The answer is A.** *(Ch. 73)* About two-thirds of patients with infective endocarditis can be managed optimally without surgical intervention. The remaining one-third are those patients who develop moderate to severe heart failure, valvular obstruction, myocardial abscesses, prosthetic valve dehiscence, persistent bacteremia, fungal infections, or at least one significant arterial emboli. These cases require prompt surgical intervention.

XII-21. **The answer is C.** *(Ch. 73)* See Table 73-12 on page 2116 in *Hurst's The Heart,* 10th edition.

PART XIII
THE HEART, ANESTHESIA,
AND SURGERY

XIII. THE HEART, ANESTHESIA, AND SURGERY

QUESTIONS

DIRECTIONS: Each question listed below contains five suggested responses. Select the **one best** response to each question.

XIII-1. Which of the following statements regarding adverse cardiac events following noncardiac surgery is true?

(A) one quarter of the deaths associated with noncardiac perioperative mortality are caused by cardiac events

(B) one out of every 500 patients suffers a myocardial infarction following noncardiac surgery

(C) there is no consistent predictor of patients who will have an adverse cardiac event following noncardiac surgery

(D) intrathoracic and intraperitoneal surgeries result in the highest number of adverse cardiac events

(E) there are more adverse effects on the heart associated with opiate-based anesthetics

(pages 2130–2131)

XIII-2. Which of the following statements regarding preoperative testing is true?

(A) the greatest risk of perioperative complications occurs in patients with left ventricular ejection fractions of less than 35 percent

(B) about 20 percent of patients undergoing noncardiac surgery are unable to achieve the necessary workload to perform exercise stress testing

(C) dipyridamole thallium testing has a higher power and accuracy for predicting adverse cardiac events than dobutamine echocardiography

(D) the use of algorithms to identify patients who need preoperative cardiac testing does not significantly increase patient mortality and should be implemented to avoid the substantial costs of testing the majority of preoperative patients

(E) preoperative stress testing has the greatest utility for those patients at high risk for an adverse cardiac event

(pages 2133–2135)

XIII-3. Which of the following statements regarding perioperative cardiovascular risk is true?

(A) the maximum risk of adverse cardiac events occurs during the surgical procedure

(B) optimal perioperative treatment of patients with cardiac disorders is to continue current medical therapy

(C) hypertensive patients should have a diastolic blood pressure less than 95 mm Hg before surgery

(D) patients with coronary artery disease should receive perioperative intravenous nitroglycerin

(E) patients with symptomatic aortic stenosis should have noncardiac procedures completed before surgery is performed on the valve

(pages 2136–2138)

XIII-4. Which of the following statements is correct regarding intraoperative monitoring and anesthesia?

(A) the use of digital pulse oximetry, capnometry, and pulmonary arterial catheters during surgical procedures is nearly universal

(B) recent prospective trials in high-risk patients have reported reduced perioperative cardiac morbidity with the use of general anesthesia compared to epidural anesthesia

(C) two studies have reported improved peripheral vascular graft patency rates with epidural anesthesia

(D) amide class local anesthetic agents are less likely to produce toxic effects than ester class agents

(E) an epidural or spinal anesthesia that reaches the T3 level can cause complete respiratory paralysis

(pages 2143–2147)

XIII-5. Which one of the following intravenous anesthetics is not a direct myocardial depressant?

(A) ketamine

(B) barbituates

(C) propofol

(D) benzodiazepines

(E) opiates

(pages 2148–2149)

XIII-6. Which of the following statements regarding inhalational anesthetics is correct?

(A) the onset of anesthesia is slower in patients with low cardiac output secondary to cardiovascular disease

(B) the alveolar concentration of a drug is generally twice as high as the brain concentration

(C) nitrous oxide is seldom used because of its cardiac depressant effects

(D) sevoflurane is the only inhaled anesthetic that is not a myocardial depressant

(E) all potent volatile agents produce vasodilation and hypotension

(pages 2149–2150)

XIII-7. Which one of the following potent volatile agents has a sympathomimetic effect?

(A) enflurane
(B) desflurane
(C) halothane
(D) isoflurane
(E) sevoflurane

(page 2150)

XIII-8. Which of the following are most frequently associated with emergence from anesthesia?

(A) sweating and hypocoagulability
(B) hypotension and hypercoagulability
(C) hypotension and bradycardia
(D) hypertension and tachycardia
(E) hypercoagulability and bradycardia

(page 2151)

XIII. THE HEART, ANESTHESIA, AND SURGERY

ANSWERS

XIII-1. The answer is B. *(Ch. 74)* Of the 40,000 perioperative deaths associated with noncardiac surgery each year, more than half are caused by cardiac events. Annually, 25 million patients undergo noncardiac surgery and about 50,000 have a perioperative myocardial infarction (about 1 in 500). The American College of Cardiology and the American Heart Association have jointly published widely accepted guidelines for predicting perioperative cardiac events. (Eagle et al., ACC/AHA Task Report: Guidelines for Perioperative Cardiovascular Evaluation for Noncardiac Surgery, *J Am Coll Cardiol* 1996;27:910–948). The surgeries that are associated with the highest number of adverse cardiac events are major emergent surgeries, aortic and other major vascular surgeries, peripheral vascular surgeries, and surgical procedures associated with large fluid shifts or blood loss. Opiate-based anesthetics generally do not affect cardiovascular function, although spinal opiates can result in sympathetic blockade.

XIII-2. The answer is D. *(Ch. 74)* Patients with significant coronary artery disease have the highest risk of perioperative cardiac events. Patients with left ventricular ejection fractions of less than 35 percent are most likely to develop postoperative heart failure. Up to 50 percent of patients who undergo noncardiac surgery cannot achieve a workload sufficient for exercise stress testing. Dipyridamole thallium and dobutamine echocardiography have similar accuracy and power for predicting perioperative cardiac events. The main problem of preoperative evaluation is to predict with sufficient accuracy which patients are at low risk for perioperative cardiac events. High-risk individuals are easy to identify. Following guidelines such as those developed by the ACC/AHA Task Force has been shown to have an acceptably small increase in perioperative cardiac events with a substantial savings in costs from avoiding unnecessary tests. Stress testing is most useful when there is an intermediate risk of perioperative cardiac events.

XIII-3. The answer is B. *(Ch. 74)* The maximum risk for adverse cardiac events occurs in the postoperative period. The vast majority of patients should be continued on their current treatment regimen, even if they must receive medications through nasogastric or intravenous routes. Surgery is contraindicated until diastolic pressures are less than 110 mm Hg. Only those patients with organic valvular heart disease and prosthetic heart valves should be given antibiotic prophylaxis before noncardiac surgery. The only preoperative medical therapy which has definitely been shown to decrease perioperative cardiac events is β-adrenergic blocking agents before peripheral vascular surgery. Patients with severe aortic stenosis are at extremely high risk for perioperative cardiac events. The valve should be surgically replaced prior to any but the most emergent noncardiac surgeries.

XIII-4. The answer is C. *(Ch. 75)* The use of digital pulse oximetry and capnometry are nearly universal, but there has been no proven benefit of invasive monitoring with a pulmonary artery catheter. Of the five prospective trials comparing general anesthesia to epidural anesthesia, two studies showed fewer perioperative cardiac complications with epidural anesthesia, and three studies reported no differences in outcomes. Three of the five studies did not report peripheral vascular graft patency rate, but the two that did found the rates to be improved in patients with epidural anesthesia. Amide local anesthetics are less rapidly metabolized and more likely to produce toxic effects. It is important to remember that sympathetic blockade extends two dermatomal segments higher than sensory anesthesia. Respiratory insufficiency, caused by interruption of sympathetic activity, can occur with anesthesia above the T1 level.

XIII-5. The answer is E. *(Ch. 75)*   Almost all of the intravenous anesthetic compounds have a depressant effect on myocardial cells. One notable exception are the opiates, making them extremely useful agents in patients with compromised left ventricular function.

XIII-6. The answer is E. *(Ch. 75)*   The onset of inhalation anesthesia is faster with lower cardiac output. The alveolar concentration of a drug is generally equal to the brain concentration. Nitric oxide has little cardiac depressant effect, but its use is limited because it is not a potent anesthetic and because it requires such high concentrations that oxygen concentrations are limited. All of the potent volatile agents are myocardial depressants and vasodilators and produce some degree of hypotension. Despite these drawbacks, potent volatile agents are the most common anesthetic technique because of low cost, reliable amnesia, brochodilation, and overall safety record.

XIII-7. The answer is B. *(Ch. 75)*   The only potent volatile agent with a sympathomimetic effect is desflurane. This effect can be blocked by fentanyl, esmolol, and clonindine.

XIII-8. The answer is D. *(Ch. 75)*   The emergence from anesthesia is associated with hypertension, tachycardia, and shivering, most frequently due to incomplete analgesia, but is also related to drug withdrawal, hypoxemia, and delirium.

PART XIV
MISCELLANEOUS DISEASES
AND CONDITIONS

XIV. MISCELLANEOUS DISEASES AND CONDITIONS

QUESTIONS

DIRECTIONS: Each questions listed below contains five suggested responses. Select the **one best** response to each question.

XIV-1. Which of the following statements regarding the adaptation of the cardiovascular system in obesity is true?

(A) adipocytes are located close to vessels with the lowest permeability
(B) adipose tissue is less impaired by hypovolemia than other tissues
(C) obese subjects have a higher cardiac output and a higher total peripheral resistance
(D) the fluid present in the interstitial compartment of adipose tissue is not readily accessible to restore intravascular volume
(E) adipose tissue has mainly β_2-type receptors

(page 2290)

XIV-2. Which of the following statements regarding frequently performed procedures in cardiology and obesity is true?

(A) one-quarter of obese patients have an associated endocrine disease
(B) complete echocardiogram studies are feasible in fewer than one third of obese patients
(C) portable bedside radiographs are excellent diagnostic tools in emergency situations for obese patients
(D) satisfactory nuclear cardiology imaging studies are extremely difficult to obtain in severely obese individuals
(E) the high rate of complications with the use of the percutaneous radial technique for cardiac catheterization limits its use in obese individuals

(pages 2291–2294)

XIV-3. Which of the following statements regarding the metabolic and structural effects of obesity is true?

(A) weight loss does not reduce blood glucose or hemoglobin A_{1c} levels in patients with type 2 diabetes
(B) weight gain in young patients has no affect on the risk of having hypertension if the weight is lost during adolescence

(C) reductions in blood pressure in patients with caloric restriction can be attributed to the resulting salt intake reduction
(D) weight gains as small as 5 to 8 kg can increase the risk of coronary heart disease as much as 25 percent
(E) normotensive obese patients have normal vascular resistance

(pages 2294–2295)

XIV-4. When extremely obese patients lose weight, they are LEAST likely to

(A) improve glucose tolerance
(B) lessen insulin resistance
(C) reduce circulating blood volume and cardiac output
(D) have regression of myocardial hypertrophy
(E) lessen blood pressure

(pages 2294–2295)

XIV-5. Which of the following statements regarding obesity and cardiovascular disease is true?

(A) the eccentric hypertrophy of the obese patient causes similar abnormal left ventricular diastolic filling patterns as seen in the concentric hypertrophy of hypertension
(B) obese subjects have impaired left ventricular diastolic dysfunction regardless of increased left ventricular mass
(C) the majority of patients with obstructive sleep apnea have pulmonary hypertension
(D) obesity is associated with increased mortality and postoperative strokes after coronary artery bypass surgery
(E) pulmonary complications are common in obese patients following cardiac surgery

(pages 2295–2297)

XIV-6. Which of the following statements regarding cardiovascular risk factors in chronically uremic patients is true?

(A) hypertension is associated with an increased cardiac output and a decreased total peripheral vascular resistance

(B) a high-sodium and bicarbonate-buffered dialysate can reduce the incidence of hypotension

(C) the goal of managing hypertension in dialysis patients by maintaining "dry weight" is realistic in most patients

(D) overactivity of the sympathetic nervous system is not affected by nephrectomy

(E) elevated low-density lipoprotein (LDL) is the most common lipid abnormality in patients with chronic renal failure

(pages 2305–2307)

XIV-7. Which of the following statements regarding the heart and kidney disease is true?

(A) coronary artery bypass grafting does not carry an increased risk for dialysis patients

(B) primary coronary intervention results in good angiographic patency

(C) pulmonary capillary permeability is reduced in uremic patients

(D) *Streptococcus viridans* is the organism that most frequently causes endocarditis in hemodialysis patients

(E) pericarditis occurs less frequently in peritoneal dialysis

(pages 2309–2310)

XIV-8. Which of the following statements regarding cardiac drugs in renal failure is true?

(A) the half-life of quinidine is approximately 3 weeks in patients with renal failure

(B) thiocyanate will accumulate when fenoldopam is given to dialysis or predialysis patients

(C) angiotensin-converting enzyme (ACE) inhibitors can cause hyperkalemia in patients who are not treated by dialysis

(D) the dosage of ACE inhibitors does not need to be adjusted in dialysis patients

(E) proximal tubular injury has been noted in dialysis patients taking β-adrenergic blocking agents

(pages 2311–2313)

XIV-9. Which of the following statements regarding the acute hemodynamics of exercise is true?

(A) resting cardiac output (CO) increases immediately after the onset of physical activity

(B) during upright exercise, stroke volume can increase to the point of approaching that seen in a recumbent position

(C) the almost instant heart rate acceleration is due to increases in sympathetic tone

(D) the increase in stroke volume accounts for a greater portion of the overall increase in CO than does the increase in heart rate

(E) blood flow to the skin, to favor body cooling, increases progressively as workload increases

(page 2318)

XIV-10. During sustained static or isometric exercise, the cardiovascular physiological response in a conditioned, healthy heart may adapt by a decrease in which of the following?

(A) heart rate
(B) cardiac output
(C) systemic vascular resistance
(D) stroke volume
(E) mean arterial pressure

(page 2319)

XIV-11. Which of the following statements regarding conditioning training is true?

(A) a heart rate of 35 beats per minute can be considered normal in a conditioned athlete

(B) current guidelines recommend that people of all ages should perform moderate intensity exercise for 20 to 30 min, 3 to 5 days per week

(C) women have a progressive increase in ejection fraction with little or no increase in end-diastolic volume

(D) left ventricular end-diastolic volume decreases with age

(E) the resting ejection fraction decreases with age, even in healthy individuals

(pages 2320–2322)

XIV-12. Which of the following statements regarding sudden death is true?

(A) men who participate regularly in high-intensity exercise are at a greater risk of sudden death

(B) there is a fairly equal distribution of sudden death in men and women

(C) the majority of cases of sudden death are due to arrhythmias, rather than mechanical abnormalities

(D) the majority of young athletes who had sudden death experienced symptoms in the 3 years prior to their death

(E) the most frequent cause of death in younger athletes (<35 years) is coronary artery disease

(pages 2323–2324)

XIV-13. Which of the following statements regarding cardiovascular structure and aging is true?

(A) left ventricular wall thickness decreases progressively with age

(B) there is a greater frequency of apoptotic myocytes in older female hearts than in older male hearts

(C) the cardiac myocyte-to-collagen ratio decreases in the older heart

(D) a reduction in myocyte number can be attributed to both apoptosis and necrosis

(E) with advancing age in healthy humans, large arteries constrict their walls

(pages 2329–2330)

XIV-14. As part of a progressive age-related cardiovascular adaptation, exercise in normal elderly individuals will cause an increase in which one of the following?

(A) use of the Frank-Starling mechanism

(B) arterial vasodilatation

(C) inotropic response

(D) chronotropic response

(E) venous pooling of blood

(page 2335)

XIV-15. To maintain cardiac output during exercise in the elderly, there is a decrease in which of the following?

(A) heart rate

(B) use of the Frank-Starling mechanism

(C) end-diastolic volume

(D) end-systolic volume

(E) contractility

(page 2335)

XIV-16. In aged cardiac muscle, there is still preservation of the inotropic response to which of the following?

(A) digoxin

(B) digitoxin

(C) calcium

(D) epinephrine

(E) isoproterenol

(page 2336)

XIV-17. Which of the following statements regarding ischemic heart disease in elderly patients is true?

(A) older patients with acute myocardial infarction are more likely to be male

(B) older patients are more likely to present with atypical symptoms of myocardial infarction such as atrial fibrillation, heart failure, confusion, or failure to thrive

(C) the extent of infarction, as measured by indices of infarct size, is the most powerful predictor of in-hospital and 10-day mortality

(D) mortality in older patients is more likely to result from ventricular fibrillation

(E) elderly patients should not be given thrombolytic therapy

(pages 2344–2346)

XIV-18. Correct statements concerning the assessment of hypertension in the elderly include which of the following?

(A) isolated systolic hypertension at rest may be considered abnormal

(B) isolated systolic hypertension during vigorous exercise is considered abnormal

(C) a resting and consistent diastolic blood pressure of greater than 90 mm Hg but less than 100 mm Hg may be considered a normal variant

(D) sympathetic hyperfunction is the underlying etiology of most hypertension

(E) beta-blockade therapy is the treatment of choice when significant hypertension is present

(page 2351)

XIV-19. Which of the following statements regarding arrhythmias in the elderly is true?

(A) elderly patients are no more likely to have myocardial ischemia as a result of arrhythmias than young patients

(B) in patients with atrial fibrillation, aspirin is superior to warfarin therapy in the prevention of stroke

(C) cardioversion should not be attempted in patients who are hemodynamically compromised

(D) the probability of a drug having proarrhythmic effects increases in patients with structural heart disease

(E) all ventricular arrhythmias need to be treated as very serious in the elderly

(pages 2349–2350)

XIV-20. Which of the following statements regarding tobacco use and women is true?

(A) tobacco is the second most important coronary artery risk factor for women

(B) it is not realistic to have a patient begin a weight-reduction program while she is simultaneously stopping cigarettes

(C) women have a lower incidence of myocardial infarction and sudden death associated with tobacco use than men

(D) women are able to stop smoking more easily than men

(E) men and women have similar withdrawal symptoms

(pages 2357–2358)

XIV-21. Which of the following statements regarding coronary artery disease (CAD) and women is true?

(A) mortality rates from CAD have decreased among diabetic women

(B) middle-aged diabetic women have lower rates of CAD than middle-aged diabetic men

(C) following myocardial infarction, diabetic women have a lower risk of death and congestive heart failure than diabetic men

(D) women are more likely than men to have controlled blood pressure

(E) in women, the strongest correlation has been observed between elevated LDL and CAD events

(pages 2359–2361)

XIV-22. Which of the following statements regarding the management of clinical CAD in women is true?

(A) men and women have similar rates of reporting angina associated with mental or emotional stress

(B) anginal symptoms in women are more predictive of abnormal coronary anatomy than those reported in men

(C) women generally present for evaluation later after symptoms began than men

(D) chronic angina has an unfavorable prognosis in women

(E) women develop at least one episode of ventricular fibrillation or sustained ventricular tachycardia more often then men

(pages 2365–2366)

XIV. MISCELLANEOUS DISEASES AND CONDITIONS

ANSWERS

XIV-1. The answer is D. *(Ch. 83)* Adipocytes are located close to vessels with the highest permeability. Adipose tissue is more severely impaired by hypovolemia than most other tissues. Obese subjects have a higher cardiac output, but a lower total peripheral resistance. The fluid present in the interstitial compartment of adipose tissue is not readily accessible to restore intravascular volume, since there is a substantial decrease in blood flow to this tissue under conditions of shock. Adipose tissue has β_1-type receptors.

XIV-2. The answer is B. *(Ch. 83)* Less than 1 percent of obese patients have any significant endocrine dysfunction. Complete echocardiogram studies are feasible in 10 to 50 percent of obese patients. Portable bedside radiography is of very poor quality in obese patients. Cardiac function can be accurately assessed in obese patients using nuclear cardiology imaging techniques. The frequency of complications with percutaneous radial technique is very low and should be contemplated when obese individuals need cardiac catheterization.

XIV-3. The answer is D. *(Ch. 83)* There is strong evidence that weight reduction reduces both blood glucose and hemoglobin A_{1c} levels in patients with type 2 diabetes. Weight gain in young people is an important risk factor for subsequent development of hypertension. Reductions in blood pressure in patients on hypocaloric diets do not necessarily result from reductions in salt intake. Weight gains as small as 5 to 8 kg have been shown to increase the risk of coronary heart disease as much as 25 percent. Normotensive obese patients have diminished vascular resistance, while hypertensive obese patients have normal vascular resistance.

XIV-4. The answer is E. *(Ch. 84)* Weight loss in obese patients with hypertension correlates poorly with the decrease in pressure. The blood pressure may drop early and then plateau as further weight is lost. Potentially desirable effects of weight loss include improved glucose tolerance, decreased insulin resistance, reduction of blood volume and cardiac output, and regression of ventricular hypertrophy.

XIV-5. The answer is A. *(Ch. 83)* The eccentric left ventricular hypertrophy in obese subjects causes an abnormal left ventricular diastolic filling pattern similar to that seen with the concentric hypertrophy of hypertension. Only obese subjects with increased left ventricular mass appear to have impaired left ventricular diastolic dysfunction. About 15 to 20 percent of patients with obstructive sleep apnea have pulmonary hypertension. Obesity is not associated with increased mortality or stroke following coronary artery bypass surgery. Obesity is, however, associated with increased risk of wound infections. Pulmonary complications are comparable in obese patients to those in nonobese patients following cardiac surgery.

XIV-6. The answer is B. *(Ch. 84)* Hypertension is associated with an increased cardiac output and an increased total peripheral vascular resistance. The overactivity of the sympathetic nervous system is reversed by nephrectomy. The goal of having dialysis patients maintain "dry weight" to control hypertension is not easily achieved. Patients often become symptomatically hypotensive or develop leg cramps before the dry weight is achieved. A high-sodium and bicarbonate-buffered dialysate, rather than acetate-buffered dialysate, should be used to reduce the incidence of hypotension. Hypertriglyceridemia is the most common lipid abnormality in patients with chronic renal failure or end-stage renal disease.

XIV-7. The answer is E. *(Ch. 84)*   The mortality rate of coronary artery bypass grafting (CABG) is about 1 percent in first-time elective patients, but this increases to 10 percent in dialysis patients, thus making it important to assure that quality of life will improve from the surgery. Percutaneous transluminal coronary angioplasty has an unacceptably high rate of restenosis. It should, therefore, be reserved only for patients who are not candidates for CABG. The role of stents in this situation has not been determined. Pulmonary capillary permeability is increased in uremic patients. *Staphylococcus aureus* is the organism that most frequently causes endocarditis in hemodialysis patients. Pericarditis occurs less frequently in peritoneal dialysis.

XIV-8. The answer is C. *(Ch. 84)*   The half-life of digoxin is prolonged to approximately 3 weeks in patients in renal failure. Thiocyanate will accumulate when sodium nitroprusside is infused in dialysis or predialysis patients. ACE inhibitors can cause hyperkalemia in patients not treated by dialysis by blocking angiotensin-stimulated aldosterone release. The doses of ACE inhibitors must be reduced by about 50 percent in dialysis patients, as such inhibitors and their metabolites are both excreted by the kidney. Proximal tubular injury has been noted in patients taking cyclosporine A and tacrolimus.

XIV-9. The answer is B. *(Ch. 85)*   Resting CO increases immediately before the onset of physical activity, due to the anticipatory changes in the autonomic nervous system. During upright exercise, the stroke volume can increase to the point of approaching that seen in a recumbent position. The almost instant acceleration of heart rate is due to vagal withdrawal, more than to an increase in sympathetic tone. The increase in heart rate accounts for a greater percentage of the increase in overall CO than does an increase in stroke volume. During light exercise, blood flow to the skin is increased to favor body cooling. However, as the workload increases, there is a progressive decrease in blood flow to the skin because the rising cutaneous sympathetic vascular tone overcomes the thermoregulatory vasodilatory response.

XIV-10. The answer is D. *(Ch. 85)*   The normal cardiovascular physiological response to isometric or static exercise is to increase systemic vascular resistance. This is mediated by a local pressor response and is exacerbated by mechanical compression of resistance vessels due to sustained muscle contraction. Thus mean arterial pressure increases, venous return may decrease, and stroke volume will actually fall. As a response to this, the heart adapts by increasing the heart rate to increased cardiac output. Static or isometric exercise may be thought of as a pressure or systolic load in contradistinction to dynamic or isotonic exercise, which is a volume or diastolic load.

XIV-11. The answer is A. *(Ch. 85)*   Heart rates as low as 30 beats per minute have been recorded in healthy athletes. The current guidelines recommend that individuals of all ages should perform moderate intensity exercise for 30 to 60 min, 4 to 6 days per week. Men have a progressive increase in ejection fraction with little or no increase in end-diastolic volume. Women, however, tend to increase end-diastolic volume without a significant increase in ejection fraction. An augmented atrial contraction ensures enhanced ventricular filling later in diastole, thus left ventricular end-diastolic volume does not decrease with age. The resting left ventricular ejection fraction (LVEF) remains stable in healthy subjects as they age.

XIV-12. The answer is C. *(Ch. 85)*   Men who participate regularly in high-intensity exercise have a lower risk of sudden death. The increase in risk during athletic training and competition is outweighed by a decrease in risk of sudden cardiac death at other times. Only about 10 percent of sudden death events occur in women. This may occur because women take part in less intensive training demands, and they do not participate as frequently as men in sports associated with the greatest risks of sudden cardiac death. The majority of cases of sudden death are due to arrhythmias, such as ventricular fibrillation. Only 18 percent of young athletes who had sudden death experienced symptoms in the 3 years prior to their death. The most frequent cause of death in younger athletes is congenital cardiac anomalies, the most common of which is hypertrophic cardiomyopathy.

XIV-13. **The answer is D.** *(Ch. 86)* Left ventricular wall thickness increases progressively with age. The observed frequency of apoptotic myocytes is higher in older male hearts than female hearts. The cardiac myocyte-to-collagen ratio in older hearts either remains constant or increases. A reduction in myocyte number can be attributed to both necrosis and apoptosis. The large arteries dilate their walls with advancing age in healthy humans.

XIV-14. **The answer is A.** *(Ch. 86)* The ability of the cardiac muscle to develop tension and the inotropic response of the muscle to direct stimulation of the myofibrils with calcium are well maintained in elderly people. However, with beta-sympathetic stimulation, as with exercise, there is a decreased inotropic response, decreased arterial vasodilation response, and decreased chronotropic response. With left ventricular loading induced by exercise and other causes, there is enhanced use of the Frank-Starling mechanism to compensate for the increased workload and lower inotropic state.

XIV-15. **The answer is D.** *(Ch. 86)* The basic factors used to maintain cardiac output in the face of stepwise increases in exercise are the same for both young adult and elderly age groups. The difference is in the degree to which each factor is used. An increase in heart rate, an increase in inotropic response, and a reduction in impedance are all used in the elderly during exercise, but to a lesser extent than in the young adult. Proportionately, the Frank-Starling mechanism is used to a greater extent as a compensatory device in the elderly. This is reflected by a progressive increase in end-diastolic volume with stress and a decrease in end-systolic volume. Because of these balanced compensatory factors in all age groups, cardiac output response to exercise is unchanged at any given level of workload in humans from 20 to 80 years of age.

XIV-16. **The answer is C.** *(Ch. 86)* In animal models of aging, studies on isolated cardiac muscle show a striking decrease in the response of tissues to inotropic factors such as catecholamines or digitalis glycosides. The inotropic response of cardiac muscles to calcium and the response of myofibrils upon direct exposure to calcium following chemical removal of the cell membrane are well, maintained with age.

XIV-17. **The answer is B.** *(Ch. 86)* Older patients presenting with acute myocardial infarction are more likely to be female, have a preexisting history of angina, and experience a non-ST-segment elevation infarction. Older patients are more likely to present with atypical symptoms of acute myocardial infarction (MI), such as arrhythmias, dyspnea, confusion, and failure to thrive. Only one-third of patients older than 75 years having an MI present with chest pain as their chief complaint. Age is the most powerful predictor of in-hospital and 30-day mortality. Mortality in older patients is more likely to result from electromechanical dissociation and a finding of cardiac rupture on autopsy, than from ventricular fibrillation. Physicians are often concerned about the risk of intracranial hemorrhage with thrombolytic therapy, but there is evidence showing a possible benefit of thrombolytic therapy in the elderly. Primary coronary intervention may be an attractive alternative.

XIV-18. **The answer is A.** *(Ch. 86)* Although aging is associated with an increase in arterial stiffness and a decrease in sympathetic arterial vasodilatory response, significant isolated systolic hypertension at rest should be considered abnormal and an indication for treatment. Isolated systolic hypertension during exercise may be considered a normal adaptation. Any diastolic pressure consistently greater than 90 mm Hg is abnormal and should be treated. Sympathetic hyperfunction is more often associated with hypertension in the young, and beta-blocker therapy is the treatment of choice in the young age group. In the elderly, there is a decrease in beta-sympathetic responsiveness and beta-blocker therapy is less effective. Vasodilator agents should be considered first.

XIV-19.   The answer is D.   *(Ch. 86)*   Older individuals experience more hemodynamic compromise from increased ventricular rate and loss of atrial/ventricular synchrony resulting from an arrhythmia. This occurs due to the age-associated changes in relaxation properties and increased dependence on atrial contribution. The benefit of warfarin anticoagulation is greater than that of aspirin to prevent embolic strokes. Cardioversion should be attempted in any patient with a reentrant arrhythmia who is hemodynamically compromised. The probability of proarrhythmic effects is increased with all drugs in patients with structural heart disease. The approach to ventricular arrhythmias in the elderly is similar to that in younger individuals. Asymptomatic arrhythmias and those not associated with left ventricular dysfunction and/or ischemia as less serious.

XIV-20.   The answer is B.   *(Ch. 87)*   Tobacco is the single most important coronary artery risk factor for both women and men. Due to the fact that middle-aged women experience less symptomatic CAD than men, they are more likely to have tobacco-associated MI and sudden death than men. Women have a more difficult time than men quitting smoking. Having patients begin weight-loss programs while they simultaneously stop cigarettes is unrealistic. It is better to encourage exercise and eating healthy snacks to counteract the weight gain that can occur during smoking cessation. Women have been shown to have greater withdrawal symptoms than men.

XIV-21.   The answer is D.   *(Ch. 87)*   Although mortality rates from CAD have decreased among diabetic men, they have increased among diabetic women. A woman with diabetes loses her "female advantage." The rates of CAD are similar among diabetic men and women. Following MI, diabetic women have a higher risk of death and congestive heart failure than diabetic men. Women are more likely to have controlled blood pressure than men. The strongest correlation has been observed in women to be low high-density lipoprotein and CAD events.

XIV-22.   The answer is C.   *(Ch. 87)*   Women have a higher rate of reporting angina with mental or emotional stress. Anginal symptoms reported in women are less predictive of abnormal coronary anatomy than those reported in men. Chronic angina generally has a favorable prognosis in women, with mortality rates of approximately 2 to 3 percent annually. Women generally present for evaluation later after symptoms began than men. Women are less likely than men to have at least one episode of ventricular fibrillation or sustained ventricular tachycardia.

PART XV
DISEASES OF THE AORTA
AND THE PERIPHERAL ARTERIES

XV. DISEASES OF THE AORTA AND THE PERIPHERAL ARTERIES

QUESTIONS

DIRECTIONS: Each question below contains five suggested responses. Select the **one best** response to each question.

XV-1. Which of the following statements regarding etiologic and pathologic considerations in aortic disease is true?

(A) medionecrosis, or the fragmentation of elastic fibers and loss of smooth muscle cell nuclei, is seen in aortic atherosclerosis

(B) advanced atherosclerotic changes are most frequently seen in the descending thoracic aorta

(C) the occurrence of cholesterol embolization in aortic atherosclerosis is mostly spontaneous

(D) replacement of degenerated tissue with interstitial collections of basophilic-staining ground substance is a feature of cystic medial degeneration

(E) penetrating atherosclerotic ulcers commonly cause aortic regurgitation and altered pulses

(pages 2375–2377)

XV-2. The characteristic pathologic aortic lesion in Marfan's syndrome is which of the following?

(A) Takayasu's arteritis

(B) Reiter's arteritis

(C) cystic medial necrosis

(D) annuloaortic ectasia

(E) diffuse atherosclerosis

(page 2377)

XV-3. Which of the following statements regarding infectious aortitis is true?

(A) bacterial aortitis most often results from infection of a preexisting aneurysm

(B) infections with many types of bacteria can cause chronic aortitis

(C) during the spirochetemic phase of primary syphilis, *Treponema pallidum* lodge in the intima of the vasa vasorum

(D) antibiotics are an appropriate treatment for infections of the aorta

(E) syphilitic aortitis is most severe in the descending thoracic aorta

(pages 2378–2379)

XV-4. Which of the following is the most common major complication of Takayasu's disease?

(A) myocardial infarction

(B) stroke

(C) aortic rupture

(D) aortic dissection

(E) heart failure

(page 2380)

XV-5. Which of the following is the most common etiology of thoracic aortic aneurysms?

(A) Marfan's syndrome

(B) syphilitic aortitis

(C) systemic arterial hypertension

(D) atherosclerosis

(E) cystic medial necrosis

(page 2382)

XV-6. Which of the following statements regarding aortic aneurysm is true?

(A) infectious endocarditis is the most frequent cause of an aneurysm of the right coronary sinus

(B) aneurysms of the arch are less likely than other thoracic aortic aneurysms to produce symptoms

(C) pain resulting from an abdominal aortic aneurysm should be seen as a threatened rupture

(D) a patient with hoarseness would most likely have an aneurysm of the ascending aorta

(E) abdominal aneurysms are most likely to be saccular

(pages 2381–2383)

XV-7. Which of the following statements regarding aortic dissection is true?

(A) aortic dissection is characterized by cleavage of the aortic intima by a column of blood

(B) aortography is an excellent diagnostic tool for all types of aortic dissection

(C) conclusive evidence of an underlying medial defect is found in most patients

(D) the discomfort of dissection generally builds in intensity from the onset of the dissection

(E) pain both above and below the diaphragm should arouse suspicion for a diagnosis of aortic dissection

(pages 2384–2387)

XV-8. A patient has a silhouette shaped like an S on chest x-ray. There is no rib notching present. What is the most likely diagnosis?

(A) abdominal aortic coarctation

(B) chronic obstruction of the terminal aorta

(C) coarctation of the aorta

(D) pseudocoarctation of the aorta

(E) acute obstruction of the terminal aorta

(pages 2389–2391)

XV-9. A patient who cannot read or name colors, but can still write and spell, has most likely had an infarct to which of the following areas of cerebral circulation?

(A) the upper division of the middle cerebral artery

(B) the inferior division of the middle cerebral artery

(C) the top of the basilar artery

(D) the posterior inferior cerebellar artery branch of the vertebral artery

(E) the left posterior cerebral artery

(pages 2399–2400)

XV-10. Which of the following statements regarding neurologic or cerebrovascular complications of cardiac surgery is true?

(A) most intellectual and behavioral changes seen after cardiac surgery are permanent

(B) hemodynamically-induced infarction related to preexisting atherosclerotic occlusive cervicocranial arterial disease is fairly common in older individuals undergoing cardiac surgery

(C) drugs are a common cause of encephalopathy following cardiac surgery

(D) the majority of strokes occur during surgery, and patients awaken with the deficits

(E) subarachnoid hemorrhages are most commonly reported in elderly individuals undergoing coronary artery bypass surgery

(pages 2404–2405)

XV-11. Which of the following statements regarding the pathology of atherosclerosis and its effects on cerebral circulation is true?

(A) in white men, the predominant atherosclerotic lesions are found at the origin of the common carotid artery

(B) a clot is much less likely to embolize 2 to 3 weeks following development of an occlusive thrombus

(C) atherosclerotic plaques at the origins of cerebral arteries differ from those seen in the aorta

(D) black men have a higher incidence of extracranial disease than of intracranial disease

(E) patients with intracranial occlusive disease have a high incidence of coronary or peripheral vascular disease

(pages 2407–2408)

XV-12. Which of the following statements regarding systemic arterial hypertension and its effects on the brain is true?

(A) lacunes are usually caused by microdissections and tiny emboli

(B) headache is often absent or not a prominent symptom in patients with intracranial hemorrhage (ICH)

(C) the majority of patients with spontaneous ICH have a history of hypertension

(D) the most common location for hematomas to develop from ICH is the thalamus

(E) patients with ICH generally have an abrupt onset of symptoms

(pages 2411–2412)

XV-13. Which of the following statements regarding subarachnoid hemorrhage (SAH) is true?

(A) SAH most often results directly from hypertension

(B) lumbar puncture may or may not show blood present in the cerebrospinal fluid (CSF)

(C) vasoconstriction does not depend on the size of the hemorrhage

(D) the most common cause of SAH is leakage from a berry aneurysm

(E) headache is occasionally seen, but is often not a prominent symptom

(page 2413)

XV-14. Which of the following statements regarding the assessment of arterial disease is true?

(A) skin ulceration is a usual presenting feature of occlusive arterial disease

(B) claudication while performing can vary from day to day

(C) the extent of occlusive disease can be quantified based on the history of claudication alone

(D) when a patient has normal pulses and no bruits before exercise and a disappearance of pedal pulses and appearance of proximal bruits after exercise, the patient has vasospastic claudication

(E) small areas of ischemic rest pain are most likely caused by thrombosis

(pages 2421–2422)

XV-15. A patient with single focal occlusion in the right lower extremity experiences claudication of the entire calf with exercise. The lesion is located in which of the following?

(A) pedal vessels
(B) tibioperoneal trunk
(C) popliteal artery
(D) superficial femoral artery
(E) common femoral artery

(page 2421)

XV-16. Which of the following statements regarding arterial diseases of the lower extremity is true?

(A) thromboangiitis obliterans (TAO) is the most common cause of lower extremity ischemic syndromes in Western societies

(B) diabetes does not seem to increase the risk of arteriosclerosis obliterans (ASO)

(C) ischemia is rare with Takayasu's arteritis

(D) secondary causes of Raynaud's phenomenon are more common than primary causes

(E) microemboli usually originate from the heart

(pages 2426–2431)

XV-17. Which of the following statements regarding arterial diseases of the lower extremity is true?

(A) amputation rates are fairly high for untreated patients with ASO

(B) livedo reticularis is associated with tobacco use

(C) any form of aerobic exercise, such as walking or bicycling, is effective in the treatment of patients with ASO

(D) TAO usually involves both upper and lower extremities to the same extent

(E) beta blockade should not be withheld from patients with peripheral ASO

(pages 2427–2429)

XV-18. Which of the following statements regarding the clinical assessment of venous disease is true?

(A) the presence of a warm, tender, erythematous, and indurated linear lesion suggests a varicose vein

(B) phlegmasia cerulea dolens is seen most commonly with advanced malignancy or severe infection

(C) patients with chronic deep venous insufficiency do not have acute episodes of pain like those seen with phlegmasia cerulea dolens

(D) central venous thrombosis usually results from benign causes such as an indwelling catheter

(E) edema of both the foot and toes characterizes the edema of chronic venous insufficiency

(pages 2433–2434)

XV-19. Which of the following statements regarding the assessment of venous disease is true?

(A) continuous wave (CW) Doppler provides qualitative but not quantitative information about the presence of a hemodynamically significant obstruction

(B) venous duplex ultrasound is the "gold standard" method for the determination of deep venous thrombosis (DVT)

(C) a patient who has slow refill of leg veins as measured by plethysomography following leg elevation most likely has valve incompetence

(D) the vein is incompetent when augmentation occurs

(E) a normal vein will increase the plethysomographic volume during exercise

(pages 2435–2436)

XV-20. Which of the following statements regarding a venous ulcer is true?

(A) it occurs on the distal portion of the lower extremities

(B) the wound edge will likely develop a callus

(C) it is usually painless

(D) it has a characteristic "cookie cutter" appearance and a serpiginous edge

(E) it often occurs over the shin

(pages 2437–2438)

XV-21. Which of the following statements regarding upper and lower extremity revascularization is true?

(A) an exercise program is the first step in the treatment of patients with claudication

(B) male gender can shift a treatment decision from revascularization to amputation in the treatment of rest pain

(C) infrainguinal bypass grafting procedures are not valid treatment for patients with claudication

(D) revascularization should be attempted in only a minority of patients with rest pain

(E) percutaneous peripheral angioplasty confers a measurable improvement in patients walking ability

(pages 2446–2448)

XV-22. Which of the following statements regarding the nonsurgical management of carotid disease is true?

(A) available data do not support the use of anticoagulant therapy for managing carotid disease

(B) ticlopidine has similar effectiveness to clopidogrel, but has a better side effect profile

(C) patients with a low risk of coronary or cerebrovascular events should be offered lipid-lowering treatments with statins

(D) restenosis is a fairly common complication after carotid stenting

(E) the routine use of ACE inhibitors has not been shown to decrease the likelihood of a subsequent cerebrovascular event

(pages 2459–2463)

XV-23. Which of the following statements regarding peripheral occlusive disease is true?

(A) embolization to the cerebral circulation is a common complication seen after endovascular treatment for occlusive lesions of proximal arch vessels

(B) endovascular intervention for renal artery stenosis positively affects the control of hypertension or prevention of renal failure

(C) percutaneous transluminal angioplasty has provided immediate successful treatment of superficial femoral arteries with a low rate of restenosis

(D) percutaneous peripheral angioplasty can provide full relief of clinically important common iliac artery stenosis

(E) endoluminal treatment is highly effective for diffuse or multifocal lesions

(pages 2471–2478)

XV. DISEASES OF THE AORTA AND THE PERIPHERAL ARTERIES

ANSWERS

XV-1. **The answer is D.** *(Ch. 88)* Fragmentation of elastic fibers and loss of smooth muscle cell nuclei, so-called medionecrosis, is characteristic of the medial changes of aging. Advanced atherosclerotic changes mostly involve the abdominal aorta, below the renal arteries. The occurrence of cholesterol embolization is rare and usually occurs as a result of intraaortic catheter manipulation, rather than spontaneously. The replacement of degenerated tissue with interstitial collections of basophilic-staining ground substance is a feature of cystic medial degeneration. Penetrating atherosclerotic ulcers do not characteristically cause aortic regurgitation or altered pulses, as they most commonly involve the descending thoracic aorta.

XV-2. **The answer is D.** *(Ch. 88)* Cystic medial necrosis was for many years considered to be the hallmark histologic lesion of medial degeneration. However, recent observations suggest that this light microscopy lesion is neither specific nor accurately named. A better descriptive term, *annuloaortic ectasia,* has been applied to reflect the anatomical findings. The defect of disease in the medial aorta lies at a biochemical and subcellular level. Annuloaortic ectasia is the characteristic aortic lesion of Marfan's syndrome. There is a prototypical "Florence flask" or "onion bulb" appearance that reflects the severity of the medial degeneration in the aortic root. Rupture of these aneurysms or aortic regurgitation secondary to root dilatation is responsible for most of the premature deaths of Marfan's syndrome. Takayasu's arteritis, a condition affecting mainly Asian females, is a nonspecific aortitis which usually involves the arch of the aorta and the subclavian and carotid arteries. Reiter's arteritis is a poorly understood diffuse inflammatory response. Diffuse atherosclerosis is not a usual complication of Marfan's syndrome.

XV-3. **The answer is A.** *(Ch. 88)* Bacterial aortitis most often presents as an infection of a preexisting aneurysm. Treponemal infection is the only one that will cause chronic aortitis. During the spirochetemic phase of primary syphilis, *Treponema pallidum* will lodge in the adventitia of the vasa vasorum. Antibiotics are not appropriate treatment for infections of the aorta. These infections almost always lead to fatal aortic rupture unless they are treated surgically. Syphilitic aortitis is usually most severe in the ascending aorta and the arch, where the vasa density is highest.

XV-4. **The answer is B.** *(Ch. 88)* Takayasu's disease is named for the Japanese ophthalmologist who first called attention to the funduscopic findings of this problem. The disease involves a nonspecific aortitis and has been labeled "pulseless" disease and aortic arch syndrome because of its predilection for brachiocephalic vessels. Cardiac manifestations may occur from aortic regurgitation, coronary artery narrowing, or severe hypertension. Dilatation of the aortic root commonly accompanies the aortic valve incompetence. Angina pectoris, heart failure, and myocardial infarction are reported. However, stroke and blindness are the most common major events. Heart failure and aortic rupture or dissection are less frequent.

XV-5. **The answer is D.** *(Ch. 88)* Aneurysms develop at sites of medial weakness. Atherosclerosis is by far the most frequent cause of aortic disease. Syphilis and cystic medial necrosis, rather than pure atherosclerosis, have a predilection for the ascending aorta.

XV-6.   The answer is C.   *(Ch. 88)*   An aneurysm of the left coronary sinus is most likely caused by infectious endocarditis. Aneurysm of the right coronary sinus is most frequent when there is congenital failure of fusion of the aortic media with the fibrous skeleton of the heart at the aortic valve ring. Aneurysms of the aortic arch are more likely to produce symptoms than aneurysms involving other parts of the thoracic aorta. A patient with hoarseness may have a compression of the recurrent laryngeal nerve and thus most likely has an aneurysm of the aortic arch. Abdominal aneurysms, as a rule, are fusiform in shape. Pain that can be attributed to an abdominal aneurysm should be seen as a threatened rupture.

XV-7.   The answer is E.   *(Ch. 88)*   Cleavage of the aortic media by a column of blood characterizes aortic dissection. Aortography may not identify intramural hematomas, as the contrast material injected into the aortic lumen cannot enter the medial hematoma. Generally, no conclusive evidence of an underlying medial defect is found. The pain of aortic dissection is most intense at onset and does not build further in intensity. Clinicians should suspect aortic dissection when pain occurs both above and below the diaphragm.

XV-8.   The answer is D.   *(Ch. 88)*   The most likely diagnosis for this patient is pseudocoarctation of the aorta. The chest x-ray is similar to that seen in coarctation of the aorta; however, rib notching is not present. This condition may be detected during investigation of a mediastinal mass or a systolic murmur.

XV-9.   The answer is E.   *(Ch. 89)*   A patient who cannot read or name colors, but can still write and spell has a left posterior cerebral artery (PCA) territory infarct. The PCA is the terminal vessel in the vertebrobasilar circuit. The hallmark of this lesion is hemisensory loss contralateral to the infarct.

XV-10.   The answer is C.   *(Ch. 89)*   Most of the changes of intellectual and behavioral changes are reversible with time. Hemodynamically induced infarction that is related to preexisting atherosclerotic cervicocranial arterial disease is a rare complication of heart surgery. Embolism that arises from cardiac and aortic sources, however, is much more common. Drugs are a common cause of encephalopathy following cardiac surgery. In general, the use of sedatives and narcotics should be limited. More strokes occur after recovery from the anesthetic, providing a strong argument favoring embolism as the cause of strokes. Intracerebral and subarachnoid hemorrhages are most commonly seen in children following repair of a congenital heart disease. These are generally caused by an abrupt increase in blood flow with rupture of small intracranial arteries.

XV-11.   The answer is B.   *(Ch. 89)*   In white men, the predominant atherosclerotic lesions involve the origins of the internal carotid artery and the vertebral artery. Atherosclerotic plaques found in these regions do not differ from those found in the aorta or coronary arteries. Two to 3 weeks following the development of an occlusive thrombi, the clot is much less likely to embolize or propagate. Blacks and individuals of Chinese, Japanese, and Thai ancestry have a much higher incidence of intracranial disease and a low frequency of extracranial disease. Patients who have intracranial occlusive disease do not have a high incidence of coronary or peripheral vascular disease.

XV-12.   The answer is B.   *(Ch. 89)*   Lacunes are usually caused by lipohyalinosis of the penetrating artery that feeds the ischemic brain tissue. Lacunes may also be caused by microdissections and tiny emboli. Headache is often absent or not prominent in patients with ICH. Many patients with spontaneous ICH do not have a history of hypertension. The most common location for hematomas to develop following ICH is the putamen/internal capsule. Patients with ICH generally have a gradual onset of symptoms.

XV-13.   The answer is D.   *(Ch. 89)*   SAH is not caused directly by hypertension in most cases. The most common lesions that cause SAH are abnormal vessels such as aneurysms and vascular malformations that are on or near the surface of the brain. The most common cause is leakage from a berry aneurysm. The absence of blood in a lumbar puncture can virtually exclude a diagnosis of SAH. Vasoconstriction of arteries is thought to be due to blood or blood products bathing the adventitia of arteries. Therefore, a larger hemorrhage would cause more constriction. Usually blood is released suddenly causing an abrupt increase in intracranial pressure. This often results in abrupt headache.

XV-14. The answer is A. *(Ch. 90)* Claudication, ischemic rest pain, and skin ulceration are the usual presenting feature of occlusive arterial disease. Claudication occurs at a predictable distance or time. When the distance to claudication abruptly decreases, thrombosis or an embolic event should be considered. The extent of occlusive disease cannot be quantified based on the history alone. Standardized treadmill testing utilizing ankle/brachial indexes at rest and after completion of an exercise protocol is necessary. It was previously thought that a patient who had normal pulses and no bruits prior to exercise and the disappearance of pedal pulses and the appearance of proximal bruits after exercise had vasospastic claudication. This phenomenon has now been shown to represent occlusive disease, usually of atherosclerotic origin, in proximal vessels. Blood is shunted to collateral arterial muscular beds during exercise, depriving downstream arteries of blood flow. Small areas of ischemic rest pain are most likely to be caused by trauma to an area with poor perfusion as a result of chronic occlusive disease.

XV-15. The answer is D. *(Ch. 90)* The site of claudication indicates the level of the occlusive process if there is a single, focal lesion. Claudication in the foot results from obstruction in the pedal and lower calf vessels. Calf and foot pain results from tibioperoneal occlusive disease. Lower calf discomfort results from popliteal occlusive disease. Superficial femoral occlusive disease causes claudication of the entire calf. Common femoral disease and external iliac occlusive disease lead to thigh and calf claudication. Aortoiliac occlusive disease can produce calf, thigh, buttock, and occasionally low back pain.

XV-16. The answer is C. *(Ch. 90)* The most common cause of lower extremity ischemic syndromes in Western societies is ASO, regardless of age. Diabetes increases the risk of ASO threefold. Ischemia is rare with both Takayasu's arteritis and giant-cell arteritis. Secondary causes of Raynaud's phenomenon are low, with a rate of only about 2 to 5 percent. Microemboli rarely originate from the heart, typically from an left ventricular aneurysm.

XV-17. The answer is E. *(Ch. 90)* Amputation rates are low for patients with ASO at about 1 percent per year. These rates do increase, however, to 15 percent within 5 years for those who continue smoking. Thromboangiitis obliterans is associated with tobacco use and is thought to be an autoimmune response to it. A walking program should be initiated for all patients with ASO. Bicycling and other forms of exercise do not provide the benefit that walking does. TAO differs from atherosclerosis in that it does not have concurrent involvement with the upper extremities. Two studies have shown that beta-blockade should not be withheld from patients with peripheral ASO.

XV-18. The answer is B. *(Ch. 90)* The presence of a warm, tender, erythematous, and indurated linear lesion suggests superficial thrombophlebitis. Phlegmasia cerulea dolens is seen most commonly with advanced malignancy or severe infection. It can also be seen following surgery, fractures, and other common causes of thrombosis. Patients with chronic deep vein insufficiency also have acute episodes of pain and swelling that can mimic new thrombosis. This is seen especially when patients are not compliant with using elastic support hose or if the limb is stressed. Central venous thrombosis results from malignancy in over 80 percent of cases. Edema of the foot with sparing of the toes is seen in chronic venous insufficiency.

XV-19. The answer is A. *(Ch. 90)* CW Doppler provides qualitative but not quantitative information regarding the presence of a hemodynamically significant obstruction. Venography is considered the "gold standard" diagnostic method for determining the presence of DVT. When a patient has slow refill of leg veins as measured by plethysomography following leg elevation, the leg veins are competent. If the vein refills quickly, this is a sign that venous incompetence is present. If there is augmentation of proximal flow in the leg veins (as measured by Doppler) while the distal portion is compressed, the veins are patent. Exercise will decrease the plethysomographic volume in a normal vein.

XV-20.   **The answer is C.**   *(Ch. 90)*   Venous ulcers are usually relatively painless. Arterial ulcers likely develop on the distal portion of the lower extremities. The wound edges of neurotrophic ulcers will often develop a callus. Arteriolar ulcers have a characteristic "cookie cutter" appearance and serpiginous edge and often occur over the shin.

XV-21.   **The answer is B.**   *(Ch. 91)*   Risk-factor modification is the first step in the treatment of patients with claudication. One study showed that percutaneous peripheral angioplasty in patients with claudication did not result in measurable improvement in walking ability. A study has shown that infrainguinal bypass grafting procedures were valid treatment in a selected group of patients with claudication. There are four variables that predict lower limb survival rates with lower extremity bypass surgery: male gender, diabetes, chronic renal insufficiency, and a history of cerebrovascular disease. Therefore, male gender may shift the treatment decision from revascularization to amputation. Revascularization should be attempted, however, in the majority of patients with rest pain.

XV-22.   **The answer is A.**   *(Ch. 92)*   Data currently available does not support the use of anticoagulant therapy for the management of carotid artery disease. Clopidogrel has a similar effectiveness to ticlopidine, but has a better side effect profile and convenient pharmacokinetics. Patients with moderate-to-high risk or coronary or cerebrovascular events should be offered intensive lipid-lowering treatment with statins. Restenosis is a long-term, but rare complication after carotid stenting. Bradycardia and hypotension are not uncommon during carotid artery stenting procedures, but they are typically transient. A recent study has shown a significant decrease in the number of subsequent events in patients with cerebrovascular disease treated with an ACE inhibitor.

XV-23.   **The answer is D.**   *(Ch. 93)*   Distal arterial dissections, vessel rupture, and embolization to the cerebral circulation along with the potential for primary lesion restenosis are rare complications of endovascular treatment of occlusive lesions of the proximal arch vessels. Questions remain whether endovascular intervention for renal artery stenoses will positively affect the control of hypertension or the prevention of renal failure. Angioplasty has been an effective treatment of common iliac artery stenosis with good long-term patency and relief of symptoms. In spite of immediate success of endovascular treatment of femoropopliteal lesions, there has been a disappointingly high rate of restenosis and a full return of symptoms. Endoluminal treatment is limited when lesions are diffuse or multifocal, and include extensive regions of the vasculature.

PART XVI
COST-EFFECTIVE STRATEGIES, INSURANCE, AND LEGAL PROBLEMS

XVI. COST-EFFECTIVE STRATEGIES, INSURANCE, AND LEGAL PROBLEMS

QUESTIONS

DIRECTIONS: Each question listed below contains five suggested responses. Select the **one best** response to each question.

XVI-1. Which of the following statements regarding determining the costs of medical care is true?

(A) overhead is an example of a direct cost
(B) bottom-up costing involves dividing all the money spent on a hospitalization or procedure by the number of episodes of care of that particular type performed
(C) indirect costs may also be referred to as productivity costs
(D) most cost and cost-effectiveness studies use marginal costs
(E) increased access to a service will most likely result in increased societal cost

(pages 2490–2492)

XVI-2. Which of the following statements regarding comparing costs with outcome is true?

(A) patient utility is often used to compare various measures of outcome
(B) patient utility does not vary with time
(C) the patient preference method of time tradeoff measures the risk of death that they are willing to take to live in perfect health
(D) life-expectancy is not included in the measure of cost-effectiveness
(E) death is often the only outcome considered in cost-effectiveness measures

(pages 2493–2494)

XVI-3. Which of the following statements regarding the cost-effectiveness in prevention, diagnosis, and therapy is true?

(A) therapy has been highly cost-effective in younger patients with elevated serum lipids
(B) the benefits of smoking cessation are most likely to be seen in the short term
(C) the elimination of smoking altogether would result in a decrease in societal costs in the long run

(D) intensive intervention for diabetes control is less expensive than conventional therapy for diabetics
(E) the cost-effectiveness ratio is unfavorable for the screening and treatment of hypertension

(pages 2595–2498)

XVI-4. Which of the following statements regarding cost-effective strategies in the treatment of heart failure is true?

(A) digoxin therapy is cost saving if the incidence of digoxin toxicity is less than 5 percent
(B) digoxin therapy in appropriate patients is cost neutral
(C) disease management programs are not cost-effective
(D) angiotensin-converting enzyme (ACE) inhibitor therapy in heart failure is cost saving
(E) the cost-effectiveness of carvedilol makes it more attractive than ACE inhibition

(pages 2504–2506)

XVI-5. Which of the following statements regarding legal actions requiring cardiac medical evaluations is true?

(A) the financial costs of work-related injuries should, to a large extent, be assumed by public funds
(B) in order to obtain compensation in a work-related injury, fault or negligence of the employer must be proven
(C) items such as pain and suffering and loss of consortium are taken into account in the determination of the award for a worker's compensation
(D) applicants under the Heart Laws need only establish existence of a disabling heart disorder or hypertension and not the causal connection to employment for compensation
(E) prior infirmity is a bar to benefits in most cardiac claims

(pages 2520–2521)

XVI-6.   Which of the following statements regarding medico-legal cardiac evaluation is true?

(A)   expert medical opinions are not subject to cross-examination in court

(B)   long-term, repetitive physical effort cannot medically be regarded as a causative element in the development of atherosclerotic coronary heart disease

(C)   if two or more etiologic bases for a person's heart disorder are present, the most likely one should be listed

(D)   the legal and medical definitions of causality are the same

(E)   continued psychological emotional stress and job demands over an extended time period are scientifically established as causative agents in the genesis or acceleration of atherosclerotic disease

(pages 2523–2526)

XVI-7.   Which of the following statements regarding behavioral medicine in the treatment of heart disease is true?

(A)   a didactic, informative method is the most effective for teaching behavioral modification

(B)   interventions that focus on the action stage are most effective

(C)   behavioral interventions are usually reimbursed by insurance companies

(D)   simply advising a smoker to quit is not effective treatment, other methods must be undertaken

(E)   smoking cessation programs are not often reimbursed by health insurance programs

(pages 2558–2559)

XVI. COST-EFFECTIVE STRATEGIES, INSURANCE, AND LEGAL PROBLEMS

ANSWERS

XVI-1. **The answer is C.** *(Ch. 94)* Overhead and business productivity are both indirect costs. Top-down costing involves dividing all the money spent on a hospitalization or procedure by the number of episodes of care of the particular type performed. Bottom-up costing involves individually costing all resources used for a service. Most cost and cost-effectiveness studies use average costs, due to the difficulties of calculating marginal costs. If access to a service increases, this may result in a decrease in societal costs.

XVI-2. **The answer is A.** *(Ch. 94)* Patient utility is often used to compare various measures of outcome. Patient utility changes over time. For example, utility may be high after a successful angioplasty, but will fall if restenosis occurs. The patient preference method of time tradeoff measures the fraction of expected survival that they are willing to trade in order to live in perfect health. Quality-adjusted life years are used to figure life expectancy into the measurement of cost-effectiveness. Death outweighs other outcome measures, including myocardial infarction, unstable angina, revascularization procedures, and so forth.

XVI-3. **The answer is B.** *(Ch. 94)* Therapy has been much less cost-effective in younger patients with elevated serum lipids than it has been for high-risk populations. The majority of benefits to be seen with smoking cessation occur in the short term. The long-term effects of the total elimination of smoking would be an increase in societal costs associated with a higher survival rate. Intensive intervention for diabetes control is more expensive than conventional therapy. The reduction in vascular events that is seen with screening and treating hypertension somewhat offsets the cost, resulting in a favorable cost-effectiveness ratio.

XVI-4. **The answer is B.** *(Ch. 94)* Digoxin therapy is cost saving if the incidence of digoxin toxicity is less than 33 percent. Digoxin therapy is at least cost neutral, and probably cost saving due to decreased hospitalization rates. Disease management programs appear to be cost-effective at reducing morbidity and improving quality of life. ACE inhibitor therapy in heart failure is cost-effective, but not cost saving. ACE inhibitors are most cost-effective than carvedilol for treatment of heart failure.

XVI-5. **The answer is D.** *(Ch. 96)* The financial costs of work-related injuries should be assumed, to a large extent, by the employer, not by the employee or by public funds. Negligence or fault by the employer need not be proven to determine the right to compensation for an injured employee. Items like pain and suffering and loss of consortium are not used in the determination of workers' compensation. Applicants under the Heart Laws often need only establish the existence of hypertension or a disabling heart disorder and not the causal connection to the employment. There is universal legal acceptance of the common law precept that prior infirmity is no bar to benefits even though the injured person would not have suffered injury if there had not been underlying heart disease.

XVI-6. **The answer is B.** *(Ch. 96)* Due to the fact that different examiners have different opinions, expert medical testimonies are subject to cross-examination in court. If two or more etiologic bases for a person's heart disorder are present, each should be listed. Medical and legal definitions for causality often differ. The physician generally searches for the basic cause or causes underlying the overall disorder, while legal professionals limit concern to one or more items under legal scrutiny as an "injury," independent of other causes. Long-term, repetitive physical effort cannot be regarded medically as a causative element in the development of atherosclerotic coronary heart disease. Continued psychological emotional stress and job demands over an extended time period are not seen medically as causative factors in the genesis or acceleration of atherosclerotic disease.

XVI-7. **The answer is E.** *(Ch. 98)* Earlier intervention studies used didactic, informative approaches, which yielded disappointing results. More recent models identify psychosocial factors. Social learning theory models that incorporate behavioral modification methods have been more effective. Behavioral change is most likely achieved through a series of stages, including precontemplation, contemplation, preparation, action, and maintenance. Many programs have focused only on the action stage. Patients need to receive counseling related to the stage they are currently in for intervention to be effective. Behavioral interventions are rarely reimbursed by health insurance companies. Smoking cessation programs are also rarely reimbursed. Just having a physician advise a smoker to quit has resulted in a quit rate increase from 7.9 to 10.2 percent.

APPENDIX
CARDIOLOGY PRACTICE GUIDELINES

APPENDIX: CARDIOLOGY PRACTICE GUIDELINES

National Guideline Clearinghouse: A service sponsored by the Agency for Healthcare Research and Quality, in association with the American Health Association and the American Association of Health Plans (see **www.guideline.gov**)

National High Blood Pressure Education Program Working Group Report on High Blood Pressure in Pregnancy. National High Blood Pressure Education Program/National Heart, Lung, and Blood Institute (U.S.), 1990 (revised July 2000), 39 pages.

Report of the Expert Panel on Blood Cholesterol Levels in Children and Adolescents. National Heart, Lung, and Blood Institute (U.S.), 1991 (reviewed 1998), 11 pages.

Quality FIRST® Coronary Artery Disease with Myocardial Infarction. Institute for Healthcare Quality, Inc., Jan. 1991 (last revised Dec. 1998), Software.

Guidelines for Electrocardiography. A Report of the American College of Cardiology/American Heart Association Task Force on Assessment of Diagnostic and Therapeutic Cardiovascular Procedures (Committee on Electrocardiography). American College of Cardiology/American Heart Association, March 1992 (reviewed 2000), 9 pages.

Practice Guideline for the Treatment of Patients with Major Depressive Disorder. American Psychiatric Association, 1993 (revised 2000), 45 pages.

Practice Guidelines for Pulmonary Artery Catheterization. American Society of Anesthesiologists, 1993 (reviewed 1998), 16 pages.

Second Report of the Expert Panel on Detection, Evaluation, and Treatment of High Blood Cholesterol in Adults (Adult Treatment Panel II). National Heart, Lung, and Blood Institute (U.S.), Sept. 1993 (reviewed 1998), 169 pages.

Hypertension in the Elderly: Case-Finding and Treatment to Prevent Vascular Disease. Canadian Task Force on Preventive Health Care, Jan. 1994 (reviewed 1999), 8 pages.

Acetylsalicylic Acid and the Primary Prevention of Cardiovascular Disease. Canadian Task Force on Preventive Health Care, March 1994 (reviewed 1999), 10 pages.

Screening for Hypertension in Young and Middle-Aged Adults. Canadian Task Force on Preventive Health Care, March 1994 (reviewed 1999), 13 pages.

National High Blood Pressure Education Program Working Group Report on Hypertension in Diabetes. National High Blood Pressure Education Program/National Heart, Lung, and Blood Institute (U.S.), April 1994 (reviewed 1998), 26 pages.

Tobacco Use Prevention and Cessation for Adults and Mature Adolescents. Institute for Clinical Systems Improvement, May 1994 (revised Jan. 2000), 24 pages.

Tobacco Use Prevention and Cessation for Infants, Children and Adolescents. Institute for Clinical Systems Improvement, May 1994 (revised Jan. 2000), 20 pages.

Lowering the Blood Total Cholesterol Level to Prevent Coronary Heart Disease. Canadian Task Force on Preventive Health Care, June 1994 (reviewed 1999), 9 pages.

Stable Coronary Artery Disease. Institute for Clinical Systems Improvement, July 1994 (revised Jan. 2000), 28 pages.

ACR Appropriateness Criteria™ for Acute Chest Pain—Suspected Myocardial Ischemia. American College of Radiology, 1995 (revised 1999), 7 pages.

ACR Appropriateness Criteria™ for Shortness of Breath—Suspected Cardiac Origin. American College of Radiology, 1995 (revised 1999), 5 pages.

ACR Appropriateness Criteria™ for Chronic Chest Pain—Suspected Cardiac Origin. American College of Radiology, 1995 (revised 1999), 6 pages.

ACR Appropriateness Criteria™ for Acute Chest Pain—Suspected Pulmonary Embolism. American College of Radiology, 1995 (revised 1999), 7 pages.

ACR Appropriateness Criteria™ for Acute Chest Pain—Suspected Aortic Dissection. American College of Radiology, 1995 (revised 1999), 5 pages.

Guidelines for Clinical Use of Cardiac Radionuclide Imaging: A Report of the American College of Cardiology/American Heart Association Task Force on Assessment of Diagnostic and Therapeutic Cardiovascular Procedures (Committee on Radionuclide Imaging). American College of Cardiology/American Heart Association/American Society of Nuclear Cardiology, Feb. 1995 (reviewed 2000), 27 pages.

Lipid Screening in Children and Adolescents. Institute for Clinical Systems Improvement, May 1995 (revised Jan. 2000), 14 pages.

Lipid Screening in Adults. Institute for Clinical Systems Improvement, May 1995 (revised Jan. 2000), 18 pages.

Hypertension Diagnosis and Treatment. Institute for Clinical Systems Improvement, June 1995 (revised Jan. 2000), 40 pages.

ACC/AHA Task Force Report. Guidelines for Clinical Intracardiac Electrophysiological and Catheter Ablation Procedures. A Report of the American College of Cardiology/American Heart Association Task Force on Practice Guidelines (Committee on Clinical Intracardiac Electrophysiologic and Catheter Ablation Procedures). American College of Cardiology/American Heart Association, Aug. 1995 (reviewed 2000), 18 pages.

Cardiac Rehabilitation. Agency for Healthcare Research and Quality, Oct. 1995 (reviewed 2000), 202 pages.

Guidelines for the Evaluation of Management of Heart Failure: Report of the American College of Cardiology/American Heart Association Task Force on Practice Guidelines (Committee on Evaluation and Management of Heart Failure). American College of Cardiology/American Heart Association, Nov. 1, 1995 (reviewed 2000), 21 pages.

Physical Activity and Cardiovascular Health. Office of Medical Applications of Research/National Heart, Lung, and Blood Institute (U.S.), Dec. 1995 (reviewed 1998), 33 pages.

Practice Guidelines for Perioperative Transesophageal Echocardiography. American Society of Anesthesiologists, 1996, 21 pages.

Screening for Asymptomatic Coronary Artery Disease. United States Preventive Services Task Force, 1996, 12 pages.

Practice Guidelines for Sedation and Analgesia by Nonanesthesiologists. American Society of Anesthesiologists, 1996, 13 pages.

Guidelines for Perioperative Cardiovascular Evaluation for Noncardiac Surgery. Report of the American College of Cardiology/American Heart Association Task Force on Practice Guidelines (Committee on Perioperative Cardiovascular Evaluation for Noncardiac Surgery). American College of Cardiology/American Heart Association, March 15, 1996, 38 pages.

Heart Rate Variability. Standards of Measurement, Physiological Interpretation and Clinical Use. European Society of Cardiology, 1996, 28 pages.

Guidelines for Risk Stratification After Myocardial Infarction. American College of Physicians–American Society of Internal Medicine, Apr. 22, 1996, 5 pages (guideline), 21 pages (background paper).

Management of Pain Using Dangerous Drugs and Controlled Substances. Florida Agency for Health Care Administration, Oct. 25, 1996, 16 pages.

Guidelines for Assessing and Managing the Perioperative Risk from Coronary Artery Disease Associated with Major Noncardiac Surgery. American College of Physicians–American Society of Internal Medicine, Oct. 25, 1996, 4 pages (guideline), 16 pages (background paper).

Aspirin Therapy in Diabetes. American Diabetes Association, 1997 (revised 1999; republished Jan. 2000), 2 pages.

Management of Stable Angina Pectoris. European Society of Cardiology, 1997, 20 pages.

ASHP Therapeutic Guidelines on Angiotensin-Converting-Enzyme Inhibitors in Patients with Left Ventricular Dysfunction. American Society of Health-System Pharmacists, Feb. 1, 1997, 15 pages.

ACC/AHA Guidelines for the Clinical Application of Echocardiography: A Report of the American College of Cardiology/American Heart Association Task Force on Practice Guidelines (Committee on Clinical Application of Echocardiography). American College of Cardiology/American Heart Association, March 18, 1997 (reviewed 2000), 59 pages.

Diagnosing Syncope. American College of Physicians–American Society of Internal Medicine, June 15, 1997, 8 pages (guideline), 11 pages (background paper).

ACC/AHA Guidelines for Exercise Testing: A Report of the American College of Cardiology/American Heart Association Task Force on Practice Guidelines (Committee on Exercise Testing). American College of Cardiology/American Heart Association, July 1997 (reviewed 2000), 51 pages.

Domestic Violence. Horizon Healthcare, Oct. 1997, 18 pages.

Management of Dyslipidemia in Adults with Diabetes. American Diabetes Association, Nov. 1997 (revised 1999; republished Jan. 2000), 4 pages.

Sixth Report of the Joint National Committee on Prevention, Detection, Evaluation, and Treatment of High Blood Pressure. National High Blood Pressure Education Program/National Heart, Lung, and Blood Institute (U.S.), Nov. 1997, 33 pages.

Lower Extremity Ulceration. American Society of Plastic Surgeons, Jan. 24, 1998, 9 pages.

ACR Appropriateness Criteria™ for Chronic Chest Pain, without Evidence of Myocardial Ischemia/Infarction. American College of Radiology, 1998, 4 pages.

ACR Appropriateness Criteria™ for Suspected Bacterial Endocarditis. American College of Radiology, 1998, 5 pages.

ACR Appropriateness Criteria™ for Suspected Congenital Heart Disease in an Adult. American College of Radiology, 1998, 6 pages.

Specialty Referral Guidelines for People with Diabetes. American Healthways, Inc., 1998 (revised 1999), 22 pages.

ACC/AHA Guidelines for Implantation of Cardiac Pacemakers and Antiarrhythmia Devices: A Report of the American College of Cardiology/American Heart Association Task Force on Practice Guidelines (Committee on Pacemaker Implantation). American College of Cardiology/American Heart Association, April 1998 (reviewed 2000), 34 pages.

Management of Hypertension in Adults. American Pharmaceutical Association, April 1998, 13 pages.

Clinical Role of Magnetic Resonance in Cardiovascular Disease. European Society of Cardiology/Association of European Paediatric Cardiologists, 1998, 21 pages.

The Pre-hospital Management of Acute Heart Attacks. European Society of Cardiology, 1998, 25 pages.

Prevention of Coronary Heart Disease in Clinical Practice. European Society of Cardiology/European Atherosclerosis Society/European Society of Hypertension/European Society of General Practice/Family Medicine/International Society of Behavioural Medicine/European Heart Network, 1998, 70 pages.

ACR Appropriateness Criteria™ for Acute Chest Pain—No ECG Evidence of Myocardial Ischemia/Infarction. American College of Radiology, 1998, 6 pages.

Practice Management Guidelines for Screening of Blunt Cardiac Injury. Eastern Association for the Surgery of Trauma, 1998, 31 pages.

Venous Thromboembolism (VTE). University of Michigan Health System, June 1998, 10 pages.

Driving and Heart Disease. European Society of Cardiology, Aug. 1998, 13 pages.

Fibrinolysis Guidelines. Mount Auburn Hospital (Cambridge, MA), Sept. 1998, 9 pages.

Management of Patients with Valvular Heart Disease. American College of Cardiology/American Heart Association, Nov. 1, 1998, 96 pages.

Fifth ACCP Consensus Conference on Antithrombotic Therapy. American College of Chest Physicians, 1998, 330 pages.

Universe of Florida Patients with Acute Ischemic Brain Attack. Florida Agency for Health Care Administration, March 5, 1999, 16 pages.

Practice Guideline for the Treatment of Patients with Delirium. American Psychiatric Association, May 1999, 41 pages.

ACC/AHA Guidelines for Coronary Angiography. A report of the American College of Cardiology/American Heart Association Task Force on Practice Guidelines (Committee on Coronary Angiography). American College of Cardiology/American Heart Association/Society for Cardiac Angiography and Interventions, May 1999, 70 pages.

Cardiac Stress Test Supplement. Institute for Clinical Systems Improvement, June 1999, 23 pages.

Guidelines for the Management of Patients with Chronic Stable Angina. American College of Cardiology/American College of Physicians–American Society of Internal Medicine/American Heart Association, June 1999, 105 pages.

Heart Failure—Systolic Dysfunction. University of Michigan Health System, Aug. 1999, 12 pages.

1999 Update: ACC/AHA Guidelines for the Management of Patients with Acute Myocardial Infarction. A Report of the American College of Cardiology/American Heart Association Task Force on Practice Guidelines (Committee on Management of Acute Myocardial Infarction). American College of Cardiology/American Heart Association, Nov. 1, 1996 (revised [via Web site] Sept. 1999), 22 pages.

ACC/AHA Guidelines for Ambulatory Electrocardiography. A Report of the American College of Cardiology/American Heart Association Task Force on Practice Guidelines (Committee to Revise the Guidelines for Ambulatory Electrocardiography). American College of Cardiology/American Heart Association, Sept. 1999, 36 pages.

Treatment of Acute Myocardial Infarction. Institute for Clinical Systems Improvement, Sept. 1999, 49 pages.

ACC/AHA Guidelines for Coronary Artery Bypass Graft Surgery: A Report of the American College of Cardiology/ American Heart Association Task Force on Practice Guidelines (Committee to Revise the 1991 Guidelines for Coronary Artery Bypass Graft Surgery). American College of Cardiology/American Heart Association, Oct. 1999, 80 pages.

ACC/AHA Guidelines for the Management of Patients with Unstable Angina and Non-ST-Segment Elevation Myocardial Infarction. A Report of the American College of Cardiology/ American Heart Association Task Force on Practice Guidelines (Committee on the Management of Patients with Unstable Angina). American College of Cardiology/American Heart Association, 2000, 93 pages.

Guidelines for the Diagnosis and Management of Blunt Aortic Injury. Eastern Association for the Surgery of Trauma, 2000, 20 pages.

Secondary Prevention of Coronary Heart Disease Following Myocardial Infarction. A National Clinical Guideline. Scottish Intercollegiate Guidelines Network, Jan. 2000, 26 pages.

AACE Medical Guidelines for Clinical Practice for the Diagnosis and Treatment of Dyslipidemia and Prevention of Atherogenesis. American Association of Clinical Endocrinologists, March–April 2000, 52 pages.

Screening and Management of Lipids. University of Michigan Health System, May 2000, 13 pages.

Treatment of Lipid Disorder in Adults. Institute for Clinical Systems Improvement, Nov. 2000, 63 pages.

NOTES

NOTES

NOTES

NOTES

NOTES